The Four Pillars

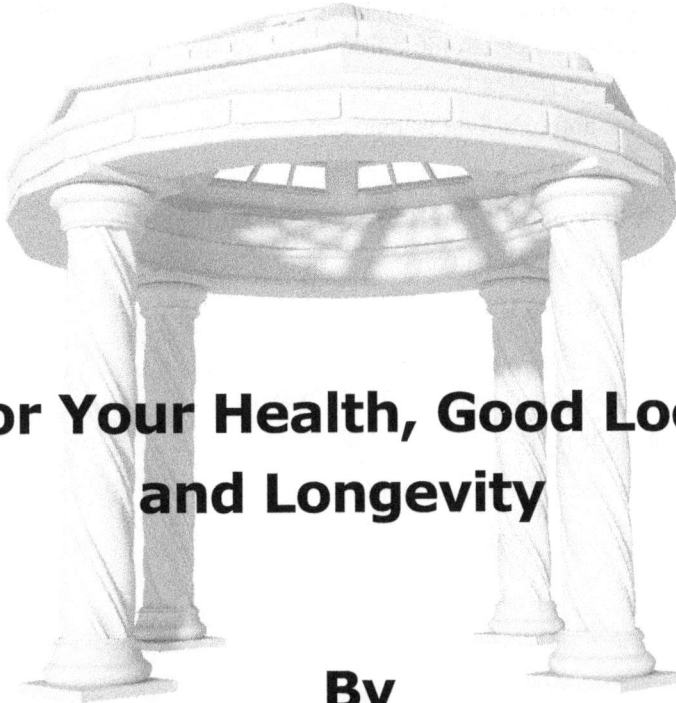

For Your Health, Good Looks and Longevity

By
Getty Ambau
Author of Alternative Health

Cover art and illustration by Philip Howe of Philip Howe Studios

Cover arrangement by Getty Ambau

Typeset by Greg Brown

Library of Congress Control Number: 2015908486

ISBN: 978-1-884459-05-4

Published by Falcon Press International

Important Note

The information contained in this book is meant to be used for educational purposes only. It is not meant to replace the advice or consultation of a trained professional. Additionally, the medicinal properties of some of the herbs and spices mentioned in this book, is not to suggest that you use these substances, in the place of exiting, scientifically-tested drugs, to treat an illness or cure disease.

Dedication

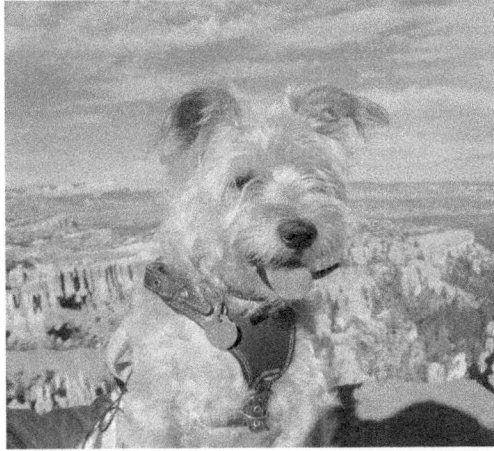

To our Scruffy who never forgets to remind me that taking
a regular walk is part of good health.

Contents

Preface   xiii
Introduction   xv

PART I
The Current Health Status
in United States   1

CHAPTER 1
Current Health Issues in the United States   3
Current Nutritional Status   7
Causes of Malnutrition   9
Optimal Nutrition—Your Answer to Health and Longevity   10

CHAPTER 2
Causes of Our Health Problems and Nutritional Solutions   13
Pillar One   17
   Vitamins: An Introduction   19

CHAPTER 3
Fat-Soluble Vitamins   21
Vitamin A   21
   Deficiency symptoms   21
   Food Sources and RDA Requirements   22
Vitamin D   23
   Deficiency symptoms   23
   Toxicity   24
   Food Sources and RDA Requirements   24
Vitamin E   25
   Vitamin E's Other Benefits   26
   Long-term Deficiency of Vitamin E and Your Health   27
   Food Sources   27
Vitamin K   28
   Deficiency Symptoms   29
   Food Sources and RDA Requirements   29
   Toxicity   29
Vitamin F   30

CHAPTER 4
Water-Soluble Vitamins   33
Vitamin C   33
   Vitamin C's Benefits   33
   Vitamin C's Other Benefits   34
   Deficiency Symptoms   35
   Vitamin C Amounts   35
The Vitamin-B Complex: An Introduction   37

Thiamine (Vitamin B1)   38
   Deficiency Symptoms   38
   Food Sources and RDA Requirements   38
Riboflavin (Vitamin B2)   39
   Food Sources and RDA Requirements   40
Niacin (Vitamin B3)   40
   Deficiency Symptoms   41
   Food Sources and RDA Requirements   41
Pantothenic Acid (Vitamin B5)   42
   Food Sources and RDA Requirements   43
Pyridoxine (Vitamin B6)   43
   Food Sources and RDA Requirements   45
Folacin   46
   Food Source and RDA Requirements   47
Cobalamin (Vitamin B 12)   47
   Food Sources and RDA Requirements   49
   Food Sources and RDA Requirements   50
Inositol   51
   Food Sources and RDA Requirements   51
Choline   52
Para-Aminobenzoic Acid (PABA)   53
   Food Sources and RDA Requirements   53
Pillar Two   55
   Minerals: An Introduction   57
   What Are Cofactors?   58
   What Are Electrolytes?   58

CHAPTER 5
Bulk Minerals   62
Calcium   62
   Food Sources and RDA Requirements   65
   Toxicity   66
Phosphorus   67
   Food Sources and RDA Requirements   67
Magnesium   68
   Food Sources and RDA Requirements   70
Potassium   70
   Food Sources and RDA Requirements   72
Sodium   72
   Food Sources and RDA Requirements   73

CHAPTER 6
Trace Elements   74
Chromium   74
   Food Sources and RDA Requirements   75
Copper   76
   Food Sources and RDA Requirements   77
Iodine   78
   Food Sources and RDA Requirements   78

Iron   79
   How Does Iron Deficiency Come About?   80
   Food Sources and RDA Requirements   82
Molybdenum   83
   Food Sources and RDA Requirements   84
Selenium   84
   Food Sources and RDA Requirements   86
Manganese   87
   Food Sources and RDA Requirements   88
Zinc   89

CHAPTER 7
Acid/Alkaline Foods   93
Pillar Three   95

CHAPTER 8
Dietary Fiber   97
   The Importance of Fibers for Your Health   98
   The Dietary Fibers in The Four Pillars   100
Pillar Four   103

CHAPTER 9
Phytonutrients   105
   Phytochemical samplers: their food sources and benefits   108

PART III
The World of Herbs and Spices   117

CHAPTER 10
The World of Herbs   119
   What are Herbs?   119
   Herbs' Function in the body   121
   Herbal Preparations and Application Methods   122
   Quantification and Standardization of Herbal Extracts   124

CHAPTER 11
Herbal Samplers   125

CHAPTER 12
Herb Tea Samplers   137

CHAPTER13
Spice Samplers   141

PART IV
The Four Pillars Recipes   151
   Introduction   153
     Suggestions and Reminders   153
   Making the Four Pillars drinks   156
   How to constitute your drinks   157

The Four Pillars—cold   157
The Four Pillars—hot   157
Four Pillars—Green   158
Four Pillars—Deep Earth   159
Four Pillars—Red   160
Four Pillars—Yellow   161
Four Pillars—Super blend   162
The Four Pillars Base Blend   163
The Master Dough   164
The Four Pillars Vegetarian Loaf   165
Kita   166
The Four Pillars Pizza   167
The Four Pillars Vegetarian Soup   169

PART V
The Four Pillars in Ethiopian Foods   171
Ethiopian cuisine   173
Nutrition Continuum   177

CHAPTER 14
Teff   178
Ethiopian spices   183

CHAPTER 15
Abesh (Fenugreek)   184

CHAPTER 16
Allspice   188

CHAPTER 17
Beso Bela (Sacred Basil)   190
Beso bela's healing properties   191

CHAPTER 18
Dimbilal (Coriandor)   193

CHAPTER 19
Inslal (Anise)   196

CHAPTER 20
Ird (Turmeric)   199
The science behind the traditional uses of turmeric   200
What contributes to turmeric's beneficial properties?   201
How to use turmeric   201

CHAPTER 21
Kewrerima (False Cardamom)   202

CHAPTER 22
Cardamom   204
Green and brown cardamom   204

Green Cardamom's nutritional profile and benefits 204

CHAPTER 23
Koseret *(Lippia Javanica)* *206*
Medical uses of koseret 207

CHAPTER 24
Kundo Berbere (Black Pepper) **208**
Kundo berbere's health benefits 209
Bioavailability 210
Cancer prevention 211
Black pepper's other benefits 211
Medicinal uses of black pepper 211

CHAPTER 25
Mitmita (Bird's Eye Chili) **213**
The benefits of mitmita 214

CHAPTER 26
Netch Azmud (Bishop's Weed aka Ajwain) **216**
Netch azmud's benefits 217

CHAPTER 27
Netch Shinkoort (Garlic) **218**
A few practical details 219

CHAPTER 28
Senafich (Mustard Seeds) **221**
Cited health benefits 223

CHAPTER 29
Shinkoort (Red, Yellow, or White Onions) **224**

CHAPTER 30
Tena Adam (Rue) **226**
Tena Adam's medical application 227

CHAPTER 31
Tikur Azmud (Black Cumin) **229**
What makes black cumin seeds and oil such versatile curative agents? 230

CHAPTER 32
Timiz (Long Pepper) **233**

CHAPTER 33
Tosign (Savory) **235**

PART VI
Selected Ethiopian Food Recipes **237**
The Super Spice Blends Found in Most Ethiopian Cooking 238
1. Berbere (the classic blend) 238
2. Mekelesha –The finishing spice for wots 241

3. Mitmita   241
4. Mitten Shiro   243
  Making the mitten shiro   244
5. Niter Kibbeh (Clarified Butter)   245
  Clarified butter's unique features: 246
Food Recipes   247
  Injera (Ethiopian Flat, Leaven Bread)   247
  Making a loaf out of teff flour   250
Meat Dishes   252
  Doro Wot (Red Chicken Stew)   252
  Sega Wot   254
  Doro Alicha (chicken stewed in turmeric sauce)   255
  Kitfo (Steak Tartar)   256
Vegetarian Dishes   256
  Shiro Wot   256
  Misir Wot (Lintel Stew)   257
  Kik Wot (split yellow peas stew)   258
  Mixed Vegetables   259
  Gomen (Collard Green)   259
  The Ethiopian Green Salad   260

PART VII
Appendices   263

APPENDIX A
Free Radicals and Antioxidants   264
Free Radicals   265
  Sources of Free Radicals   267
  Antioxidants   268
Food-Derived Antioxidants   269
  Beta Carotene—Precursor of Vitamin A   269
  Vitamin C   270
  Vitamin E   270
The Mineral Antioxidants   271
  Selenium   272
  Cysteine, Glutathione, Methionine and Lysine   273
Herbal Antioxidants   274
  A Team of Antioxidants for Maximum Health   274

APPENDIX B
The Importance of Good, Clean Water to Your Health and Longevity   276
  What Could Be Wrong With Your Drinking Water   277

APPENDIX C
The Importance of Physical Exercise   283
  Understanding Exercise   283
    How it Works   284
    Nutrition and Exercise   288

APPENDIX D
Losing and Managing Your Weight 291
Causes of Obesity   291
Things You Can Do About Obesity   293
What is the best exercise?   297

APPENDIX E
The Importance of Good Digestion   298
Proper Digestion: The First Step to Good Health   298
The Digestion and Absorption of Nutrients   299
Digestion Disrupters   301
Your Solution   302
Digestion Disturbances   303

APPENDIX F
Enzymes: The Keys of Life   305
Enzymes   305
The Importance of Enzyme Supplements for Our Health   306
Glossary   310

PART VIII
References   327
Ethiopian Spice and Teff flour suppliers   347

PART IX
Index   349

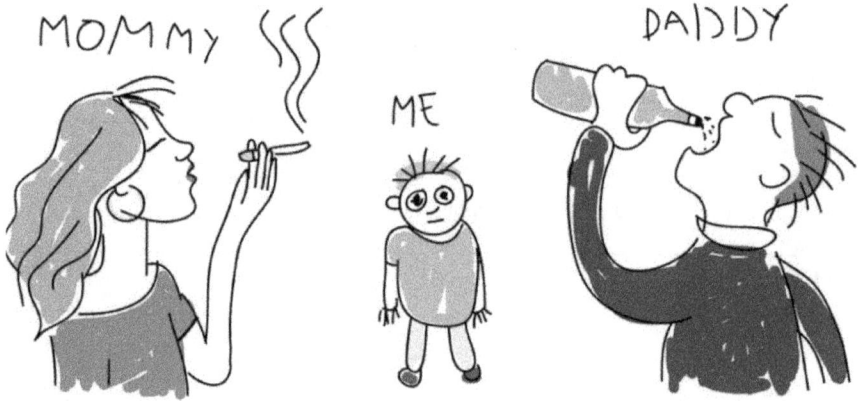

Health Risk Factors

Preface

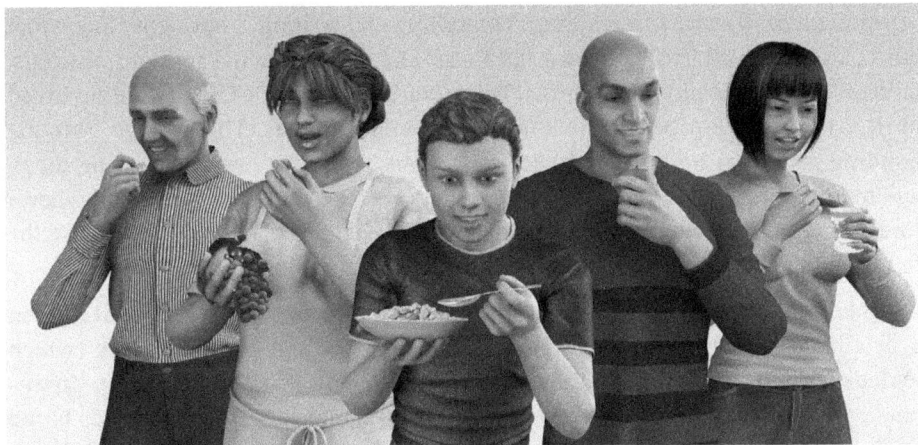

The idea of eating good food to nourish and keep our body healthy is not novel. Nearly 2,500 years ago, Hippocrates, the father of Western medicine, advised us "to make food our medicine; our medicine our food." But the practice of choosing and organizing our foods according to their maximum nutritional benefits and disease-preventing properties may be new, because most of us eat merely to kill an appetite or satisfy hunger. Most of us don't even have a rudimentary knowledge of nutrition. The subject was neither a part of our academic training nor our family upbringing. Our doctors don't receive more than one semester of training on diet and food in medical school, hardly enough education to expect them to be our purveyors of good health through proper nutrition. They are trained mainly to prescribe drugs. For most of us, good health or wellness means taking pills when we get sick or going under the knife when we have a cancer, blocked artery or any other ailments to remove or fix the disease.

But these diseases happen largely because we have abused our bodies by engaging in risky behavior and overeating. Smoking, using drugs, consuming excessive alcohol and sexual promiscuity are risky behaviors. A life-long consumption of foods rich in fats, sweets, and salts are the other causes. Some of us may live or work in a polluted or stressful environment.

Proper nourishment of our bodies, so they can heal themselves when they get sick or prevent diseases, should be in our everyday, conscious thoughts. Our bodies are made to take care of themselves if we avail them the right nutrients. The fundamental law of nature for most life is to live out its genetically programmed lifespan. No life is created to self-destruct or die prematurely. As you will see in this book, most diseases and premature deaths happen because of the suboptimal quality of our foods, our poor nutritional habits, our sedentary lifestyle and as it is the case for some of us, our engagement in activities that are both disease inducing and life-shortening.

From all of my years of reading, researching and writing, I have concluded that our health and wellness rests on what I call The Four Pillars. These are vitamins, minerals, fiber and phytonutrients. These four components of health are involved in nearly all of the processes that take place in our bodies. These range from the building and repairing of our tissues and organs, to protecting and healing them, and to the proper processing and elimination of waste from our system. It's therefore important for every human being to understand the basic functions of the foods and their contribution to his or her health and wellness.

To help all those who may be in the same position as I once was, I have given a detailed account of the vitamins, minerals, fibers and phytonutrients (which include herbs and spices) and the various roles they play in our well-being. In this book, you will also find recipes for making drinks, soups, stews and breads based on these four pillars of health.

I am originally from Ethiopia and knowing how popular Ethiopian foods are becoming in the United States and other countries, I have researched and written several chapters on Ethiopian food ingredients. These foods are nutritious and healthy and I thought people would appreciate and enjoy them even more, after they learn about the benefits of all the spices and other ingredients that go into the creation of the Ethiopian cuisine. These food ingredients maybe one of the reasons why degenerative diseases, such as cancer, heart diseases, diabetes and others, are rare in that country.

In the appendices, I have given a brief account of free radicals, antioxidants and enzymes for those who may wish to know the role they play in our health. Exercising regularly and drinking purified water are important components to our health and longevity. I have covered these topics as well. Nearly 68% of the population in the United States is either obese or overweight. For those for whom weight maybe an issue, I have a long article on how one can lose or manage weight through normal means—without dieting or being on a weight-loss program.

Finally, having all the healthy foods at our table means nothing unless their nutrients are properly processed and absorbed by our digestive system. For those who may wish to know about this system, I've addressed the significance of keeping our digestive tract healthy and properly functioning so we fully realize the role foods can play in our health, good looks and longevity.

-GTA

Introduction

I feared my fingers and toes would char and shrivel as if singed with fire, my skin would be covered with blisters and lesions and my feet and hands would become numb and tingle with pain. My kidneys would fail, my eyes would become blurry and my blood vessels would get damaged, leading to many complications, including wounds and cuts that are slow to heal. These were some of the symptoms my diabetic sister-in-law experienced in the late stages of her disease. But I was not diabetic, although I had the early symptoms of a diabetic person. As discussed on Page 13, mine appears to be a result of poor circulation, which can be caused by a number of things—not getting enough exercise, eating too many fat-filled foods, and chronic smoking. Although I'm guilty of the first reason because of the sedentary aspect of my work, I had neither of the other potential problems. Yet, if unchecked, I still had a potentially life-threatening situation on my hands. Having nutritional knowledge can help.

I had never valued or consciously connected the food I eat to my own health and well being, until about twenty years ago. To me, as is probably true with a lot of people, food was there merely to satisfy my hunger or to kill an appetite. I consumed just about anything I was accustomed to eating. That meant meats, white bread, white rice, pasta, alcohol and soft drinks. In general, foods that were rich in fat, sweets and salt were my favorite. I was overweight. I had problems with my lower back (because of the added pounds in the front), and I never felt quite up to par mentally. Some afternoons I was drowsy or I felt out of sorts. But I never connected all these problems to the types of foods I was eating.

Then I joined a company that manufactured and sold nutritional supplements. In my academic background I have studied molecular biophysics and biochemistry and economics in college. At meetings, distributors used to come up and ask me what benefit the ingredients had to the human body. I didn't know the answers to their questions other than the commons ones, like Vitamin A helps with night vision, Vitamin C wards off scurvy and Vitamin D prevents children's bones from bowing and that calcium and magnesium are good for the growth of bones and teeth.

Most of the distributors knew these answers, and my responses were not adequate enough for them. The shortcomings of my own knowledge about these food components inspired me to study the benefit of all of the ingredients found in the company's products—vitamins, minerals, and herbal extracts. Then I focused on nutrition in general. I read just about any book and journal article I could find on the value of proper nutrition to human health.

I discovered that

1. there is a high level of malnutrition in this country—not the classical type but the modern type. (See Chapter 2). Because the foods we eat are highly processed—white rice and white flour, all forms of pasta—which have little of their vitamins and mineral content.

2. stress and pollution increase our need for the key nutrients: vitamins, minerals and large doses of anti-oxidants compounds.

3. every chemical reaction, including the conversion of proteins into amino acids, and the synthesis of these amino acids into tissues, such as hair, skin, nails and thousands of other proteins, are helped by vitamins and minerals. These nutrients are critical to life.

4. the colors in fruits and vegetables are not solely for our visual enjoyment. They have many health benefits, from serving as antioxidants to boosting the immune system and preventing degenerative diseases.

5. the agricultural soils in this country have been depleted of their mineral reserves. The nutrient content of the fruits and vegetables may vary depending where they are grown. Certain parts of the country are rich in certain minerals more than others.

6. our body is constantly challenged by chemical fragments called free radicals that are produced in our bodies or come from outside sources. These are found to be one of the major causes of the degenerative diseases, such as cancer, cardiovascular disease, and macular degeneration that affect us as we get older. Free radicals may be made harmless if we eat the right foods.

7. as we get older our nutritional needs are higher because nutrients are no longer processed and absorbed efficiently.

I realized that I was not just a skin-bound bundle of blood, muscle and bones. Within each of my 60 trillion cells, amazing chemical processes take place, all without my conscious control. Nature had given them intelligence to act on their own. It is my responsibility to give these cells proper foods so that those processes can work smoothly and keep my body healthy.

Those biological processes involve the conversion of foods into the energy, that is keeping us moving, talking, thinking and doing a great number of things every day. They also use certain nutrients to build tissue and organs. A great many chemicals help to run our bodies as smoothly as possible. All of these processes are made possible by the foods that we eat. If we want our bodies to do their job efficiently and to function optimally, not just *any* food is acceptable.

Our bodies are also equipped with a defense system that tries to ward off harmful viruses from the outside and thwart the formation of diseases like cancer from within. This system functions to full capacity if the body is supplied with the quality nutrients it needs. In normal circumstances our sleep pattern and mental state can be greatly influenced by the types of foods or drinks we consume.

As a result of all these findings, I began treat my body with respect and responsibility. I changed my eating habits completely, cutting out all fats, sweets and soft drinks and replaced them with fruits and vegetables. I drank distilled or filtered water and fresh juices.

I wrote my first book about the company's products as well as the value of good nutrition in general. This book became a world-wide bestseller among the distributors. Later, I followed it with a more comprehensive general nutrition book called, *The Importance of Good Nutrition Herbs and Phytochemicals for Your Health, Good Looks and Longevity*. This, too, became popular with the distributors as well with the general public, including the physicians.

I have detailed how my learning and writing experience in nutrition and health issues that my wife and I were having, led to the creation of the recipes for the Four Pillars drinks that appear in Part IV. Before I begin, let me first give you a background about our health and nutritional status in this country.

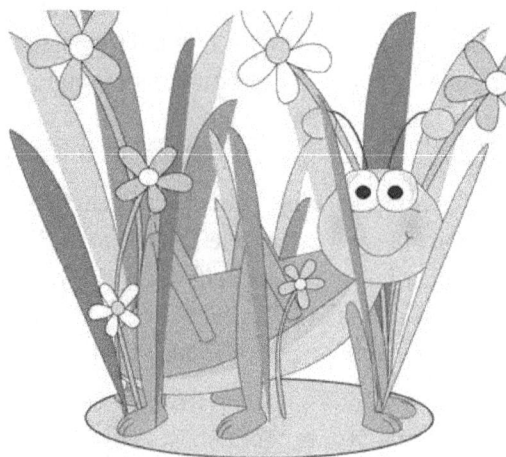

**The grass hopper is the Chinese symbol of longevity,
good health, happiness, good luck, abundance, fertility and virtue.**

PART I

The Current Health Status
in United States

CHAPTER 1
Current Health Issues in the United States

Increasingly, people are living longer today. This is particularly so when you realize that two-thirds of the people who have ever lived past 65 years of age are alive today. This piece of information is astounding in another way. Over a hundred years ago, people did not expect to live past 40 years of age. As of 2014, the average man can expect to live to 76.4 years of age and the average woman to 81.2 years of age or a combined average age of 78.8 years.

These figures are far less when compared to the life expectancies of other nations. From the top three ranking countries, Monaco has a life expectancy of 89.57 years, Macau 84.48, and Japan 84.46. United States is 42nd. Guinea-Bissau with 49.87 years, South Africa with 49.56 and Chad with 49.44 are the bottom three in the list.

The future of human life is even more impressive. According to experts on aging, not only will there be a greater number of people living past 100 years, but some may even live as long as 120 years, the current maximum biological age for humans. How you care for yourself is what will determine how many years you can expect to live. See Figure 1.1 for past, present and future survival curves.

Nowadays, venereal diseases, influenza and tuberculosis are not the main killers in the United States and other industrialized societies. Instead, the main killers are cardiovascular diseases and cancer. These two diseases account for over 50% of the top ten causes of death in this country. These diseases were relatively unknown in the early part of the previous century and a great percentage of them are preventable.

For example, in 2014, thirty percent or 176,000 of the 585,720 estimated cancer deaths were tobacco related. The other thirty-three percent are caused from being obese or over weight. Of the remaining thirty-seven percent, infectious diseases, such as the hepatitis B and C virus, HIV or human immunodeficiency virus and skin cancers are the causes of these deaths. These, and those caused by tobacco, are preventable, if people did not smoke or took precaution in their sexual encounters.

Cancers, derived by heredity, are small. It's believed that even these cancers happen when people, who are genetically predisposed, subject themselves to unhealthy lifestyle such as smoking, an excessive use of alcohol and drugs, and environmental risks, such as polluted air or water, radiation or hazardous waste.

Relatively speaking, smokers are 23 times more likely to get cancer than those who do not smoke. A woman who has a mother with a history of breast cancer is twice as likely as the woman who doesn't have the familial connection to the disease. Interestingly, seventy-seven percent of all diagnosed cancer occurs in persons 55 years and older.

Most of the cardiovascular diseases are caused by fatty deposits or are due to sedimentation of cholesterol-bound calcium along the arterial walls. When these fats collect there, they block the flow of blood, and this can lead to heart attack. Calcium and cholesterol deposits, on the other hand, cause the blood vessels to become rigid and brittle. This condition can result in a breakage or rupture of the blood vessels as well as a stroke if the blood vessels are in the brain. Both these outcomes are largely caused by fatty, sweet foods and our sedentary lifestyle.

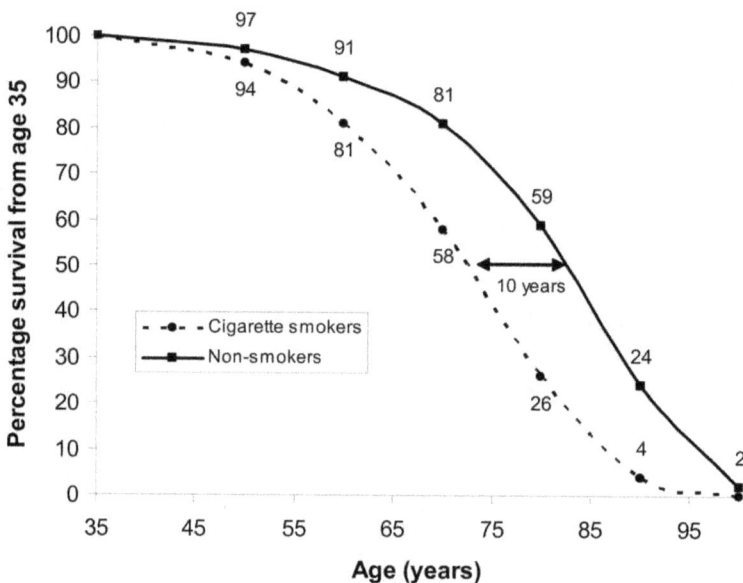

Figure 1.1 Survival Curves for the U.S. Population

These Life Expectancy Curves show past, present and future U.S. population life span profiles. Average life expectancies at a 50% survival rate are shown below:

1900   44 years

1950   60 years

1990   76 years

2040   89 years[1]

The other nutrition-related circulatory disorder is one that comes from electrolyte imbalance. Both the heart muscles and nerves need certain minerals like sodium, calcium, potassium, and magnesium for their normal functioning. Severe shortage of these minerals can lead to spasms and even sudden death.

The best solution to any of these health hazards is to avoid or minimize the consumption of foods that are rich in saturated fats and cholesterol. Foods that are rich in saturated fats, such as red meat, whole milk and coconut and palm oils, can be some of the major culprits. Lowering stress level and exercising regularly can also help you clear up some of these circulatory problems. Making and including the Four Pillars drinks with at least two of your meals can your body to manage and care for itself reliably.

---

1   The National Institute on Aging projects that by the year 2040, the life expectancy for men will be 86 years and for women 91.5 years; the average of these two number is roughly 89 years.

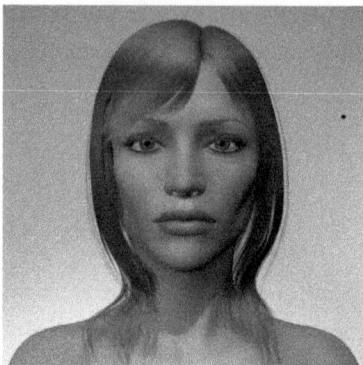

Subclinical (harder to detect)

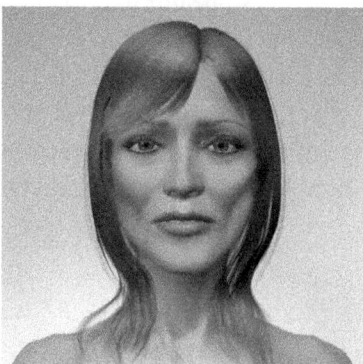

Marginal (sometimes observable)

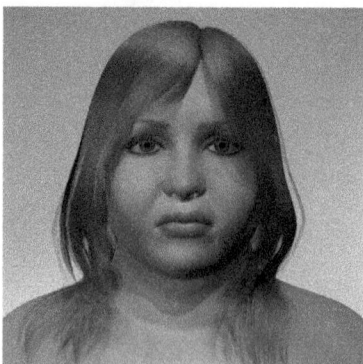

Obesity(observable)

Figure 1.2 Malnutrition Examples

Current Nutritional Status

Given the present health problems, Americans are far from getting what would be considered optimal nutrition for good health, vigor and well-being. Malnutrition or some form of nutritional deficiency is common in this country. However, the kind of malnutrition that exists in the United States and most industrialized nations today is not your classical type where children's stomachs become bloated and people end up with protruding bones and emaciated faces.

More often, the malnutrition that exists in Western countries is of the subtle, undetectable type, referred to (see Figure 1.2) as subclinical. In this type of nutritional deficiency, you may have nourished yourself just enough to meet all your body's minimum requirements but not sufficiently enough to give you that extra zest in life.

Subclinical malnutrition is not observable, because for all practical reasons you feel OK. The problem with this form of malnutrition, as with the other two discussed below, is that in the long run, your health will be seriously compromised. Like subterranean termites that slowly eat away at the wooden foundation of your home and finally bring the house tumbling down, a subclinical type of malnutrition could do the same to your body. Often, like those hidden termites, you would not notice that something is amiss until it's too late. Particularly predisposed to this type of nutritional deficiency are pregnant women, infants, teenagers and the elderly.

Marginal deficiency (also shown in Figure 1.2) is another type of malnutrition. With this, your body might be low in one or more nutrients, but you go on living without any outright sign of sickness, except perhaps for slight behavioral changes you might be experiencing from time to time.

People who have the third kind of malnutrition, obesity, can have the marginal or subclinical type in addition to being overweight. The problem with obese people is not that they get enough nutrients, but more often that they get too much of the wrong food. For example, if you gorge on fat-laden meals similar to those you find in fast-food outlets and some restaurants, or drink too much beer and eat too many processed foods, you will be malnourished. The fat, alcohol and sugars in these foods have no nutritional value for your body. They merely make you fat.

In addition, over time, fat begins to clog the arterial walls, alcohol starts to erode the health of your liver and brain cells and sugar undermines the proper function of the pancreas. You now become a strong candidate for cardiovascular diseases, diseases of the liver, diabetes and premature aging and death. At the moment, cancer and cardiovascular diseases account for more than 50% of the deaths or 1.3 million people in this country.

Ironically, in the United States, the above nutrition problems are not necessarily a condition of the poor, the homeless or a particular class or race of people. Several government surveys have shown that they are problems that affect people of all socioeconomic classes. According to one expert, "Everyone who has in the past eaten processed sugar, white flour, or canned food has some deficiency disease, the extent of the disease depending on the percentage of such deficient foods in the diet." That means practically everybody.

The chart below and Figure 1.3 show what could happen to the body as a result of chronic malnutrition. As you can see in these illustrations, nutritional deficiency can come about as a result of either inadequate diet or from the body's inability to process the food properly due to physiological or metabolic disorders. In either case, when this happens, nutrient stores in the body begin to decline. This problem leads first to abnormal function of tissues and organs, then to outwardly expressed symptoms or diseases such as scaly or coarse skin, cracking or ridging nails and thin and weak hair or scurvy, pellagra or rickets. To determine the causes of these symptoms or diseases, a health care professional first assesses a person's diet and medical history. These assessments are followed by a series of laboratory tests and physical examinations and measurements.

Series of events that could take place in one's body from chronic malnutrition

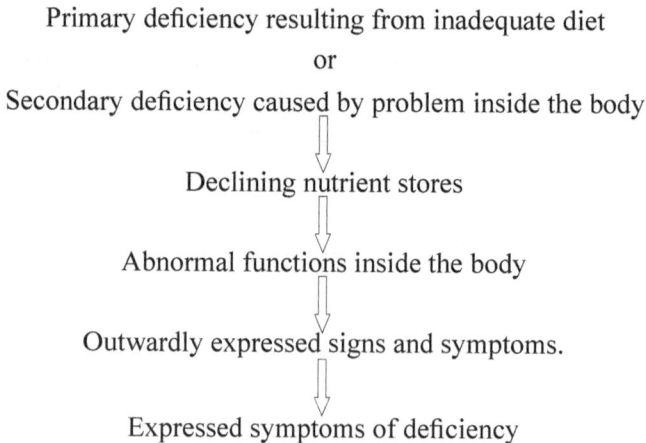

Primary deficiency resulting from inadequate diet

or

Secondary deficiency caused by problem inside the body

⇓

Declining nutrient stores

⇓

Abnormal functions inside the body

⇓

Outwardly expressed signs and symptoms.

⇓

Expressed symptoms of deficiency

Causes of Malnutrition

Besides having a problem with processed foods, Americans have had a great love affair with dairy and meat products. These foods are rich in saturated fats and protein, which may contribute to cardiovascular diseases, obesity, and a number of other problems. Milk, for example, could interfere with proper absorption of foods, and in infants, it could cause diarrhea and iron deficiency anemia. Furthermore, the high protein content in milk, could, among other things, lead to the depletion of a number of vitamins and minerals from the body, including potassium, calcium, magnesium and B vitamins.

More often than not, the food you eat is naturally nutritionally sparse because of over-farming. The agricultural lands of this country have long been depleted of their minerals, and the fertilizers used today have no more than three or four nutrients in them. A high concentration of these few nutrients may help plants to grow big and attractive, but these plants are far from being nutritionally balanced and complete. This is proven when you realize that plants need as many as 16 essential nutrients to grow well. There is a great variation in the nutritional content of vegetables grown in the United States.

The other major problem of malnutrition is simply a practical one. In these days of working couples and single men, single women and single parents, people don't seem to have the time, the desire, the discipline or the know-how to prepare well-balanced meals. These folks often opt for TV dinners, fast food or restaurant meals. The food from these sources either is not nutritious or has too much of the wrong things, such as fat, white bread, excess sugar, additives, and a number of other unhealthy substances.

Whatever the causes or the reasons—subclinical, marginal or obesity-malnutrition will definitely shorten the path to your grave. If you are serious about your health and quality of life, you need to take important steps right now! Since nutrition is the basis of it all, one of the first things you can do is to eat a well-balanced meal and incorporate the Four Pillar drinks as part of your everyday meals. As a margin of safety you also may want to take supplements: vitamins, minerals, amino acids and other nutrients. Your goal is not to have just normal nutrition but rather optimal nutrition.

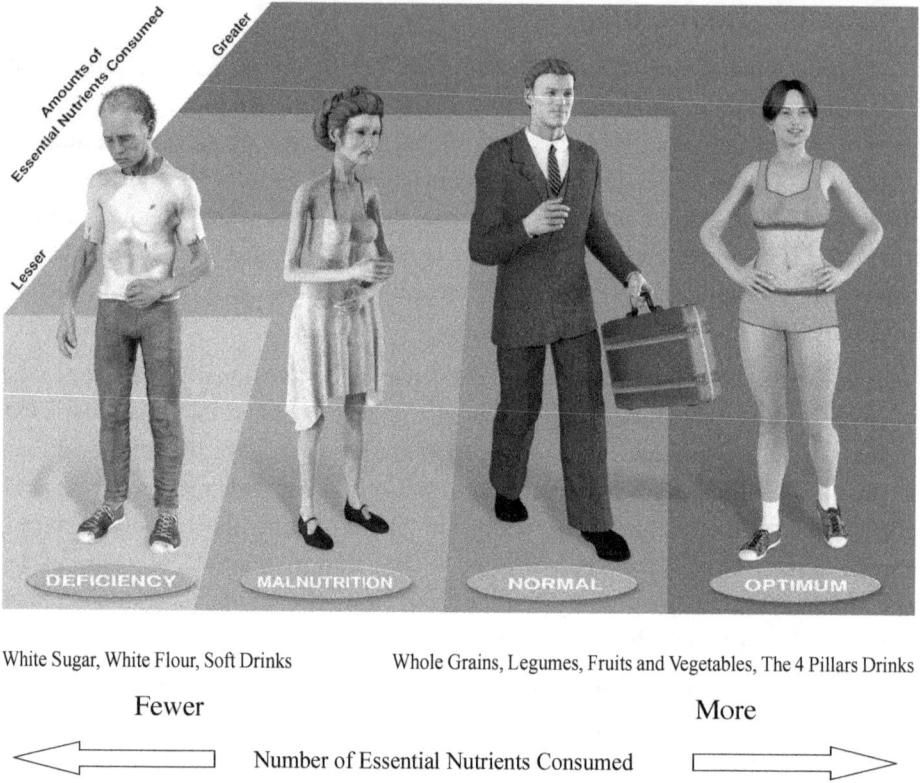

White Sugar, White Flour, Soft Drinks   Whole Grains, Legumes, Fruits and Vegetables, The 4 Pillars Drinks

Fewer   More

Number of Essential Nutrients Consumed

Figure 1.3 Nutrition Continuum

This nutrition continuum illustrates the four possible levels of nutrition and serves as a model that accommodates individual differences and nutritional need variabilities among humans.

Optimal Nutrition—Your Answer to Health and Longevity

As we mentioned earlier, current estimations put the maximum human biological age in the 115-year to 120-year range. Among many factors that influence your chance of reaching this range, nutrition ranks on top. To illustrate this point, we'll call that nutrition level that may help us reduce the gap between our current life expectancy of 76 years and the biological limit, the "optimal" nutrition.

However, because of the biological, physiological and gender variations among people as their age, stress level, physical conditions or types of work they do, people's nutritional needs will vary accordingly. This variability will create a problem for us to come up with a single nutritional or optimal standard.

Moreover, researchers have so far shown that we need at least 45 to 50 essential nutrients—nutrients that our bodies are not capable of producing. These include two essential fatty acids, eight essential amino acids, fifteen vitamins, twenty minerals and another five that are not conclusively known to be essential. Researchers have also shown that quantities higher than current RDA values of these nutrients can help us deal with many health-related issues, some of which are described below.

One, since your body depends on the food you eat for practically everything it does, the greater availability of the above nutrients in the tissues, the more effectively and vigorously it accomplishes its tasks or activities. For example, with optimal nutrition, your immune system can marshal its forces (immune cells) quickly and efficiently to defend your body in times of invasion by foreign elements like virus, bacteria or parasites. It can equally quickly suppress or destroy potential dangers (such as the growth of cancer) from within the body.

Two, if you are one of those people with special circumstances—e.g., have a stressful life-style, live or work in a polluted environment, are pregnant, are elderly or have a certain genetic defect—your need for nutrients may consequently be higher than most people's. Similarly, if you have surgery, are undergoing drug treatment or are having therapy, your need for nutrients may also be higher than most people's.

Three, certain nutrients when taken in higher doses do things that normal RDA amounts may not do for you. For example, when Vitamin A (as beta carotene) is taken in higher quantities, it protects the body from the destructive side effects of chemotherapy. Higher-than-RDA amounts of Vitamin E improve circulation. In women with premenstrual syndrome, Vitamin E also may help reduce breast tenderness. Similarly, higher amounts of Vitamin C and zinc speed up recovery from wounds and infection.

According to recent reports, greater amounts of Vitamin C (300 to 400 mgs per day) can prolong the life of men by six years. The current RDA for Vitamin C is 60 mgs. Similarly, higher-than-RDA amounts of Vitamin E were found to reduce the risk of heart disease..

Thus, to accommodate nutrient needs and quantity variabilities, we have to treat nutrition as a continuum. This means that in Figure 1.3 the two variables can be adequately represented. In this graph, office workers, physically active or sick people, as well as others with special nutritional needs, will also have their places. Let's see exactly what this graph tells us.

The horizontal axis represents the number of essential daily nutrient intakes. The vertical axis represents the amount of those intakes. The results of combining these two describe the nutritional conditions that we have labeled *deficiency, malnutrition, normal* and *optimum*. The figures in the chart represent each one of these conditions, or the z-axis of coordinate geometry.

Thus, as we go from left to right on the continuum, we are moving from nutritionally low foods (such as white bread, candy, pastries and soda pop) to those that are nutritionally dense[2] and balanced (such as The Four Pillars, liver and fish), which may bring you closer and closer to optimal health. How far along and how wide you are in the "optimal" range will depend on your own individual needs. If you are a person who is concerned about your looks or well-being, or the appearance of your hair and skin, you want to be as far along the continuum and as high up on it as your individual needs dictate.

If you are a growing person, elderly, sick, athletic or physically or emotionally stressed, you need nutrients and nutrient levels that can adequately help you meet these conditions. Are you a smoker, heavy drinker or other drug user? If so, your nutritional needs will be equally high and further to the right and higher up on the continuum. In this manner, as you provide your body with all the good nutrients it needs, all the organs (heart, lungs, liver, brain, etc.) should function to their maximum efficiency and capacity.[3]

Good nutrition, simply speaking, means eating a well-balanced diet, rich in vitamins, minerals, proteins, fibers, essential fatty acids and carbohydrates. Such a combination of nutrients and in higher concentrations may bring peace and order to your body. In the end you may feel a heightened sense of well-being, contentment and happiness.

---

2 Nutrient density is defined as the amounts of proteins, carbohydrates, vitamins and minerals contained in 100 kilocalories of any food. The health value (or desirability) of the food depends on the density of the nutrient per kilocalorie. This means, the greater the density, the more valuable (or desirable) the food. White bread has few nutrients, and therefore it is the least valuable. The Four Pillar drinks have a lot of nutrients and they therefore should be the most desirable.

3 This assumes, of course, that you have no genetic abnormality or other complications in pour body.

CHAPTER 2
Causes of Our Health Problems and Nutritional Solutions

As I indicated in the introduction, five years ago I began to experience numbness and tingling sensations in the two little fingers of my left hand. At the same time, my feet began to feel cold at night. So much so that I had to sit before a heater and warm them or bathe them in warm water, dry them and quickly go to bed. If I fell asleep right away, I was good. If I was awake for any length of time, I still could feel the coldness down there. Again I would get up and warm them for a while and then try to go to sleep once more.

When this problem persisted, I bought heavy wool socks and started wearing them shortly after I warmed my feet and right before I went to bed. This was a good temporary solution to my problem.

However, what the symptoms portend was rather alarming. We have heart problems in my family. My father and two of my older brothers died of heart attacks. My sister-in-law, who died of diabetes complications, had similar problems. But I was not diabetic. Mine was a case of poor circulation, because of possibly clogged arteries. What I couldn't get out of my mind was the image of my sister-in-law.

As mentioned earlier, in the final stage of her disease, my sister-in-law watched her body die by degrees right before her own eyes. Her toes and fingertips became black and shriveled as if they were singed with fire. Blisters appeared all over her body and she became progressively weaker and sicker.

I knew this was going to happen to me if I didn't take care of the problem immediately. At the time I noticed these troubles I didn't have a doctor and was away from a hospital where I could go to get checked. To allay my concerns, I called a cardiologist friend in New York City and explained the situation to him. He thought I might have some sort of blockage in my arteries and suggested that I should get checked as soon as I can.

I know it's foolhardy and I won't suggest to anybody to do this. I more or less guessed what the doctor would recommend as an ad hoc fix to the problem: give me a blood thinning pill.

I have never been a pill taker, not even Tylenol or aspirin. I always prefer to try natural remedies first. I knew ginger is one of the good natural remedies recommended for thinning blood and improving circulation. I began to take ginger tea—two to three times a day. I also began to exercise more often. I went on a longer walk and rode a stationary bike. Doing these things helped me quite a bit. I felt the tingling less often and the coldness in my feet was not as severe. I knew, however, this was only a band aid to a potentially worsening situation. I needed a systemic fix.

I theorized that the main cause of my poor circulation was my slowed metabolism due to my sedentary life. Before the onset of this condition I was writing the first volume of the *Desta* series where I sat at my computer for long hours at a time. Although I was not visibly overweight, still fat was manufactured and stored in my body, and some of it was beginning to clog the blood passages.

I also knew vitamins and minerals are critical for the processing and utilization of the food I eat—both as fuel and its conversion into my body tissues.

Phytonutrients—the bright colors in fruits and vegetables—have many beneficial properties. They serve as antioxidants and help fight cancer and heart diseases, including the aging of our bodies. Dietary fibers remove excess fat, toxins and many other harmful substances from the bod y. They also improve the function of the gastro-intestinal (GI) tract.

To take advantage of all these benefits, I wrote down a list of fruits, vegetables and herbs I thought would be helpful for my condition and went shopping. You will see many of these items in the Four Pillars recipe section of this book. In all, there were twenty-two. My wife and I had to play with the proportions until we achieved a good-tasting drink. We made enough of this to last us a week.

To our amazement, by the time we finished our first batch, I no longer had the problem with my circulation. No tingling sensation in my little fingers or coldness in my feet. We continued to make and drink the concoction. We noted something else happening in our bodies. Our skin became soft, healthy and vibrant. I used to have bleeding in my gums. This problem stopped. I also used to have throat irritation where I had to constantly clear it as if something was stuck in there. I have no more of this problem, either.

My wife had equally surprising results. She used to have severe allergies—itchy eyes, throat and ears, and her eyelids felt dry. To find relief from these conditions, she took daily allergy pills. Now since she has been on The Four-Pillars drink, all those problems stopped and she no longer takes the pills. Our skins improved significantly, becoming smooth and translucent. Our hair became thicker, healthier and more vibrant. We also noticed faster growth in our nails and hair. In addition to all these results, we have had a great sense of well-being and vitality since we have been on these drinks.

What we have observed with these foods is a true testament to Hippocrates' ancient dictum: "Make food thy medicine, medicine shall be thy food."

Precaution: The results we got may not be true with every person who wishes to make their own Four Pillars drinks, using the recipes given in this book. If you're on medication or have any health problems, you should check with your doctor first before incorporating these foods into your daily regimen. All we suggest is you try them and see if they work for you.

Now let's talk about the components of The Four Pillars: vitamins, minerals, fiber and phytonutrients.

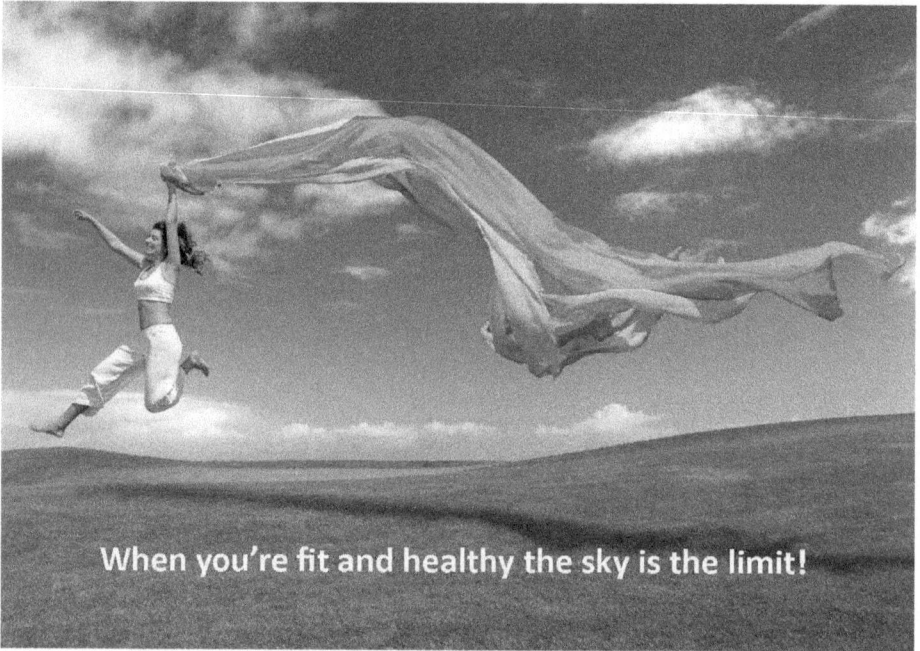

When you're fit and healthy the sky is the limit!

Pillar One

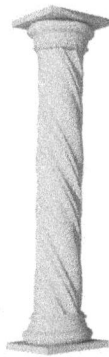

Vitamins

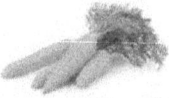

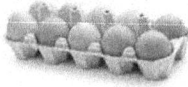

Vitamin A is also called retinol. It is necessary for healthy vision and also helps create strong bones and teeth, as well as a strong immune system.

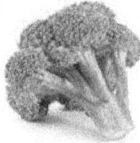

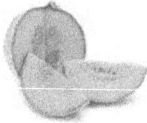

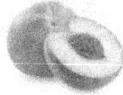

Vitamin B is a group of vitamins that help the body turn food into energy. They are also needed to make red blood cells and the genetic materials DNA and RNA.

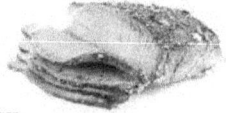

The vitamin B group includes:

- °B1 (thiamin)
- °B2 (riboflavin)
- °B3 (niacin)
- °B5 (pantothenic acid)
- °B6 (pyridoxine)
- °B9 (folic acid)
- °B12 (cobalomin)
- °BIOTIN

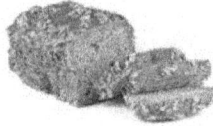

Vitamin D is made by the body when it is exposed to the sun. The vitamin is also found in certain foods. Vitamin D helps the body absorb the mineral calcium. It also helps build strong bones and teeth.

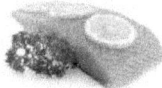

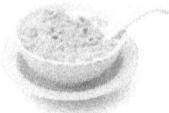

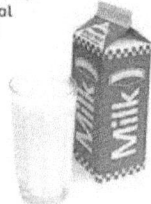

Vitamin C, also called ascorbic acid, is necessary for making collagen, which holds body cells together. It also aids in the healing of wounds and burns and helps build strong teeth and bones.

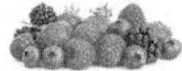

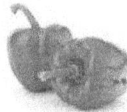

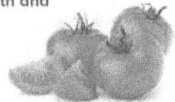

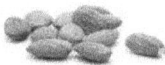

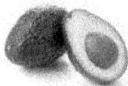

Vitamin E helps maintain healthy red blood cells and muscle tissue.

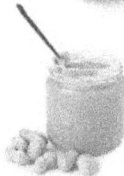

Vitamin K is necessary for blood to clot when you get a cut. Half of the vitamin comes from the food you eat; the other half is manufactured by bacteria in your intestines.

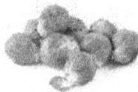

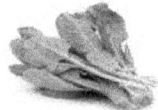

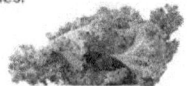

WWW.KIDSDISCOVER.COM

Sample foods and their vitamin contents

Vitamins: An Introduction

Vitamins are a group of organic compounds that have critical metabolic functions in the body. They are essential for the conversion of food into energy and the repair and growth of body tissues. In fact, all the carbohydrates, proteins and oils you eat would mean nothing to your body if you didn't have the necessary vitamins in your diet. Simply speaking, if you have a deficiency of one or more of the vitamins, your physical, intellectual and emotional activities will be all compromised.

Two types of vitamins:

• Fat soluble ones: A, D, E and K

• Water soluble ones: Vitamin C and the nine B-complex vitamins.

The fat-soluble vitamins require fat in the diet to be picked up by the lymphatic fluid and delivered into the bloodstream. You don't have to consume extra fat for this reason. What you obtain from your normal diet is usually sufficient.

Once in the body, any excess amounts of the fat-soluble vitamins are stored in the liver and the fat tissues of the body. Therefore, your need for this group of vitamins is not as frequent as for those that are water soluble, which get flushed out of your body with urine and perspiration. This latter group may stay, at the most, four days in the body. The only exception is Vitamin B12, of which the liver stores in large enough supply to last you three to five years.

Vitamins are required in minute amounts. Although they don't become directly involved in metabolic processes (as fuel or structural components), they are responsible for the proper functioning of those processes as well as the general well-being of your body.

Biochemically speaking, vitamins function as cofactors or coenzymes, enabling the various chemical processes in your body to take place efficiently and smoothly.

In this regard, vitamins resemble the oil or lubricating fluids in your car. Just as your car would begin to show problems and eventually come to a grinding halt if you didn't have a sufficient amount of lubricating oil in it, so would your body if you didn't give it the necessary vitamins. The absence or shortage of vitamins in your body can lead to deficiency symptoms. For instance, bleeding and easy bruising can be a sign of Vitamin C deficiency, while listlessness, weight loss and heart failure can indicate a shortage of thiamine (Vitamin B1).

With the exception of Vitamin B12 and vitamin D, which can be synthesized by some animals, all the vitamins must be obtained from plant sources. Theoretically, if you choose your food from a wide variety of sources—whole grains, fresh vegetables and fruits and meats like liver and chicken—you should get all the vitamins and other necessary nutrients. This, according to several surveys, is far from being the norm.

As I indicated earlier, people in this country are nutritionally impoverished. There are several factors leading to this problem, including the food-processing industry, the lifestyles and habits of people and the long depleted soils. Processing, canning and storing foods deplete or destroy nutrients. Added to this are the lifestyles and eating and working habits of people: skipping meals, eating on the run, working and living in stressful environments, smoking, drinking too much coffee and alcohol and consuming too much junk food.

If you are a teenager, a workaholic, an older person or an athlete or are pregnant, your need for complete and balanced meals is much greater than average. Just as a teenager or a fetus needs all the necessary nutrients to develop and grow properly, so does a workaholic or an athlete who depletes his/her body's nutrients from too much exertion. When one grows older or consumes excessive alcohol and coffee or when one is stressed, the absorption of nutrients from the intestine is decreased.

From national surveys, the most commonly deficient nutrients are vitamins A, C, D and E and the minerals calcium, potassium, magnesium, zinc, iron, copper, chromium, fluoride and selenium, as well as nearly all the Vitamin B-complex series. What is the solution to this dire problem?

The first thing you can do is watch what you eat and drink. Minimize or eliminate your intake of sweets, alcohol and coffee and select whole grains, fruits, vegetables and legumes as your primary foods and meats and dairy products as your secondary foods. With regards to the fruits and vegetables, the most effective way to make your Four Pillar drinks, using the recipes given later in this book. If you don't have a ready-made supply of this drink or are traveling, you may want to include quality supplements with some of your daily meals.

The following chapters can help you understand the significance of each vitamin in your health and factors that may aid or hinder their absorption through the intestinal wall.

CHAPTER 3
Fat-Soluble Vitamins

Vitamin A

There are two common forms of vitamin A. Beta carotene (a member of the carotenoid pro-vitamins), which you find in yellow, red and green vegetables as well as eggs and dairy products, is the precursor of vitamin A. This form is the safest in terms of toxicity because once it gets into the body the liver converts it into Vitamin A as the need arises. You can consume a massive amount of beta carotene without having to worry about overdosing. The form of Vitamin A found in fish oil and organ meats is known as retinol. Because it is fat soluble, if taken in excess for a prolonged period, it can build up in the body and become toxic.

Vitamin A is important for the health and appearance of your skin, hair and eyes and the lining of your digestive tract. It is also important for healthy formation of nails, bones and teeth and for growth and maintenance of tissues and organs. In addition, this important vitamin is involved in wound healing, as well as the healthy development and maintenance of intercellular tissues and mucous membranes. When you have sufficient amounts of Vitamin A in your body, nerve cells transmit information faster, hence enhancing your ability to recall and think clearly.

Women who suffer from menstrual problems find Vitamin A to be helpful in reducing flow and discomfort. For those who are pregnant, this vitamin contributes to full and healthy development of their fetuses. This vitamin is equally important for children and lactating women. Vitamin A is a great antioxidant and it helps fight infections and other diseases by strengthening the immune system.

Deficiency symptoms

A deficiency of Vitamin A is often manifested as poor tooth formation and gum problems, susceptibilities to allergies and infections, night blindness and dry, scaly skin and hair. Furthermore, in children, Vitamin A deficiency can lead to growth retardation and poor muscular and skeletal development. In adults, Vitamin A deficiency can cause the mucous membranes of the mouth and the respiratory and gastrointestinal tracts to dry out. This can lead to a loss of taste and smell as well as vulnerability to colds and microbial infections.

Food Sources and RDA Requirements

All the colored vegetables, dairy products and organ meats, such as liver, kidney, beef and eggs are excellent sources of vitamin A. However, most people don't get sufficient amount of this important vitamin from their normal diets. Several studies have shown that most Americans suffer from a deficiency of vitamin A. However, if you take your Four Pillar drinks daily, you should get a healthy amount of this important nutrient.

The RDA for Vitamin A is 5000 I.U. (international unit), as retinol. To have the dosage necessary for some of the powerful effects of vitamin A, you may need to consume large amounts of the vegetables mentioned above. For example, to use Vitamin A as a weapon against cancer and aging, you need to have a daily intake of four to five times the RDA. For most people, this is an impractical situation. This is where the Four Pillars recipes come in handy.

Finally, depending on your age, health and stress level, you may also need more of this vitamin to fortify you from infections and diseases or to assure your fast recovery from illness. As you age, the body also tends to generate more free radicals, chemical fragments believed to be the causes of cancer, heart diseases and the aging of our bodies. This, combined with daily emotional or physical stress, can require larger amounts of this vitamin.

You have two options. 1. You can make your own Four Pillars drinks and have a glass of it with your meals every day. 2. Find a good supplement that can give you four to five times the RDA of vitamin A—preferably as beta-carotene. Option 1 would be your best choice. Besides vitamin A, you get many other nutrients, including fiber and phytonutrients. Of course, you can still supplement for the times you have not made your drink or when you're traveling.

Absorption Suppressors: Alcohol, coffee, Vitamin D deficiency and sometimes excessive iron.

Absorption Facilitators: Vitamins C, D, E and F (the essential fatty acids), zinc, calcium and the Vitamin B-complex.

Vitamin D

Nicknamed the "sunshine vitamin" because it can be produced in the body with the help of the sun's ultraviolet light, Vitamin D has several benefits to your health. These range from its function in the proper development of the skeletal system in growing children to the maintenance of adequate calcium levels in adult bodies to its use in the treatment of certain skin conditions and even to the suppression of some cancer cells.

There are ten different compounds that are grouped together as vitamin D, but the ones that are most important are Vitamins D2 (ergocalciferol—found in plants such as yeasts and fungi) and D3 (cholecalciferol-found in animal products such as liver). Both of these vitamins can be formed in the skin and used by the body.

Historically, Vitamin D deficiency has been linked to the malformation of bones in children and to the softening or hollowing of bones in adults. Vitamin D regulates the absorption and utilization of calcium and phosphorous—minerals responsible for the construction and growth of strong bones and teeth.

Deficiency symptoms

The absence or lack of Vitamin D in the body often leads to rickets in children and osteoporosis (hollowing of the bones) and osteomalacia (softening of the bones) in adults. Normally, these conditions can be avoided if one gets sufficient amounts of sunlight and minerals regularly.

Naturally, Vitamin D is synthesized in the skin from the sun and cholesterol. After conversion into active form in the liver and kidneys, it enters the bloodstream where it functions as a hormone and a vitamin. As mentioned above, Vitamin D promotes the absorption of calcium and phosphorous through the intestinal wall into the blood. When the availability of these minerals in the diet is limited or there are absorption problems, Vitamin D induces the mobilization of calcium from the bones. This event can lead to osteoporosis or osteomalacia in adults if it occurs over prolonged periods.

In recent years, Vitamin D has been found to help in the treatment of psoriasis when taken internally or used in skin lotions. This white crystalline substance has also been shown to reduce the replication or duplication of certain cancer cells. Cancers that afflict the lungs, cervix, colon, breast and blood were shown to respond to Vitamin D supplementation. According to one study, people who spent a great deal of time indoors were more prone to get colon and rectal cancers than those who spent time outside.

The absence of Vitamin D in the body even seems to contribute to bilateral (both sides) deafness in humans. Since the cochlea in the inner ear is made up of bones, anything that affects the structural integrity of these bones (like increasing porosity) can affect the normal transmission of information from the outer to the inner ear. Although there has not been conclusive evidence to indicate whether Vitamin D supplementation can help reverse the problem, preliminary findings show it to be promising.

One thing to remember is the fact that as you get older, less and less of the available minerals will be absorbed by the intestine. By increasing your intake of calcium and phosphorous as well as Vitamin D, you help minimize the problems associated with its deficiency.

Toxicity

Because Vitamin D is fat soluble, it tends to collect in the fatty tissues of the body. When there are excess amounts of Vitamin D in your system, calcium and phosphorous begin to accumulate in the wrong places—such as the blood vessels, the heart and even the lungs and kidneys.

The reported toxicity threshold is in the range of 500 to 600 mcgs/k of body weight per day consumed over a period of several weeks. The resulting symptoms from Vitamin D overdose vary from headaches, nausea, loss of appetite and thirst to excessive urination and lethargy.

Bear in mind that Vitamin D toxicity can come only from food sources. It seems that the Vitamin D produced in your body is monitored by keratin and melanin synthesis that block the ultraviolet rays.

Food Sources and RDA Requirements

The RDA requirement for Vitamin D varies from 7.5 micrograms for infants to 10 micrograms for children, adults (up to 24 years of age) and pregnant and lactating women. For adults above 25 years of age, the dietary requirement for Vitamin D drops to 5 micrograms.

Study after study bears out the fact that there is widespread Vitamin D deficiency in the adult population in this country. This is another indication of the inadequacies of the RDA as a nutritional guideline. As you get older, your need for vitamin D, calcium and phosphorous is increased because of intestinal malabsorption and reduced exposure to the sun. With age, the body doesn't readily convert Vitamin D into its active forms.

Fish such as salmon, herring, sardines and tuna as well as cod liver and fish oil extracts are good sources of vitamin D. Other food sources include egg yolk, liver, butter and fortified milk. Plants, in general, are very poor sources of vitamin D.

Absorption Suppressors: Mineral oil.

Absorption Facilitators: Phosphorus, vitamins A, C and F, choline and calcium.

Vitamin E

From its early discovery, Vitamin E has been associated with something near and dear to everyone's heart: sex. Researchers who established the importance of this vitamin in our health also observed a correlation between the fertility of experimental animals and the presence of Vitamin E in their diet. For example, rats that were fed food that lacked Vitamin E failed to have offspring but the reverse happened when they were given a diet with known sources of the vitamin. From this connection, early discoverers of this vitamin coined its scientific name: tocopherol. Tocopherol is a combination of two Greek words, tocos and phero, which means "childbirth" and 'to bring forth," respectively. For a long time, Vitamin E has been dubbed as the "sex vitamin" much to the wary minds of the researchers who came later.

Although you shouldn't expect to improve your sexual prowess by taking heavy doses of vitamin E, you can be assured that the reasonable level of the vitamin will enhance your fertility level. If you are a woman, you can also count on this vitamin to help reduce menopausal symptoms of "hot flashes" and headaches. If you are a man, you'll benefit by an adequate level of Vitamin E in your diet; it plays a role in the proper functioning of the sexual glands.

Vitamin E is divided into several related compounds that, depending on their molecular structures are called alpha, beta, gamma, etc., tocopherols. There is also a synthetic version, which is prefixed as dl-tocopherol. The one that is natural and which people commonly refer to as Vitamin E is the alpha-tocopherol. This is the most biologically active. The synthetic version is not as effective as the one that is natural.

The pure form of Vitamin E is a yellowish oil that is very sensitive to light and oxidation. Vitamin E's primary function in the body is to protect the tissues and other vitamins such as A, C, D and F. Free radicals formed from unsaturated fatty acids and during metabolic processes have been linked to the genesis of various cancers and aging.

Vitamin E, by interfering with the damaging effects of these biological rene-gades, can help slow down the aging process and the onset of cancers in the body. For example, the testes and the brain cells are rich in unsaturated fatty acids. Vitamin E helps protect these organs from free radical damage and consequently can help prevent loss of fertility or brain tissue damage.

In other areas, Vitamin E is found to help in the maintenance of healthy muscles and nerves as well as to protect the functional integrity of blood vessels. Your skin and hair and the lining of the mucous membranes also benefit from a proper level of Vitamin E in the body. In addition, Vitamin E was found to lower overall cholesterol levels while increasing the HDL (the good cholesterol) in the body. This versatile vitamin is also found to help in healing wounds and in improving circulation.

Vitamin E's Other Benefits

Vitamin E has many other important benefits, some of which are directly or indirectly related to its ability to fight free radicals. Our immune system, for example, declines with age, and it's believed that this is attributable to free radical damage to the immune cells. When you protect these cells by supplying an adequate amount of Vitamin E and other antioxidants, you improve their effectiveness and protective power.

Vitamin E helps protect the structural and functional integrity of red blood cells. Because this group of cells is critically involved in transporting the life-giving oxygen in your body, the presence of a sufficient level of Vitamin E in your blood will improve your energy level and well-being.

Those who engage in a strenuous physical activity (for example, athletes and construction workers), can greatly benefit from this vitamin. During physically stressful activities, the body produces many free radicals. Drinking a glass of your Four Pillars drink along with quality multi-vitamins supplement can help protect the damaging effect of these harmful substances.

In addition, Vitamin E is known to help with a host of other health-threatening situations. The aggregation of platelets that obstructs the normal flow of blood is one of the causes of heart attacks. Vitamin E has been shown to minimize this problem by keeping the platelets fully dispersed in the blood.

One physician has used Vitamin E to effectively control the fibrocystic breast disease, a precursor to breast cancer. A dosage of 600 I.U. of the vitamin was used in this particular experiment.

This multipurpose vitamin has also been shown to help fend off the deleterious effects of some noxious chemicals in the air and damage from radiation and toxic industrial/agricultural chemicals, such as food additives, herbicides and insecticides. Furthermore, Vitamin E has been shown to help with osteoarthritis, muscular dystrophy and something as common as tartar buildup on the teeth.

Women using birth control pills often hear of a common side effect: internal blood clots. This could lead to a serious heart problem if allowed to persist. The pill interferes with the adequate absorption of Vitamin E into the intestinal tract. At higher doses of vitamin E, however, this problem was shown to be reversed.

Long-term Deficiency of Vitamin E and Your Health

Unlike the other two vitamins discussed above, which have been associated with specific diseases when severe deficiency exists, no particular disease has been attributed to a lack of vitamin E. Nonetheless, a serious shortage of the vitamin can lead to multitude of symptoms—from anemia (resulting from premature deaths of red blood cells) to the degeneration of the muscular, nervous and vascular system, as well as to the atrophying of brain, spinal cord and endocrine glands.

It is now believed that a long-term, subclinical deficiency of Vitamin E can also lead to cancer, heart disease, senility, premenstrual syndrome and even premature aging.

RDA Requirements

The current RDA requirements range from 3 milligrams for infants to 12 milligram for breast-feeding women. As was stated earlier with the other vitamins, one needs to take considerably higher amounts than the RDAs to realize the full benefits of Vitamin E. Some experiments used as high as 1,600 I.U. of this vitamin without any complications. Continuous usage of extremely high doses (in excess of 1,200 mg), however, has been reported to cause a number of ailments, including diarrhea, headaches, nausea and palpitations of the heart.

Food Sources

There are a variety of food sources for vitamin E. These include whole wheat, brown rice, oatmeal, rye, molasses, sesame and alfalfa seeds, potatoes, organ meats and nuts like almonds, walnuts and peanuts. Nearly all the green vegetables are other good sources, but the richest sources by far are foods such as wheat germ, soybean oil, sunflower seed oil, cottonseed oil and corn oil.

There are a number of reasons, however, why you would not get adequate levels of Vitamin E from the above food sources.

One, because a great percentage of the food in this country is processed, Vitamin E is destroyed or eliminated during processing. What is available in processed foods is not sufficient to give the level of protection we discussed above, including fighting free radicals. As mentioned earlier, you need at least 600-1,200 mg of the vitamin to realize all its healing and protective benefits.

Two, canning and long storage of foods, a common practice, can also destroy this rather fragile vitamin.

Three, although Vitamin E is found in greater quantities in oil-based foods, it is destroyed during the heat-extraction process. Cold-pressed oils tend to retain much of their vitamin E.

The Solution

Consume your Four Pillars foods and drinks. Have supplements handy for the time you don't make your drinks or are traveling.

Absorption Suppressors: Chlorine, heat, air-damaged oils and mineral oil.

Absorption Facilitators: Selenium, manganese, phosphorous, vitamins A, C and F and the B-complex group.

Vitamin K

This vitamin is one of the unsung heroes because although its known function in the body is a critical one, it does not have the prominence or versatility of usage the other vitamins discussed so far bear. Vitamin K , whose name was derived from the Scandinavian equivalent for "coagulation" (koagulation), has one primary but critical purpose in the human diet: *it is responsible for stopping the flow of blood when you get cut.*

Prothrombin is a precursor protein to thrombin, which enables the blood to coagulate and stops the flow of blood when you bleed. Vitamin K is the agent responsible for the synthesis of prothrombin in the liver and indirectly for blood clots.

There are three forms of Vitamin K. K1 is derived from alfalfa. K2 is synthesized by bacteria within the intestinal tract of mammals, and Vitamin K 3 is man made and, functionally, has twice the potency of the natural forms.

Deficiency Symptoms

Although Vitamin K deficiency is relatively uncommon in adults, since the body can produce its own from the bacteria inside the intestine, newborns and infants experience Vitamin K deficiency at a relatively high frequency. When the deficiency does occur, the associated symptoms are the appearance of blood in the stool, in urine and in vomit.

When the deficiency occurs in adults, it is usually a result of poor diet or the destruction of the Vitamin K-producing bacteria in the intestine by antibiotics, barbiturates and sulfa drugs. Even aspirin, food, air pollutants and radiation can lead to the depletion of Vitamin K in the intestinal tract.

In addition, since Vitamin K is fat soluble, anything that interferes with the absorption of fats (such as poor production of bile and pancreatic juices, mineral oil, steatorrhea or celiac disease) can also interfere with the availability of the vitamin to the body.

Food Sources and RDA Requirements

Vegetables like cauliflower, cabbage, kelp and spinach are excellent sources of Vitamin K . Soybeans, liver, egg yolk, fruits, cereals, yogurt, fish oil and dairy products are also known to have a sufficient level of the vitamin. Since your body naturally produces the vitamin, these food sources serve mainly as a security blanket.

For the first time, we now have an RDA for Vitamin K . It ranges from 5 mcgs for newborns to 95 mcgs for lactating women, 80 mcgs for normal adults.

Toxicity

Although there is no known full-blown toxicity from Vitamin K overdose, a condition known as hemolytic anemia (resulting from excessive breakdown of red blood cells) has been observed in premature and low-birth weight infants.

Absorption Suppressors: Mineral oil, aspirin, oxidized fats, x-rays and radiation.

Absorption Facilitators: None.

Vitamin F

These are group of molecules called Essential Fatty acids or EFAs. The most critical ones of these molecules are alpha-linolenic acid (an omega-3 fatty acid) and linoleic acid (an omega-6 fatty acid). They were discovered in the early 1920s and found to be essential for good health and were called Vitamin F. Later, because of their molecular properties they were classified as fats. I resurrect their former name here for convenience and emphasize their importance. Only omega-3 and omega-6 are considered essential but there are two more fatty acids that can become essential under certain circumstances.

The EFAs in and of themselves are no more significant than ordinary fats. They serve as fuel, used to build tissues or get converted and stored as body fat. Their essentialness lies in their serving as the raw materials for the synthesis of an intriguing group of molecules called Prostaglandins. Isolated from the prostate gland (thus their name) in the early 1930s, Prostaglandins perform many critical functions in our bodies.

There are roughly 30 known prostaglandins, but of these, only about three have been extensively studied. Prostaglandin El is one of those on which we have an impressive amount of information. Formed from omega-6 fatty acid, Prostaglandin El has many benefits to your health. They function like hormones in that they control the activities of enzymes, cells and organs. Yet unlike hormones, prostaglandins are more localized and short-lived-lasting, at most, a few seconds after being synthesized.

The influence they have on our bodies during these fleeting moments, however, is pretty astounding. By enabling the blood vessels to dilate and platelets to remain fully dispersed, El can help you minimize the incidence of cardiovascular diseases. When platelets stick together, they tend to form clots, which can obstruct blood vessels, causing heart attack or stroke. In the liver, El limits the production of cholesterol, which is equally important to the health of your circulatory system. Prostaglandin El similarly inhibits the production of potentially cancerous cells in the body.

Insulin, which helps us metabolize sugar, is empowered in the presence of prostaglandin El. This is a bit of good news for diabetics. Those who suffer from arthritis can find relief with El, because it has an ability to inhibit the production of inflammatory chemicals in the joints and elsewhere in the body. In the brain, El can increase the activities of the neurons that help elevate your mood and bring you a sense of well-being.

Your immune and reproductive systems are also greatly benefited by prostaglandin El. Outwardly this versatile molecule can also improve your skin and hair because it has an influence on the production of sebum and other chemicals that keep the skin healthy.

Unfortunately, as much as there are health-providing prostaglandins like El, there are also others that have the opposite action on our bodies. One particular culprit, called prostaglandin E2, can instigate many unwanted problems. These range from causing inflammation in the joints to making the platelets to stick together and fluid to build up in the tissues, which are all not good.

Fortunately, the production of E2 is inhibited as long as you have more of El. It has been found that although both El and E2 have the same parent, the production of El is normally favored over E2. As it turns out, this is dependent on the amount of essential fatty acids you have in your body. Flaxseed and evening primrose oil are the best sources of these series of prostaglandins. The availability of the necessary vitamin and mineral cofactors is also very important for the conversion of the fatty acids into prostaglandins.

The third, very well documented prostaglandins are the E3 series. These molecules can be derived from omega-3 fatty acids, but they also can come from eicosapentaenoic acid (EPA) found in fish oil. Considering E3's role in the proper functioning of the nervous system and its use in the synthesis of brain cells, the folklore about the importance of fish to the brain is not without basis.

In terms of their benefit to our health, E3s have many functions similar to Els. These included their ability to reduce heart attack and stroke by lowering the production of cholesterol and triglycerides (fats) and their ability in helping to boost the immune system and in lowering the incidence of cancer. Prostaglandins, E3 as well as El, are also involved in alleviating mental disorders such as depression and schizophrenia.

In another area, these prostaglandins are essential for protection of the gastric mucosa (the mucous membrane) against the extreme acidity found in the stomach. The gastric side effects of drugs like Motrin happen because the levels of prostaglandins in the gastric mucosa are also reduced (not just those in the uterus), and hence one can get irritation of the gastric mucosa.

As you can see, the conversion of these important foods into those key endproducts is not often an easy one. There are many factors that can impede, as well as aid, the processes. The key is to distinguish those that aid your cells to manufacture the prostaglandins from those that block their synthesis.

Food sources: salmon, Herring and Mackerel from fish and flax, hemp, walnut and almond, from nuts and such, and dark greens such as broccoli and spinach from vegetables. Olive oil, whole grain foods and eggs can be a good source as well.

CHAPTER 4
Water-Soluble Vitamins

Vitamin C

From your health science classes, you probably remember a disease called scurvy that afflicted sailors in the British Navy until James Lind discovered the cure for it, the juice of citrus fruit. Scurvy is a Vitamin C deficiency disease that manifests itself in a variety of ways, including hemorrhaging, gum inflammation, loosening of teeth, swollen joints, weakness, weight loss and difficulty in healing soft tissues after a bruise or trauma.

This disease is perhaps now no more than a medical curiosity, something akin to the bubonic plague, smallpox or cholera. When medicine was in its infancy and people didn't know much about health and nutrition, such afflictions were disastrous.

Today you hear more about the benefit of Vitamin C and orange juice when you are sick with the common cold or the flu than you hear of its benefits in preventing scurvy. "Drink a lot of orange juice" is the classic response as soon as someone finds out about your malady.

Vitamin C's Benefits

Vitamin C, also known as ascorbic acid, has many important and critical functions in your body. These range from lowering the incidence of cancer and heart disease to helping you cope with emotional and physical stresses. This nutrient is truly a wonder of nature. There is no other vitamin that contributes as much to the overall structural and functional integrity of your muscles, bones, teeth, skin and connective tissues as vitamin C. Simply put, if you had a severe deficiency of vitamin C, you could literally fall apart!

Collagen is the scaffolding protein that holds everything together from your connective tissues to your bones and teeth, to your skin and tendons. It will not function or form properly without an adequate level of Vitamin C in your tissues. The adrenal, pituitary and thymus glands and the metabolically active tissues, like your muscles, also depend on the availability of Vitamin C in the blood for their proper development and function.

Vitamin C helps in the growth and repair of cells, blood vessels and gums. If you have a wound, a burn or a cold, Vitamin C speeds your recovery from these sicknesses. By fortifying your immune system, Vitamin C can also help your body protect itself against viral infections and many cancer-causing agents.

In addition, this wonder vitamin is known to assist in alleviating tension by inducing the production of stress-reducing hormones in the body. For example, whenever you suffer emotional or physical stress, your body is drained of its Vitamin C supply. Increased Vitamin C intake during this time will help you cope better with your condition. Researchers have also observed the benefit of Vitamin C in lowering blood cholesterol and triglycerides (fats) and the reduced incidence of clots in blood vessels. One British study showed that a high level of Vitamin C significantly increases the HDL (the good) cholesterol while it lowers the LDL (the bad) cholesterol. This role of the vitamin consequently reduces the incidence of heart attack and stroke.

Vitamin C's Other Benefits

This great vitamin has many other roles in your health. For instance, sufficient amounts of Vitamin C in your body will enhance your mental ability as well as improve your sleep patterns. The absorption of iron, calcium and certain essential amino acids from the intestinal tract, as well as the removal of toxic metals such as mercury, cadmium, lead and aluminum, is greatly aided by the presence of a sufficient amount of Vitamin C in the body. Smokers and older persons have a higher need for vitamin C. Athletes and all those who engage in strenuous physical exertion will be benefited if they take a 500 mg - 1,000 mg of Vitamin C before and after activity.

Do you have lower back problems? Are you recovering from surgery or trying to heal a wound? Take higher doses of Vitamin C more frequently. Its ability to help in the formation of collagen plays an important role in speeding up the healing process as well as in strengthening your tissues.

Diabetics often suffer from easy bleeding and bruising because of weak and fragile capillaries. Vitamin C along with bioflavonoids can strengthen the collagen matrix and help reduce the problems.

People suffering from arthritis, fatigue, herpes or even schizophrenia find Vitamin C to be very helpful in lessening the effects of their illnesses. Vitamin C also improves fertility in both men and women and does a great job in mopping up the toxins and pollutants that may find their way into our bodies through the air, water and food we consume.

Incidentally, smokers need more than the RDA amounts because each cigarette destroys 25-100 mg of vitamin C. Perhaps this is one of the reasons why smokers have such a high incidence of cancer. Carbon monoxide also has the same effect on the vitamin C. These people, in addition to making and consuming their Four Pillars drinks, are encouraged to take a good Vitamin C supplement.

Deficiency Symptoms

Some of the associated symptoms arising from Vitamin C deficiency are swollen joints, muscular weakness, slow healing wounds, easy bruising and bleeding as well as low resistance to colds and infections.

Vitamin C Amounts

For many of the above benefits, you need considerably higher than the RDA, which is 60 mg for adults. In many of the experiments that showed significant improvements, patients were given levels of more than 1,000 mg, and some as many as 3,000 mg daily.

Obviously, you are not going to get these amounts of the vitamin from your morning orange juice or even from individual vegetable sources such as broccoli, peppers, cabbage, tomatoes, Brussels sprouts, collards and cauliflower or even from your Four Pillars drink. All these are known to be rich in Vitamin C and may only help you to achieve three to four times the RDA. Because of vitamin C's water solubility, canning, cooking, soaking and storing these vegetables will further diminish their content of vitamin C.

If you are depending on frozen orange juice, chances are you may not even be getting enough Vitamin C to meet the RDA. Vitamin C is highly oxidizable, and during processing and freezing much of the vitamin found in natural form is destroyed. Fresh fruits and vegetables as found in the Four Pillars drink are best, but to attain the beneficial levels (1,000 mg or more), you would have to consume a large number of these fruits or vegetables daily—obviously not much of an option.

The Solution

The first option would be to make your Four Pillars blend out of all the sources of Vitamin C mentioned above and drink it as juice with your three meals. That way you can get a substantial amount of the vitamin, together with all the other nutrients. However, if you are physically active, a smoker or elderly or work at a stressful job, you may want to complement your Four Pillars drink with a well-formulated Vitamin C supplement. This would be the second option.

Both generic and brand-name products abound at your local health food or drug store. You need to be watchful of the type of supplement you take, however. Some of the supplements you find in your local health food or drug store can be of poor quality and low potency. Regardless of what form (tablets or capsules) they come in, most of the supplements don't have even the RDA amounts.

You also have to be concerned with the quality of the supplements. If tablets are pressed too hard or are constituted with fillers and binders that don't easily dissolve in the stomach, the Vitamin C in them will simply pass through without getting absorbed by your body. Such tablets may also settle in the stomach lining while dissolving and cause local inflammation. Most manufacturers don't tell you what binders and fillers they use in their products. Look at the labels. Those suspended in natural cruciferous fibers are usually the better binders. Capsules are perhaps the best. You also may want to know with what the vitamin is formulated, i.e., whether it's an Ester-C© which is one of the best forms of Vitamin C or regular ascorbic acid, which is not as good.

Food Sources and RDA Requirements

Your food sources range from citrus fruits, strawberries, tomatoes and canta-loupes to green and leafy vegetables, cauliflower and potatoes. The adult RDA for vitamin C, as mentioned, is 60 mg.[4]

Absorption Suppressors: Stress, cigarettes, aspirin, cortisone and viral infections.

Absorption Facilitators: All other vitamins, and minerals such as calcium and magnesium.

---

4   Vitamin C is a harmless nutrient regardless of dosage. Its water solubility causes excess amounts to be flushed out of the system. One study reported that quantities of more than 10,000 mg (far more than anybody is likely to get) could result in kidney stones, but even this claim seems groundless. The possible side effects include gas, gastritis and diarrhea. Be aware that agents like cigarettes, aspirin, cortisone, antihistamines and barbiturates deplete your system's vitamin C.

The Vitamin-B Complex: An Introduction

There are a total of eight B-complex vitamins. The B vitamins as a group have many important functions in the body. They are necessary for the conversion of the food you eat into energy, the building and repair of tissues, the transmission of nerve impulses, the metabolism and transportation of cholesterol in your blood and many other important biochemical reactions. In fact, your body's processes can be seriously compromised if you have a severe deficiency in even one of these vitamins.

Like the other vitamins covered in the previous chapters, the B vitamins function primarily as coenzymes in metabolic processes. Enzymes are highly specialized workers that cannot do their job effectively without help from vitamins and minerals.

As an analogy, you might want to think of enzymes as engineers or architects and the B vitamins as laborers at a construction site. If anything of value is to be built or constructed, these two groups have to work in close cooperation. Just as laborers are needed to transport and deliver materials to the construction site, the B vitamins are needed for ferrying food molecules to reaction sites within the cells.

Perhaps you can imagine how terribly slow and inefficient the project would be if the engineers or architects were not only to plan the design but also to actually pick up and deliver the necessary construction materials. What happens to your body if you don't have enough of the B vitamins is a lot more severe, but this gives you some idea of what could happen if you have a deficiency of the key B vitamins.

The carbohydrates, fats and proteins you eat will accumulate in the cells with very little happening to them. As a result, your nerves, brain and the immune system begin to malfunction and your overall health and appearance will be in jeopardy. Some of the symptoms could be subtle (if the deficiency is marginal), while others can be outright sickness. The expressed symptoms of Vitamin B deficiency can vary from mild depression, irritability, fatigue and forgetfulness to confusion, loss of muscular coordination, insomnia and nervousness. In an extreme case, coma and death can occur.

All the B vitamins are water soluble. This means they get flushed out of the body regularly. Unless you eat foods that are rich in these vitamins on a regular basis, your chance of being deficient in any of them is quite high. Any situation that encourages the loss of water will also remove these vitamins from the body.

More specifically, let's look at the individual vitamins in this group.

Thiamine (Vitamin B1)

Thiamine—also known as Vitamin B1—serves as a facilitator in the conversion of sugar and starch into energy. Simply put, it is the spark plug that ignites these fuels to keep you going smoothly. Without a sufficient amount of this vitamin, partially "burned carbohydrates (like pyruvic and lactic acid) can accumulate in the body to cause muscle cramps and nervous and digestive system disorders. The health and appearance of your skin, hair and eyes also depend on having an adequate amount of this vitamin in your diet.

In general, any situation or process that requires the expenditure of very much energy will also require increased amounts of thiamine in the body. These can be such activities as athletic competition, mental concentration and surgery. Pregnant and lactating women also have a greater need for this vitamin. Alcoholics use up quite a bit of thiamine and, as a result, often suffer from a deficiency of this vitamin. The resulting symptoms involve loss of memory, confusion, lack of muscular control and delusion and, if severe, can even lead to paralysis and death.

Deficiency Symptoms

The classic dietary disorder arising from thiamine deficiency is known as beriberi. It was first noticed in the Far Eastern countries where polished rice was the staple food among some of the natives. The most typical characteristics of this disease are a loss of appetite, fatigue, digestive disorders and feeling of numbness in the arms and legs. If deficiency persists, a gradual degeneration of the skeletal and heart muscles as well as of the nervous system will take place. Excessive fluid (edema) can also accumulate in the ankles and feet with thiamine deficiency.

In children, in its mildest form, thiamine deficiency can stunt growth and impair their nervous system and learning ability. At its worst, beriberi can lead to a progressive hearing failure and death.

Food Sources and RDA Requirements

Some of the best sources of thiamine are organ meats (liver, heart and kidneys), beef, whole grains, eggs, beans and peas. Green vegetables such as spinach, broccoli, Brussels sprouts and asparagus and dried foods such as raisins, prunes and nuts are also good sources of thiamine.

When you look at the list above, it seems that thiamine deficiency in this country should be nonexistent. You would think that there would be no problem getting enough thiamine since it is found in such common everyday foods. Surprisingly, according to some of the national surveys, thiamine deficiency is among the most common deficiencies in this country.

Considering the fact that more than 60% of the food consumed is processed and that processing removes much of the nutrients, the high incidence of thiamine deficiency in the U.S. should perhaps come as no surprise.

Moreover, in such a fast-paced society where stress is an integral part of one's daily life, this vitamin can get depleted from the body quite easily. Coffee, alcohol and tea are some of the most frequently consumed drinks in the U.S. These beverages are the worst enemies of thiamine in the body. Since this vitamin is water soluble, daily loss can be quite high, but if you make your Four Pillars meals and drink daily, you should get proper nourishment of this nutrient.

The RDA figures for thiamine range from 0.3 microgram for infants to 1.6 microgram for pregnant and lactating women and in between these figures for children and other adult men and women. Since there is no known toxicity of this vitamin, however, and there is a great need for it in our bodies, getting more than the RDA amounts may be of benefit.

Absorption Suppressors: Alcohol, cigarettes, coffee, tea, stress, fever and surgery.

Absorption Facilitators: All the other B vitamins, manganese, vitamins C and E, sulfur and niacin.

Riboflavin (Vitamin B2)

Speaking in lay terms, riboflavin is the agent responsible for helping your cells to breathe efficiently by providing them with the correct mixture of fuel and air. Without this key vitamin, they would suffocate and operate sluggishly. Riboflavin is also the power behind the mobilization and conversion of proteins, fats and carbohydrates to energy and structural components.

Several of the intracellular enzymes, as well as the adrenal hormones and the other B vitamins, depend on riboflavin for their production and proper function in the body. In addition, this vitamin is important for the formation of red blood cells and antibodies that are part of your body's main line of defense. In some instances, Vitamin B2 was found to help in removing toxic chemicals from the body.

Since riboflavin is very important in the body's fundamental functions (the extraction of energy from foods and the utilization of foods for building tissues and other biochemical components), the lack of a sufficient amount of this vitamin can create major health problems. Biochemically, a deficiency of Vitamin B2 can lead to a poor utilization of carbohydrates, proteins and fats. This means proteins (in the form of amino acids) will be excreted unprocessed, fats will accumulate in the wrong places (blood vessels, liver and kidneys) and carbohydrates will be burned sluggishly.

Often, the expressed symptoms of riboflavin deficiency are inflammation of the eyes, mouth, tongue and lips and skin conditions such as scaly, oily and dry spots around the nose, ears, hairline and eyes. In some instances, mental disturbances that manifest themselves as anxiety, depression and lack of concentration can be some of the other symptoms. The most typical examples of Vitamin B2 deficiency however are amblyopia (poor visual acuity) and photophobia (abnormal sensitivity to light).

Food Sources and RDA Requirements

The best sources of riboflavin are dairy product, organ meats, fish, eggs, brewer's yeast, nuts, legumes, leafy green vegetables and whole grains. Riboflavin can be destroyed if exposed to light (but not heat), oxygen or acid.

The RDA requirements range from 1.2 to 1.7 mg daily, but lactating and pregnant women require slightly more than these amounts. Considering its importance in energy production, athletes, people who are physically active, sick people and stressed people can use substantially higher amounts of this vitamin.

Riboflavin deficiency is one of the most common vitamin deficiencies in this country. If you eat healthy and also make and consume your Four Pillars blend, you should get sufficient amount of the nutrient. On the other hand, if you are one of those people with higher than normal needs, you may want to augment your diet with a good supplement of the vitamin. As a water-soluble vitamin, riboflavin gets flushed out of your body in a short time.

Absorption Suppressors: Sulfa drugs, estrogen, alcohol, coffee, excessive sugar and cigarettes.

Absorption Facilitators: All the B vitamins and vitamin C.

Niacin (Vitamin B3)

Niacin, or Vitamin B3, has a multitude of functions. As a coenzyme, it functions in biochemical reactions that involve the metabolism of carbohydrates, amino acids and fatty acids. Niacin also plays an important role in the synthesis of sex hormones, cortisone, insulin and thyroxine. All these are essential in energy production and the metabolism of proteins, carbohydrates and fats and in dealing with stressful situations.

Niacin has also been found to be beneficial in lowering cholesterol and in improving blood circulation. Regarding its benefit in lowering cholesterol, niacin was shown to be more effective than clofibrate, a successful drug used in treating high cholesterol problems. In other area, Niacin is necessary for the healthy functioning of the nervous and digestive system.

Several doctors, including one from Canada by the name of Abram Hoffer (who has been using niacin for over 20 years to treat patients with schizophrenia), feel strongly about the beneficial effects of this vitamin when given to certain mentally ill patients. Another doctor, William Kaufman, has also used a form of niacin to treat patients who suffer from arthritis. These treatments have not been without controversy, however. It's sufficient to say that this versatile vitamin is something you should enjoy having as part of your daily meals.

Deficiency Symptoms

When you lack Vitamin B3, the traditional deficiency symptoms are dermatitis, diarrhea and dementia (also known as the "3D's"). In dermatitis, exposed areas of the skin (such as the arms, legs, face and hands) become dry, scaly and itchy with dark pigmentation. The mucous membranes and the digestive tract will also be affected. The tongue may be swollen and bright red in appearance.

A malfunctioning gastrointestinal tract and a malabsorption of nutrients, which lead to diarrhea, are some of the other associated symptoms of niacin shortage in the diet. Symptoms associated with dementia are nervousness, irritability, depression, memory loss, sleeplessness and, in extreme cases, delusion, convulsion and death.

Pellagra was first noticed in the rural and poor areas of the South where corn was the staple food of the people. Since niacin can ordinarily be made from tryptophan (an amino acid), and corn is a poor source of tryptophan, those who lived mainly on corn suffered the worst. An exception to this are Mexicans, who consume lots of corn without any deficiency symptoms. This is because the lime water they use to soak the corn makes the tryptophan available for the body to convert to niacin.

Food Sources and RDA Requirements

The RDA requirements vary from 5 to 6 mg for infants to 18-20 mg for men and 13-1 5 mg for women. Add to these 2 and 3 mg of the vitamin for pregnant and lactating women, respectively. Niacin is not toxic except when taken as nicotinic acid and in doses over 100 mg per day. The resulting symptoms are itching and a burning sensation in the skin.

The best natural sources of niacin are milk, lean meat, liver, kidney, fish, poultry, eggs and legumes. Whole grains, roasted peanuts, dates and figs are also good sources of niacin. Eggs and milk have some of the highest concentrations of tryptophan and are the best, while processed foods like white bread and white rice are the worst. In this last group of foods, milling removes up to 90% of the niacin.

Absorption Suppressors: Alcohol, coffee, sulfa drugs, sleeping pills, excessive consumption of water and sugar.

Absorption Facilitators: All the B vitamins and phosphorus.

Pantothenic Acid (Vitamin B5)

Vitamin B5—also known as pantothenic acid or pantothenate—is an important nutrient that helps you cope with all kinds of stressful situations. These could be emotional, like the loss of a loved one, or physical, like athletic competition. It could also be environmental stress, such as cold weather, pollution or confinement in unusually crowded places.

Pantothenic acid enables you to withstand any of these situations because it stimulates the adrenal cortex to produce the hormones necessary for you to deal with stress. These are your "fight or flight" hormones, and they depend greatly on pantothenic acid to function effectively.

To show the importance of Vitamin B5 in dealing with stress, three groups of rats were given "excess," "standard" and "less than the standard" amounts of the vitamin and made to swim in cold water until they became exhausted. Interestingly, those that were given "less than the standard" amount swam for only 16 minutes, those that were fed the "standard" amount swam for 29 minutes and those that were given the "excess" amounts swam for an amazing 62 minutes.

In a different experiment which tested deficiency response in humans, subjects who were fed a synthetic diet with Vitamin B5 antagonist agents in it showed mental, physical and psychological disturbances within a few weeks. These varied from fatigue, irritability and loss of muscular coordination to vomiting and total exhaustion.

Metabolically, pantothenic acid's function in the body is in the conversion of sugars, proteins and fats into energy. In fact, pantothenic acid is a precursor (the raw material) of coenzyme A—a very important molecule needed by every cell in the body during energy production. Pantothenic acid is also essential in the synthesis of antibodies, hemoglobin, cholesterol and bile acids. Neurotransmitters like acetylcholine and sphingosine also depend on Vitamin B5 for their production and function.

In other areas, pantothenic acid is known to help heal wounds and reduce the incidence and/or the adverse effects of allergies and radiation. According to some researchers, this vitamin may even help alleviate the pain and stiffness in joints that is associated with rheumatoid arthritis.

Although this should not lead you to rush out and buy a jar full of Vitamin B5 supplements, in some animal experiments, pantothenic acid was shown to prolong life by as much as nearly 20%.

Food Sources and RDA Requirements

Some of the known sources are whole grains, all organ meats, brewer's yeast, chicken, eggs, saltwater fish, nuts, potatoes, milk, legumes and green vegetables. You might consider obtaining these foods as fresh as possible. Canning, cooling and storing, as we have said often, remove many of the valuable nutrients, including pantothenic acid.

The National Research Council (RCA) recommends from 5 to 10 mg of the vitamin for adults. To get the most of its beneficial effects (like reducing the pain associated with rheumatoid arthritis) you may be advised to take doses of more than 500 mg a day. There are no known pantothenic acid toxicities.

Absorption Suppressors: Alcohol, coffee, sleeping pills, sulfa drugs.

Absorption Facilitators: Folic acid, Vitamin C and all the B vitamins.

Pyridoxine (Vitamin B6)

Pyridoxine, or Vitamin B6, is perhaps the most versatile and highly beneficial vitamin of the B-complex group. In women, it helps minimize birth defects and alleviate PMS[5]-related problems such as moodiness, depression and irritability. This important vitamin is also known to benefit those who suffer from arthritis, heart diseases, cancer and diabetes as well as those who have asthma, anemia and seborrheic dermatitis. The list goes on.

Biochemically speaking, pyridoxine enables the body to convert foods such as fats, proteins and carbohydrates into energy. These foods, in turn, are responsible for the health, growth, repair and proper functioning of your tissues and organs. For example, many of the amino acids that are used in the repair and building of tissues are also important precursors to many of the brain chemicals (neurotransmitters) that control your memory and thoughts, as well as your moods, appetite,

---

5   PMS stands for premenstrual syndrome. Somehow the premenstrual syndrome seems to deplete the vitamins women get from their normal diet.

sexual desires, sleep and breathing patterns. Pyridoxine is the key vitamin that controls the conversion of these amino acids into neurotransmitters.

An insufficient amount of this vitamin in a person's diet could lead to nervousness, irritability, confusion and depression at the least, or convulsion, mental retardation and even death at worst. A salient example of this is what happened to babies who were fed an infant formula brand called SMA in the early 1950s. For no apparent reason, babies who were on this formula went into sudden convulsions. Curiously, when these babies were fed a different formula or milk, their maladies disappeared. It was later discovered that what was missing in the SMA formula was pyridoxine.

Adults, particularly the middle aged, pregnant women, PMS sufferers and those who are on the pill, sometimes experience a neurological disorder that affects their hands.[6] It is called carpal tunnel syndrome. The associated symptoms are pain, numbness and a tingling sensation in the hands. People who have rheumatoid arthritis also have this problem. In some studies; when such people were given pyridoxine, their condition was reduced or eliminated.

People with diabetes and cancer also seem to have a greater need for Vitamin B6. Tests have shown that these people have a low level of the vitamin. For some unknown reason, their conditions seem to use up most of the Vitamin B6 they get from their normal meals.

Pyridoxine's importance in diabetes and heart disease is largely due to its function in collagen formation. Collagen is the structural protein found in the heart and skeletal muscles, blood vessels and others tissues. When you have a strong heart and durable blood vessels, you can minimize some of the problems associated with heart failure. The red blood cells and immune cells also depend on Vitamin B6 for their production and proper function.

In other areas, pyridoxine is the key nutrient involved in the conversion of tryptophan to niacin. Niacin is the parent molecule to Vitamin B5. As was discussed earlier, niacin is one of most powerful vitamins and is involved in a multitude of reactions in the body.

---

6 It is reasoned that somehow, in the presence of the pill or with rheumatoid arthritis or hormonal changes, pyridoxine's effectiveness has been blurred or that the body needs this vitamin in higher amounts.

In addition, pyridoxine helps remove or reduce the side effects of toxins like those in cigarettes and certain chemicals and drugs such as those used for sedation and psychiatric treatments. This versatile vitamin even has a place in dentistry. In one study, children taking supplements of the vitamin had a 40% reduction in tooth decay when compared to those who were given placebo or "dummy" pills.

Food Sources and RDA Requirements

The RDA figures range from 0.3 mg for infants to 1.6 and 2.0 mg for women and men, respectively. The requirement for pregnant and lactating women is about 2.2 mg. These may be far too low, however, to get all the beneficial effects of this great vitamin.

To cite an example, in one experiment when animals were fed a diet that consisted of a pyridoxine level found in the normal American diet, they had more tooth decay than those that were supplemented. As mentioned above, individuals with certain health conditions have a higher need of pyridoxine. Furthermore, the many physical and emotional stresses people experience daily raise the requirement of this nutrient. As a solution to all these problems, you need to include top quality Vitamin B6 supplements with your daily meals.

One word of caution: although pyridoxine has not been shown to have toxic side effects, daily doses of over 2,000 mg could lead to some neurological disturbances.

Good food sources are organ meats, whole grains, soybeans, poultry, fish and yeast. Cabbage, bananas, potatoes, prunes, avocados, peas and green peppers are also well-regarded sources. Poor sources range from refined and processed food to egg white, lettuce and milk.

Pyridoxine is soluble in water, so much so that the longest it can stay in your body after you consume this vitamin is eight hours. Thus, canning and cooking pyridoxine-containing foods in water can deplete a major portion of the vitamin. Fiber-rich foods also tend to trap the vitamin and make it unavailable for absorption by your system.

Absorption Suppressors: Alcohol, contraceptives, cigarettes, light, fiber, radiation exposure and coffee

Absorption Facilitators: All the B-complex team, sodium, Vitamin C and magnesium.

Folacin

Folacin, also known as folate, folic acid or Vitamin M, is part of the B-vitamin group. Although it doesn't have the versatility or the prominence of Vitamin B6, folacin has a few known crucial functions without which life would not be possible.

The first one of these is its role in the synthesis of proteins and the genetic materials DNA and RNA. Of course, without these two, life would not be possible.

In this regard, you might say that folacin is life itself. From the moment of conception to your death, folacin is necessary for cells division and replication. It's also necessary for the repair and maintenance of your body, enabling you to look and feel your best.

Human life begins from the union of two cells: an egg and a sperm. After several divisions of the genetic materials and differentiation, the whole organism comes to being. The process of cell division is continuous from conception to birth and adulthood.

Think of the basal cells of your skin, hair and nails and those cells that line the nasal passage and digestive tract. All these cells are continually born and replaced after they reach maturity. The cells of the male reproductive organ and the immune system also continuously divide to replace those that are dead or dying. Cell division goes in other parts of the body as well but at a slower pace.

This means that if you want to have beautiful skin, hair and nails and overall good health, you need a sufficient amount of folic acid in your diet. The production of red blood cells in the bone marrow and the synthesis of the oxygen-carrying hemoglobin greatly depend on folic acid.

A deficiency of this vitamin leads to a rather tongue-twisting condition called megaloblastic anemia. When the red blood cells are born in the bone marrow, they go through several stages of development. Megaloblasts are abnormally large cells that never went past one of those stages due to folic acid deficiency. This could also happen when there is a Vitamin B12 deficiency.

The nervous and immune systems are affected by a folate deficiency. Ordinarily, brain and spinal fluids contain the highest concentration of folic acid.

This is because, among other things, folic acid serves as a coenzyme for the synthesis of norepinephrine[7] (a hormone/neurotransmitter) and methionine (an amino acid that serves as an antioxidant in the brain).

---

7 Norepinephrine1s also produced by the medulla of the adrenaline gland. Its primary function there is to constrict small blood vessels and to increase blood pressure and flow through the arteries while slowing the heart rate. It's secreted largely in fright, fight and flight situations. In the brain norepinephrine increases alertness.

The expressed symptoms of foliate deficiency are irritability, forgetfulness, weak- ness in legs and feet and poor reflexes. Some of the other symptoms include depression, numbness in the extremities, insomnia, paranoia and dementia. Because of correlations, doctors have used large doses of folic acid to ameliorate certain congenital conditions such as some forms of retardation, schizophrenia and other psychological disorders. A sore and inflamed tongue, weight loss, digestive disturbances and diarrhea are also common with people who lack a sufficient amount of folic acid in their diet.

In other areas, folic acid has uses in dealing with hypoglycemia (low blood sugar) psoriasis, gingivitis and even heart disease.

Food Source and RDA Requirements

Not surprisingly, folic acid deficiencies are very common, particularly among pregnant and lactating women, alcoholics and the elderly in those who use all kinds of drugs, including the prescribed and contraceptives.

The RDA for folic acid varies from 25 mcg for infants to 400 mcg for pregnant women. The interesting thing is that although the RDA for adult males and females is 200 mcg and 180 mcg, respectively, what people often end up getting, due to poor absorption, is only 20% to 50% of these figures.

You must also realize that up to 90% of the vitamins contained in foods are destroyed during cooking, storing, canning and processing. Thus, considering that the RDAs on the whole are marginal and high losses can be encountered during food preparation, your consumption of folic acid should be much greater than the RDA figures to assure yourself of good health.

Folic acid is found in many different sources. These include dark green vegetables (broccoli, cabbage, asparagus, collard green, etc.), beets, cauliflower, whole grains, yeast, orange juice, beans and peas, organ meats, wheat germ and others.

Absorption Suppressors: Alcohol, drugs, stress, coffee, intestinal bacterial infections and cigarettes.

Absorption Facilitators: All the B vitamins, biotin and vitamin C.

Cobalamin (Vitamin B 12)

Vitamin B12, or cobalamin as it's sometimes called, is unique of all the vitamins in that it contains a mineral (cobalt). Vitamin B12 is also unique in another way: it is the largest and the most complex of all the vitamins and it comes strictly from animal sources.

In the human body, cobalamin has so many crucial functions that if you didn't have this vitamin for a prolonged time, you could encounter a serious health problem. For example, the syntheses of proteins, DNA and RNA cannot be adequately accomplished without this vitamin. Cobalamin is also important for the development and proper function of nerve cells and red blood cells. Like folacin, B12 is intimately involved in the health and development of the fetus.

In children, B12 promotes growth and enables them to have better appetites, memory and concentration. In adults, B12 functions as a provider of energy by enabling them to properly metabolize proteins, fats and carbohydrates. Cobalamin also has fortifying function in the nervous and immune systems, for a deficiency of this vitamin can lead to mental disorders and susceptibility to diseases.

Cobalamin is required only in extremely minuscule amounts--something like one millionth of a gram. Even so, there is a fatal disease called pernicious anemia associated with the deficiency of this vitamin. The related symptoms are irritability, disorientation, nervousness, impatience, forgetfulness, poor muscular coordination, a sore and inflamed tongue, lethargy, weakness, depression and diarrhea.

One group who can be prone to pernicious anemia is strict vegetarians. As we said above, cobalamin is the only vitamin that comes from an animal source. However, even these people are not entirely without help if they watch what they eat.

Certain seaweeds, like spirulina, kombu and wakame contain organisms that synthesize the vitamin. Artificially, this vitamin can also be made by growing yeast (like brewer's yeast) in a cobalt-rich medium. Unpasteurized milk, fermented soybean (miso) and soybean paste (tempeh), tamari soy sauce, fish and pickles can also be a good source of the vitamin. Then, of course, there are supplements you can take.

Another group that can be affected by B12 deficiency is people past middle age. As you get older, not only do you have problems with malabsorption, but you also have more frequent gastrointestinal disturbances that can lead to deficiency symptoms of certain vitamins, including B12.

Sometimes, deficiencies can result even if you are taking a sufficient amount of a vitamin. For example, the absence of cofactors—calcium for Vitamin D and iron for Vitamin C—can cause vitamin deficiency symptoms. Vitamin B12 requires one such cofactor known as an "intrinsic factor," an organic substance produced by the stomach that assists in the absorption of B12 in the intestine. Depending on your health, with age, the secretion of the intrinsic factor can be diminished.

Interestingly, some of the crankiness, depression, nervousness and even psychosis that sometimes come about with old age are thought to be nothing but a result of B12 or other vitamin deficiency. There exist many documented cases in which patients with unexplainable mental disturbances were treated with cobalamin injections. (Please bear in mind though that every time you have the above symptoms, it is not necessarily because you have a Vitamin B12 or other vitamin deficiency.)

If you eat a well-balanced diet and are healthy, you may not need to worry about deficiency problems. This water-soluble vitamin manages to stay in the body for a long time: up to five years. The liver serves as a storehouse for B12. Be that as it may, this vitamin has no known toxicity.

Food Sources and RDA Requirements

Other than the vegetarian sources mentioned above, for carnivores, liver, kidney, beef, pork and lamb are very good sources. In addition, fish such as mackerel and herring, oysters, clams, eggs and tofu contain sufficient amounts of cobalamin.

Although Vitamin B12 survives moderate cooking, agents such as acids, alkali and light can easily destroy it. This means that it would be of great benefit to you to minimize exposure of the aforementioned foods to those destructive elements.

The RDA for this vitamin range from 0.2 mcg for infants to 2.0 mcg for adults, with extra requirements for lactating and pregnant women. Supplements up to 2,000 mcg are available.

Absorption Suppressors: Cigarettes, alcohol, coffee, estrogen, sleeping pills and laxatives.

Absorption Facilitators: All the B vitamins, inositol, vitamin C, calcium, sodium and potassium.

Biotin (Vitamin H)

Biotin is one of those quasi-vitamins that is not well understood. It is required by the body, yet the body can make some of its own with the help of bacteria in the intestinal tract. There are also definite, though not common, deficiency symptoms associated with biotin, which therefore make it an essential vitamin.

Like most of the B vitamins, biotin plays an important role in the metabolism of proteins, fats and carbohydrates. The synthesis of proteins, fatty acids and nucleic acids is also aided by the availability of this vitamin in the blood. As a coenzyme, it assists many enzymes to perform their duties effectively.

Those glands directly involved in the metabolism of carbohydrates, such as the thyroid and adrenal glands, as well as the skin and the nervous system, are also the beneficiaries when there is sufficient biotin in the body. Adequate amounts of biotin contribute to healthy skin, hair, nails and muscles.

Unless you have an intestinal disorder or eat a very restricted diet, which includes the consumption of raw eggs, your suffering from a biotin deficiency is unlikely. There are many sources of biotin, and as mentioned above, your body also produces its own. In the event you wonder what is wrong with raw eggs, a protein-carbohydrate compound called avidin (found in egg white) combines with biotin in the intestine and renders the vitamin unavailable to the body. When you cook eggs the heat deactivates avidin.

The resulting symptoms when deficiency occurs are many, but some of the obvious ones are severe skin abnormalities such as eczema and seborrheic dermatitis, loss of appetite, anorexia, depression, fatigue, numbness of the hands and feet, insomnia and anemia. Other symptoms such as improper function of the heart, high blood cholesterol, muscular pain and increased susceptibility to infections and diseases can occur.

Food Sources and RDA Requirements

Many plant and animal foods contain biotin, so much so that it is believed that the average American gets between 150 and 300 mcg of biotin per day. Some of the common food sources are organ meats, pork, beef, whole wheat, brown rice, nuts, fruit, molasses, cheese, milk, chicken, soybeans, fish and eggs.

The RDA requirements range from 10 mcg for infants to 100 mcg for adults. Bear in mind, however, that although these requirements are less than what people are thought to get every day from their meals, you should not be lulled into believing that everything is fine with you regarding this vitamin. Even though we don't know a great deal about this vitamin (since it is relatively new), there is also evidence to show that people such as alcoholics, the elderly, pregnant women and athletes often have inadequate levels of biotin in their systems. There is no known toxicity of biotin.

Absorption Suppressors: Alcohol, raw egg white, coffee, sulfa drugs and antibiotics.

Absorption Facilitators: Folic acid, B2, B6, niacin, B12, pantothenic acid and vitamin C.

Inositol

This is another of those B vitamins not completely studied. According to preliminary findings, inositol is believed to have a number of benefits. These range from its role in enhancing the appearance of the skin, hair and nails to its function in the metabolism of fats and cholesterol. The nervous system and vital organs like the liver, heart and kidney, as well the skeletal muscles seem to benefit from inositol as well.

This new member of the B family has also been shown to enhance nerve impulse transmission (thus giving you good muscular coordination) and aids in suppressing cancer of the bladder. Since the brain is one of the areas where there is a high concentration of inositol, this vitamin purportedly has a calming or sedative effect during anxiety. In the circulatory system, inositol helps minimize the accumulation of fat in the liver and blood vessels.

Food Sources and RDA Requirements

Some of the best sources are organ meats (heart, liver, beef brain, lungs), cantaloupe, grapefruit, oranges and cabbage. Raisins, peanuts, cooked beans, limes, green beans, whole wheat bread, nuts and brewer's yeast are some of the other sources.

Since it is new, the RDA for it has not been figured out yet. In practice, doses ranging from 100 to 500 mg are being used by some doctors. There is no known toxicity with inositol.

Absorption Suppressors: Coffee, alcohol, excessive sugar, antibiotics, food processing, sulfa drugs and estrogen.

Absorption Facilitators: All the other B-complex vitamins, phosphorus and linoleic acid.

Choline

Here is another inadequately studied, borderline vitamin. Choline is classified as part of the B-complex. Because the body can make some of its own choline and there are no known deficiency symptoms associated with it. It has so far been relegated to a quasi-vitamin status. Be that as it may, what choline does in the body and the kinds of diseases it has been linked to would make you think twice before you disregard this nutrient and assume it is a nonessential vitamin.

Choline's primary function is as a precursor to acetylcholine, a very important chemical messenger in the brain involved in memory and thought processes. Choline is also used as a structural component by nerves and brain cells. Myelin, the sheath that covers and protects nerve fibers and the membranes in brain cells, is composed of phosphatidyl choline. Elsewhere in the body, choline is involved in the metabolism and transportation of fats and in the proper functioning of the gallbladder and the thymus gland. It is also good for hair.

Regarding its role in memory and thought processes, choline is the raw material from which acetylcholine is made. Acetylcholine serves as a transmitter of electro-chemical signals from one nerve cell to another. This relaying of information across a synapse enables you to think clearly and retrieve stored information quickly. There are many neurotransmitters like choline in the brain. Any abnormalities that lead to an imbalance of these chemicals can lead to depression, confusion, and aggressive and compulsive behaviors, including excessive drinking, substance abuse and eating disorder.

Such degenerative diseases as Parkinson's disease, tardive dyskinesia and Huntington's disease (all of which are characterized by loss of muscular control that leads to tremors and shaking) are often observed in some elderly people and are believed to have nutritional bases. Alzheimer's disease is also one of those degenerative diseases affecting memory in this group of people.

Several experiments performed to test the effect of choline on patients suffering from Alzheimer's disease have shown some promising results. A similar test done on college students, though not conclusive, was found to be encouraging. Although all these are preliminary studies and we should not draw any conclusion from them, the notion that there could be a nutritional basis for many of our ailments is a tantalizing fact that should make all of us be selective in what we eat.

Food Sources and RDA Requirements

Most foods contain only a tiny amount of choline. The best source is lecithin, found mostly in seed oils, soybean oil, brewer's yeast, flax, whole grains, cereals, legumes, egg yolk, liver, green leafy vegetables and fish.

There are no established RDA amounts for choline. Some nutritionists believe 20 to 300 mg would be optimal for both men and women. The average diet is thought to contain many times more than these figures. Choline has no known toxicity.

Absorption Suppressors: Alcohol, coffee, cigarettes and excessive sugar.

Absorption Facilitators: Linoleic acid, inositol, vitamin A, folic acid and all the B-complex vitamins.

Para-Aminobenzoic Acid (PABA)

You probably have seen PABA more often on sunscreen products than on food labels. For many years, PABA has had a reputation as one of the best chemical compounds for protecting you from the sun's cancer-causing ultraviolet rays. Now, its use as a vitamin is getting more attention than its former role.

PABA, or paraaminobenzoic acid, is categorized as one of the B-complex vitamins, albeit a quasi one. There has not been extensive, controlled research done on PABA to show its essentialness. What is known so far, however, is sufficient enough to include it in food ingredients.

PABA, like all the other B vitamins, works as a coenzyme for the breakdown and utilization of proteins. For example, with pantothenic acid, PABA is purported to restore or delay graying of hair. PABA also helps bacteria in the gastrointestinal tract in their production of folic acid and in the bone marrow with the formation of red blood cells. In other areas, PABA has been found useful as an antioxidant, protecting tissues from ozone-a damaging, poisonous gas found mostly in the upper atmosphere. Aesthetically, PABA is known for its function in maintaining healthy skin and hair and in retarding wrinkle formation.

Food Sources and RDA Requirements

The best food sources of PABA are liver, kidney, brewer's yeast, wheat germ, molasses and whole grains. There are no RDAs for PABA, but some nutritionists recommend 25 mg and up for most common uses. There is no known toxicity for PABA.

Absorption Suppressors: Sulfa drugs, coffee and alcohol.

Absorption Facilitators: Vitamin C, folic acid and all the B vitamins.

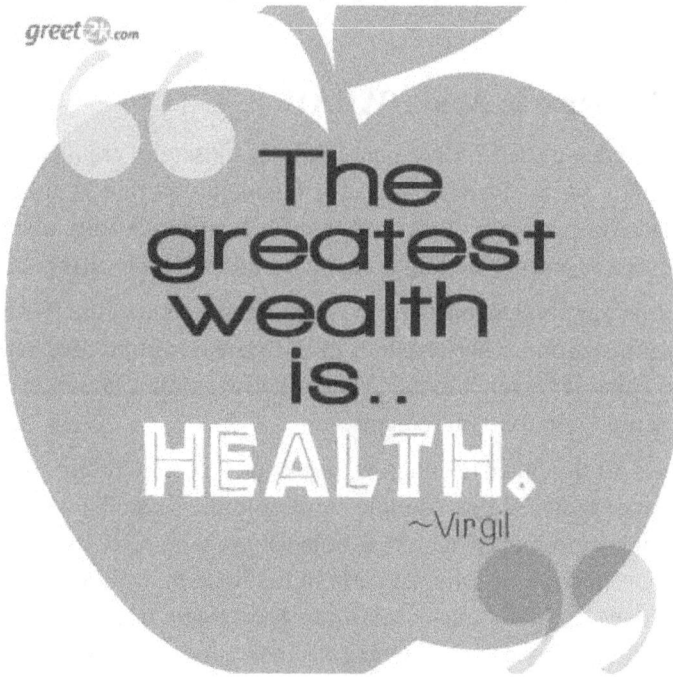

The greatest wealth is.. HEALTH.

~Virgil

greet2k.com

Courtesy: greet2k.com

Pillar Two

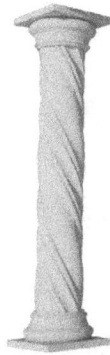

Minerals

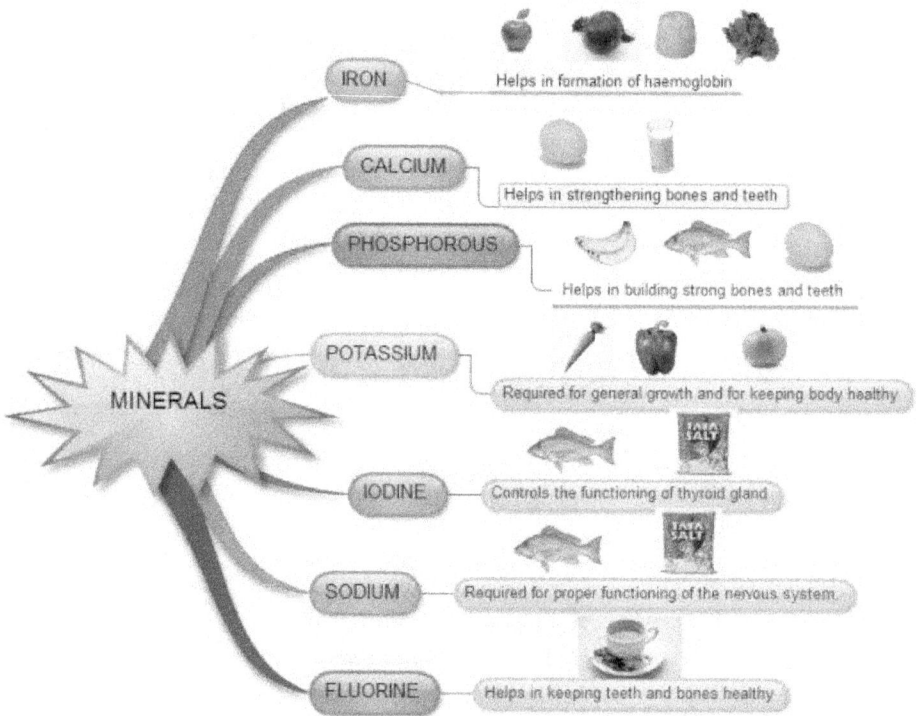

IRON — Helps in formation of haemoglobin

CALCIUM — Helps in strengthening bones and teeth

PHOSPHOROUS — Helps in building strong bones and teeth

POTASSIUM — Required for general growth and for keeping body healthy

IODINE — Controls the functioning of thyroid gland

SODIUM — Required for proper functioning of the nervous system.

FLUORINE — Helps in keeping teeth and bones healthy

MINERALS

Minerals: An Introduction

Like vitamins, minerals have many crucial functions in our bodies. Whether serving as structural components and cofactors of many biochemical processes or functioning as electrolytes, minerals are some of those essential nutrients you can't live without. If you don't get all the necessary minerals for a long time, your bones and teeth begin to disintegrate, your heart and skeletal muscles become weak and your brain malfunctions.

There are many different minerals found in the body, but over 70% of these consist of calcium, phosphorus, sodium, potassium, magnesium, chlorine and sulfur. These are called macro (or bulk) nutrients because your body uses them in large amounts. In our discussion of individual minerals, in this group all but chlorine and sulfur will be covered. There are no known deficiency symptoms associated with chlorine and sulfur.

The others that are needed in small amounts (the so-called trace elements) are chromium, manganese, zinc, iron, molybdenum, iodine and selenium. Bear in mind, though, the quantities have nothing to do with their essentiality. The trace elements are just as important to the body as the macro minerals. Be aware also that there are still other trace elements found in the body, and they include cobalt, fluorine, nickel, silicon, vanadium, tin, and bromine. In fact, you can pretty much expect to find nearly every element found in the earth's crust in the body, albeit in tiny amounts. By weight, minerals account for about 4% of your body mass.

When you think of minerals as structural components, perhaps what you think of is calcium, because for years milk commercials have touted it as the mineral that strengthens your teeth and bones. Phosphorus and magnesium do the same, but you probably have never seen commercials about these minerals or iron, which is very important for the synthesis of hemoglobin, a critical life-supporting protein.

There are many other minerals (although in smaller amounts) that are part of the skeletal system, body tissues and fluids. What you also don't hear about are these minerals' roles as cofactors of many enzyme systems and their function as electrolytes that regulate your heart rhythm or thought processes. Furthermore, minerals are essential for the maintenance of acid-base neutrality and the regulation of body fluids across cell membranes (also known as osmotic pressure).

Before we discuss the individual minerals, let's briefly define a few terms.

What Are Cofactors?

Cofactors are similar to enzymes, and they help other components (like enzymes) speed up certain chemical reactions and bring them to completion. For example, calcium is a cofactor in the synthesis of blood-clotting protein, and chromium helps the hormone insulin to bring sugar to the cells. Without each of these minerals, bleeding cannot be stopped and sugar cannot be metabolized. Copper is another mineral that serves as a cofactor for several enzymes in the body. The generation of energy from fuel and the formation of elastin, collagen and melanin (the skin and hair pigment) all need the availability of copper to the enzymes that accomplish these processes. Copper is also involved in the synthesis of superoxide dismutase (SOD—the powerful antioxidant enzyme that protects the body from the aging and tissue-damaging effects of oxygen free radicals). Manganese and zinc are also involved in this.

In short, the hundreds of metabolic processes that convert proteins, carbohydrates and fats into energy, water and carbon dioxide in your body, or those that catalyze the synthesis of muscle tissues, hormones and countless other biological molecules, are dependent on minerals. Even the absorption of food from the intestine and into the individual cells is facilitated by minerals. For instance, sodium and magnesium assist in the uptake of carbohydrates. Calcium assists the absorption of Vitamin B12. The enzymes that catalyze the breakdown of food in your stomach and intestine also use minerals as their cofactors.

What Are Electrolytes?

An electrolyte is a substance, or a group of substances, that dissociates into two (positively and negatively) charged ions when melted or dissolved in water. For example, when you dissolve table salt in water you get free sodium and chloride ions. Such ions are often capable of conducting electrical charges or impulses. There are many other minerals and organic molecules that have this property (see Table 5.1). In the body, these substances serve as regulators of fluids (osmotic pressure) between the internal and external environment of the cells. Minerals are also important in the maintenance of an acid-base balance of body fluids and in the conduction of electrical impulses along nerve fibers.

In your body, there are three defined spaces or compartments: intercellular (exist inside the blood vessels), intracellular (found inside the cells) and interstitial (spaces outside the blood vessels and between cells). The distribution of water and nutrients among these spaces is regulated by a process called osmotic pressure. In this process, particles or fluids move across a semipermeable membrane from where they are highly concentrated to where there are fewer of them or none at all. On the basis of this simple principle, food is able to get past the intestinal wall into the bloodstream and be delivered to various tissues and organs. In turn, waste material is removed from the blood by the kidneys and lungs.

Minerals also facilitate in the conduction or transmission of nerve impulses along a nerve fiber. If you recall from your biology classes, a nerve cell consists of a body, a long tube-like structure (axon) and tiny fingerlike projections called dendrites. The transmission of a nerve impulse along the axons and dendrites (nerve fibers) is accomplished by a change in the electrical properties of the fluid that bathes the nerve cells when stimulated by the impulse.

This change, which creates a temporary electrical charge on the cell membrane, is caused by the exchange of sodium and potassium ions across the cell membrane when stimulated by a nerve impulse. This process facilitates the transmission and propagation of the nerve (electrical) signals down the axon. At the juncture of the dendrites and the next neuron are tiny gaps called synapses.

Acetylcholine is the chemical that serves to bridge these gaps so that the electrical impulses can continue their journey to the next series of nerve cells. In less technical terms, this means that when you have healthy and properly functioning nerves, an abundance of acetylcholine and the necessary minerals, you can think clearly and remember things more quickly.

Similarly, the contraction and relaxation of muscles are influenced by the presence of an adequate amount of certain minerals in the fluids that bathe these tissues. Calcium, for example, is responsible for the muscle contraction, while sodium, potassium and magnesium are necessary for its relaxation. The proper functioning of all the body muscles, including the heart, depends on these minerals.

It is apparent from the above information that anything that upsets the balance of minerals in your body severely compromises your health and well- being. Tetany, for instance, is a muscular condition characterized by spasm and twitching of the face, feet and hand muscles. This problem is often caused by a drop in the calcium level in the body fluid (due to an improper functioning of the parathyroid gland), calcium deficiency or rickets. Calcium rigor is a condition induced by an excessive presence of the mineral in the blood. Similarly, magnesium deficiency can lead to muscle weakness, depression and disturbance of muscular contraction.

Table 5.1 Major Electrolytes Found in Body Fluids

Positive ions	Extracellular Fluid (from blood plasma) mEq/l	Extracellular Fluid (in muscles) mEq/l
Sodium (Na+) 145 10	145	10
Potassium (K+) 5 150	5	150
Calcium (Ca++) 3 2	3	2
Magnesium (Mg++) 2 15	155	15
Total	155	177
Negative ions		
Chloride (CI-)	105	5
Bicarbonate (HC03-)	25	10
Phosphate (PO4 ---)	2	
Organic Acids	6	120
Proteins	17	42
Total	155	177

mEqll = milliequivalents per liter
Source: J.R. Robinson "Water and Life," *World Review of Nutrition and Dietetics.*

Minerals also influence the alkalinity of the bile and the acidity of the stomach juices as well as the acid-base balance of the blood. The proper strength of the bile and stomach juice is important for efficient digestion and processing of food. Blood acid-base neutrality which must be kept within a pH range of 7.35 to 7.45 is also important. Any deviations from these values can lead to acidosis or alkalosis, conditions that arise from an increase in the acidity (lower than pH 7.35) or the basicity (higher than pH 7.45) of the blood.

The mineral salts, or rather, the electrolytes generated from them, play a major role in monitoring the movement of fluids in the different body spaces. For example, an increase in electrolyte concentration on one side of a semipermeable membrane raises the osmotic pressure on that side of the membrane. This differential in osmotic pressure encourages fluid to move from low to high electrolyte concentration. This movement of fluid between the two sides of the membrane will go on until the osmotic pressure is even on both sides.

From the above synopsis you can see that minerals are a very important part of your health. You should provide your body with sufficient amounts of these nutrients daily to experience good health and well-being. Since minerals are water soluble, they don't get stored in the body unless they are part of tissue structures like calcium and phosphorus in the bones and teeth. Moreover, the body tissues are constantly broken down at varying rates, and you need to have all the necessary nutrients to help rebuild or repair them.

In the body, electrolytes control much of the fluid movement across the capillaries into the cells, and vice versa. The biological significance of this is that water and other nutrients are able to get into the cells. Any major increases or decreases in the electrolyte concentration will cause a shift in the homeostasis of the body.

Now let's discuss the individual minerals.

CHAPTER 5
Bulk Minerals

Calcium

Calcium is the king of all minerals. It is the most abundant and the most funda-mental mineral nutrient in the body because our teeth and skeletal system are built largely from this mineral. Calcium, in addition to being important for the proper functioning of the muscles, including those of the heart, can help facilitate the reactions of many metabolic processes in the body.

The enzymes that catalyze the conversion of food into energy and body tissues and those involved in blood clotting all require the presence of a sufficient amount of calcium in the blood. The absorption of Vitamin B12 from the intestine and the synthesis and breakdown of the neurotransmitter acetylcholine are also aided by this mineral.

We receive many other benefits from calcium. Calcium can help lower blood pressure. It can help prevent colon cancer and heart disease. For women, the most important of all its functions is in deterring the onset of osteoporosis and osteo-malacia. In other areas, calcium is known to block the absorption of poisonous metals like strontium, cadmium and lead. As was discussed in the previous pages, calcium's role in nerve impulse transmission and muscle contraction is equally important to the health and well-being of an individual.

About 30% of bone is a rather flexible and porous material composed of colla-gen, mucopolysaccharide, carbohydrates and glycoprotein. These substances are formed during fetal development, and shortly after birth they begin to gain hard-ness as calcium compounds are deposited in the porous collagen matrix. For the next 20 years or so, the whole human skeleton forms and grows by this gradual deposition of calcium in the bones and teeth. In the end, the body can accumulate roughly 2-1/2 pounds of the mineral. About 99% of the calcium in the body is located in bones and teeth. The other 1% circulates in the bloodstream.

Bear in mind, though, that calcium deposition is never a one-way process. During the growth process and throughout life, bone (and therefore calcium) is continuously resorbed and rebuilt to replace older, stressed bone. Bone is also broken down when there is a drop of the mineral found in the blood. For survival, the presence of an adequate amount of calcium in the blood is more important than having strong bones and teeth.

There are quite a few factors that limit the availability of calcium in the blood. One of these is simply not having enough calcium in your diet. The other may be not getting enough sunshine or Vitamin D (which helps in the absorption of calcium). It may also be that you have a problem with your parathyroid gland, which produces hormones that regulate the calcium level in the blood. Your emotional state, the amount of exercise you get, the level of phosphorus in your blood and the acid-alkaline balance in your digestive system also determine calcium absorption.

Other interfering factors are the consumption of too much protein, cereals, vegetables and fruits like rhubarb, cranberries, spinach and beets and tea. These foods contain chemical compounds called physic acid and oxalic acid that combine with calcium in the gastrointestinal tract, thus making it unavailable for absorption. Vomiting, diarrhea and even excessive fat and fibers can be some of the other culprits. When too many of these agents are limiting the availability of the mineral, microscopic segments of the bone begin to break down to release more calcium to meet such life-sustaining needs as keeping your heart beating.

The most common of the above situations is not having enough calcium in the diet. Milk is often the best and easiest source of calcium, but most people don't drink milk once they are past their formative years. The estimated optimal daily requirement for calcium ranges from 1,000 to 1,500 mg. To meet these requirements, you may need to drink four to six glasses of milk a day. There are two problems with this option.

One, the average adult does not commonly drink even one glass a day, let alone four to six. Two, drinking this much milk a day can bring along with it the problem of excess calories, saturated fat, cholesterol and too much protein. All of these are thought to encourage the loss of calcium from the bones as well as the incidence of other health-threatening diseases.

As a result the average adult American doesn't get even half of the adult RDA (800 mg) a day. Add to this the fact that on the average, only 35% of that amount gets absorbed into the blood. In some cases, some nutritionists think that it might even be as low as 2%. The requirement for lactating and pregnant women and those under 24 is 1,200 mg. A quick computation will tell you that 35% of the RDA for lactating and pregnant women is 420 mg; and 35% of the general adult RDA is 280 mg. Considering that the average person can lose up to nearly 400 mg of calcium a day, this figure is not even sufficient enough to replace what is being removed from the bones daily.

No wonder, then, that some nutritionists once called osteoporosis a 20th-century epidemic. It is a very subtle disease causing the bone to become thin and brittle like a pane of glass, and neither x-rays nor regular blood tests can show its existence. It takes a loss of 35% to 40% bone mass before it becomes apparent. It is estimated that roughly 12 million adults suffer from osteoporosis in this country—9.1 million are women and 2.8 million are men. Women are more prone to osteoporosis because they can lose up to 15% of their bone mineral density in the 5 to 7 years after menopause. Certainly calcium deficiency is not the only cause of osteoporosis, particularly in menopausal and postmenopausal women but it is important to remember that chronically low levels of calcium in the diet will undermine the structural integrity of your skeleton.

Two more factors that can contribute to osteoporosis are the overconsumption of phosphorus and the undersupply of magnesium in the body. These two minerals are integral parts of the bones and teeth. For the body to use calcium properly, phosphorus and magnesium must combine with calcium in the right proportions.

While the required calcium to phosphorus ratio is 1:1, that of calcium to magnesium is 2:1. Any deviations from these figures often lead to an improper utilization of calcium. As you may well be aware, phosphorus-containing foods and drinks are available everywhere in Pepsi, Coca Cola, some meats, canned foods, cheeses, salad dressings, bread and many other processed foods that use phosphate compounds as preservatives.

As a result, the average American consumes far too much phosphorus, exacerbating the already bleak problem concerning calcium consumption and absorption. Incidentally, whole milk is said to have a 1:5 calcium-to-phosphorus ratio, and for this reason some experts advise us not to rely solely on whole milk as the calcium source. Low-fat milk, on the other hand, is supposedly a much preferred alternative.

The case with magnesium is more a problem of undersupply. Far too many people in this country get less than 50% of the recommended levels of magnesium. As a result calcium absorption and utilization are affected.

As shown above, the incidence of osteoporosis is much greater in women than men. By the age of 70, the average woman can lose up to 25% of her bone mass. The shrinkage in height and the hunched back so characteristic of some older women (and, to some extent, older men) are a result of more bone breakdown than bone formation, for whatever reason (mineral deficiency, lack of hormones, etc.).

For most women, it usually begins by about age 35, although some say even at a younger age, and continues into old age. There are several reasons advanced for the difference between men and women regarding calcium loss.

One of these reasons is the drop in the production of the hormone estrogen as women get past menopause. It is believed that this hormone helps prevent the net loss of calcium from the bones while it encourages its formation. Another reason is low calcium intake and poor absorption. During pregnancy women have a tendency to use up the calcium from their bones to meet the needs of the fetus as well as their own needs. Moreover, women lose a lot of blood during their reproductive years, and this tends to rob the calcium store in the bones and set the stage for osteoporosis in later years.

Another very common disease associated with calcium deficiency is one that affects the teeth and the alveolar (jaw) bone that supports them. It's called periodontal disease, and it affects over three-quarters of the people in this country. This disease is a slow one that becomes more apparent as a person ages. It is said that 50% of the population loses some teeth by the age of 60.

Please bear in mind there are also other causes of periodontal disease. These include the growth and action of bacteria on food debris that collect under the gum, which turns into a hard plaque. If left untreated, this condition eventually grows to become gingivitis. Later, as it spreads under the periodontal membrane and the alveolar bone, it causes the teeth to become loose and ultimately fall out. This often is a prelude to chronic periodontal disease.

Besides preventing or reducing the incidence of osteoporosis and periodontal disease, calcium has been shown to help in lowering cholesterol levels (particularly the LDL). Calcium is also believed to prevent colon cancer. In one study, the administration of 1,200 mg of calcium daily for three months to people who had colon cancer showed a reduction in the growth of the cancer. In addition, calcium was found to help normalize high blood pressure. In one study where patients were given 1,500 mg of calcium carbonate supplement daily for an extended period, they were shown to have a significant improvement in their blood pressure.

Food Sources and RDA Requirements

The best food sources for calcium are dairy products. Others include soybeans, salmon, sardines and green vegetables, such as cabbage, collard greens, kale and broccoli. Peanuts, dried beans, walnuts, sunflower seeds, oysters, clams and shrimp are also good sources of the mineral.

The RDA for calcium starts at 400 mg for infants and goes to 1,200 mg for young adults and pregnant and lactating women. Considering the low level of absorption and high rate of daily loss, some experts think that these figures are misleadingly low. Raising them by 50% may help reduce the onset of osteoporosis and other diseases. You may wonder if it's necessary to drink six glasses of milk each day to meet even the RDA for calcium.

Your alternative is, of course, to find a good supplement. In the marketplace, calcium supplements come in many different forms. There are tablets made from bonemeal (crushed bones) and dolomite (naturally found in the earth as calcium-magnesium carbonate). Then there are calcium gluconate and calcium lactate, which come from vegetarian and milk sources, respectively. These two are known to be safer and better absorbed than dolomite or bonemeal supplements, which can contain lead contaminants. Don't forget that the RDA of 1,200 mg means 1,200 mg of *elemental* calcium: 1,200 mg of calcium gluconate contains only 9%, or 108 mg, of elemental calcium. So be careful to calculate your calcium supplement needs, bearing in mind that it must be the amount of elemental calcium you need.[8] Because the Four Pillars drinks contain various vegetables and fruits, herbs and spices, many of which are known calcium sources, these foods can be good supplemental sources as well.

Absorption Suppressors Excessive amounts of fat, vegetable-derived acids like physic, oxalic and tannic acids, stress and lack of exercise, Vitamin D and magnesium.

Absorption Facilitators vitamins A, C and D, iron, manganese, magnesium and phosphorus.

Toxicity

It is reported that the consumption of over 2,000 mg of elemental calcium for a prolonged time could lead to hypercalcemia, which in infants can lead to mental disorder. In adults, it can contribute to atherosclerosis (hardening of the arteries due to calcium and fat deposits).

---

8   Here are some common calcium compounds and their elemental calcium percentages: Calcium glubionate contains 6.5%, calcium gluconate *9%*, calcium lactate 13%, calcium citrate 21%, calcium acetate 25%, calcium carbonate 40% of elemental calcium. Hence, in the above example, 9% of 1,200 mg of calcium gluconate contains only 108 mg of calcium. You can use the above percentages to compute elemental calcium in a supplement that contains these calcium compounds.

Phosphorus

Since phosphorus is the second most abundant mineral in the body, it is only logical that we discuss phosphorus as our next essential mineral. In the bones and teeth, phosphorus is found at a 1:2 ratio with calcium. The amount found in these tissues is roughly 80% (or 560 grams). The other 20% is distributed throughout the body, fulfilling many other metabolic as well as biochemical requirements.

Some of its roles are the production and storage of energy, the synthesis of nucleic acids (DNA and RNA) and the metabolism and transportation of fats, proteins and carbohydrates. It is also an integral part of the cell membrane and a number of enzyme systems. The function of the heart and kidneys and the growth and repair of cells, as well as the assimilation of niacin, are aided by phosphorus. Additionally, this versatile nutrient serves as a buffer in body fluids. This relates to the maintenance of neutrality in these fluids in order for the body to carry out its numerous metabolic processes efficiently.

Because phosphorus has so many critical functions, you would ordinarily be concerned about its adequacy in your diet. As it turns out, this is one of the few minerals you need not worry too much about. Phosphorus is just about everywhere. If anything, most of the concern is that we may be getting too much of it. This is because whenever there is excess phosphorus, calcium absorption is depressed while the latter's resorption (its removal from the bone) is increased. Therefore, if osteoporosis is a major concern to you, watch what you eat and drink.

Food Sources and RDA Requirements

The RDA for phosphorus ranges from 300 mg for infants six months and under to 1,200 mg for young adults and pregnant and lactating women. Phosphorus deficiency is not common in men. It's important to remember, however, that to maximize its benefit as a structural component, you need to take an equal amount of calcium with it. Like calcium, phosphorus is constantly resorbed from the bones and teeth.

Legumes, milk and milk products, poultry, meat, fish, whole grains, bonemeal, nuts and seeds are all good sources of phosphorus. There is no known toxicity associated with phosphorus, and the only known deficiency is in animals that graze on phosphorus-poor land.

Absorption Suppressors: An excessive intake of iron, magnesium, aluminum and white sugar.

Absorption Facilitators: Calcium, thiamine and vitamin E.

Magnesium

Magnesium is the third most abundant mineral in the bones and teeth, and its content in these tissues accounts for roughly 60% of the mineral found in the body. Its function in these tissues is clearly to produce strong, hard bones and teeth.

The remaining 40% of the mineral is found in cells and extracellular body fluids, where it's involved in so many critical functions. In the cells, it facilitates the production of energy as well as its release from ATP—the universal carrier of energy in the body. This energy is used to synthesize proteins and nucleic acids (DNA and RNA), to transport nutrients around the body and to perform many other functions. A number of enzyme systems depends on magnesium for their function and activation.

Magnesium's role in the muscles is purely "mechanical" but a very important one nevertheless. It enables these tissues to relax, while calcium (magnesium's antagonistic partner) empowers them to contract. It is evident that life could be quite miserable without a sufficient amount of this mineral in your body. As you can see below, magnesium deficiency can be quite harrowing, too.

Magnesium also assists nerve cells to conduct electrical impulses efficiently. This feature of the mineral enables you to think quickly and clearly and maintain a well-balanced and integrated body and mind.

In addition, magnesium has other healthful functions you might appreciate knowing about. These range from its role in the maintenance of your heart and normal blood pressure to fighting kidney stones, diabetes and osteoporosis. Magnesium's importance for keeping a healthy heart has so far not been fully understood. It has been found that people who live in areas of the world where the water's content of the mineral is high have less incidence of heart attack than those who live where the magnesium content in the drinking water is low. The scientific basis of this information has yet to be fully explored.

Its function in controlling blood pressure seems to stem from the fact that it helps keep the blood vessels in proper working condition. Just as you need a flexible and elastic water hose to accommodate any changes in water pressure, you need blood vessels that have similar properties. Magnesium is able to relax not only the blood vessels but also the tissues that surround them. This dilating and relaxing effect helps you maintain normal blood pressure.

In other areas, magnesium helps diabetics by increasing their tolerance for sugar. In women with PMS, it helps reduce the tension and depression that is often associated with this malady. Its significance in minimizing osteoporosis is related to the fact that it's an integral part of bones and teeth. When used with the vitamin pyridoxine (Vitamin B6), magnesium can be an effective treatment for kidney stones. This excruciatingly painful complication often results from a lodging of crystallized calcium oxalate in the urinary tract. It's believed that magnesium helps keep the offending compound fully dissolved in the urine. Food sources of oxalic acid (the precursor to calcium oxalate) are rhubarb, leafy vegetables and coffee. If you are susceptible to kidney stones, it helps to avoid these substances.

Magnesium has also been used in treating certain mental disturbances such as schizophrenia, nervousness, insomnia, depression and similar conditions. During diuretic therapy (administered to help patients remove excess fluids), magnesium is one of the minerals that gets depleted. During this time it's important that you take extra amounts of the mineral to keep its normal presence in the body fluids.

Although there reportedly exists no magnesium deficiency in this country, the average daily magnesium intake of Americans is not something one can write home about. In a nationwide survey, it was found that 50% of Americans get less than two-thirds of the RDA of magnesium. Certain groups such as alcoholics, bulimics, diabetics and those that use certain therapeutic drugs are known to have low levels of magnesium in their bodies.

When magnesium deficiency does occur, the experience can be quite dreadful. The associated expressed symptoms vary from muscle weakness, irritability, confusion and dizziness to outright convulsions, tremors, delirium and even seizures and coma. These are, of course, extreme situations. What may be common, however, are the marginal or subclinical conditions. You feel there is something wrong with you, but you and your doctor can't figure out what it is. Such subtle symptoms may serve as a clue to your dietary magnesium imbalance, for otherwise there are plenty of food sources that can provide you at least the minimum amount of magnesium. What you want, of course, is maximum health and well-being, and this is where your Four Pillar drinks and meals come in handy. As a bonus, you may also consider taking multi-vitamin supplement.

Food Sources and RDA Requirements

The best sources of magnesium are meat, dairy products, fish, tuna, molasses, soybeans, nuts and seeds. Other good sources are brown rice, honey, bran, oatmeal and green vegetables. Remember, anytime a food is processed, it loses its mineral content—in some cases as much 90% of it.

The RDA starts at 40 mg for up to six-month-old infants and goes to 355 mg for lactating women.

While we are talking about requirements, it's important to discuss briefly the importance of magnesium to athletes. Because this mineral is involved in energy generation and utilization, as well as in muscular activities, athletes around the world have come to realize the beneficial effects of magnesium and magnesium supplements. So, whether you are a football jock, marathon runner or weekend jogger, make sure you have plenty of the mineral in your diet. Studies have shown that people who engage in intensive physical activities utilize oxygen more efficiently when they have extra magnesium in their foods.

Absorption Suppressors: Alcohol and diuretics.

Absorption Facilitators: Calcium, phosphorus, Vitamins B6, C and D and protein foods.

Potassium

The majority of the body's potassium-nearly 98%-is found in the cells. It serves to maintain the osmotic pressure (fluid balance) as well as the acid-base neutrality of the cell. Potassium also functions as a cofactor to many enzyme systems that are involved in the breakdown of energy-providing foods (carbohydrates, proteins and fats). The synthesis of proteins and the conversion of glucose into glycogen (the tissue's stored fuel) are also accomplished with the help of potassium.

Together with sodium, potassium enables the heart to work in a steady, regular rhythm. Potassium helps you to think clearly by facilitating the transportation of oxygen to the brain.

In other areas, potassium is involved in nerve-impulse transmission and muscular contraction. It works antagonistically with sodium, which is found predominantly outside the cells. As was explained previously under "Electrolytes," in the presence of a nerve impulse, the potassium from within the nerve cell migrates outward, thus altering the electrical potential of the cell and allowing the impulse to be transmitted down the axon. This is critical for the proper functioning of the brain and the rest of the nervous system.

Potassium's role as a muscle relaxer, along with magnesium, is equally important because some of the life-sustaining muscles-such as the heart, intestinal and respiratory muscles-won't function effectively without a sufficient amount of Potassium. Magnesium and potassium enable your heart to beat steadily and rhythmically.

Potassium has also been found to alleviate hypertension or high blood pressure in some cases. To the 50 million people who suffer from hypertension this may be a little bit of good news. The mineral sodium is very common in the American diet, and this mineral also has a high water retentive capacity that can lead to high blood pressure. Since sodium and potassium are antagonistic partners, the presence of a large amount of the latter tends to normalize the former. In this regard the presence of high amounts of calcium and magnesium, also have a blood pressure-lowering effect.

The explanations advanced for potassium's effectiveness in lowering sodium are manifold.

One, because the two minerals compete for reabsorption in the kidneys, the higher the potassium in the renal fluids the less sodium will be reabsorbed (i.e., it will leave more sodium to be eliminated).

Two, potassium's muscle-relaxing effect enables blood vessels to dilate and thus helps lower blood pressure. Catecholamines are a group of stress-induced chemicals that are capable of increasing blood pressure. Potassium can reduce the secretion of these hormones.

One little caveat relating to this effect of potassium on blood pressure is the fact that it's somewhat controversial. Some scientists have questioned the efficacy of the mineral on hypertension, although there are those who believe that it has an influential role. The research that is being done in various labs will, one would hope, prove it one way or the other, but until then there is nothing wrong with being optimistic about what potassium does for this particular purpose.

There are roughly 250 grams of potassium in an average-sized body, and any substantial drop from this level usually leads to serious health problems. The first associated symptoms of potassium deficiency are general muscle weakness, irritability, confusion, pulse irregularity, lethargy, loss of appetite, muscle cramps and constipation. In severe cases, paralysis, a drop in heart rate and even death can occur.

Food Sources and RDA Requirements

The estimated RDA for potassium is 500 mg for six-month-old infants, 700 mg for one-year-olds, 1,400 mg for age two to five, 1,600 mg for age six to nine and 2,000 mg for teenagers and adults. Certain drugs, as well as excessive sweating can cause a substantial loss of potassium. For this reason, and the fact that potassium has a beneficial effect on hypertension, the NCR suggests that a daily intake of up to 3,500 mg can satisfy the need for the mineral.

Amounts of more than 25 grams consumed on a daily basis, however, can lead to acute toxicity. Sometimes kidney failure or other complications such as infection or severe acid-base imbalances can be the cause. Some of the associated symptoms are confusion, lethargy, weakness and paralysis of muscular tissues. One could also experience an erratic heartbeat, which, if prolonged, can lead to cardiac arrest. Some of these symptoms are similar to what happens when there's a deficiency of the mineral.

Potassium is found in many foods, such as legumes, vegetables, fruits, meat and milk. Bananas, potatoes, broccoli, cantaloupe, dried apricots, peanuts, avocados and lima beans are some of the great sources of the mineral. Remember, however, that potassium is one of those minerals that are lost in cooking water. For this reason, steaming or microwaving the foods is strongly recommended. For those of you who are making and consuming your Four Pillars drink, this problem shouldn't be an issue.

Absorption Suppressors: Coffee, alcohol, sugar, diuretics, stress and cortisone laxatives.

Absorption Facilitators: Vitamin B6, sodium and magnesium.

Be aware, also, that any substantial drop in your potassium level because of the aforementioned suppressors can be the cause of many of your mood changes. Coffee drinkers, alcoholics and sweet eaters often become hyper or jittery. This may be due to the loss of potassium from the blood as much as from the effect of these products on your system.

Sodium

Sodium is potassium's antagonistic partner. Most of the body's potassium is found inside the cells. Most of sodium bathes the outside of the cells. (See Table 5.1.) This relationship is the key to their function in tandem to coordinate muscle contraction and nerve impulse transmission, which are important for the mechanical movements of the body parts, as well as for processing thoughts.

By itself, sodium's primary purpose is to regulate the in-and-out flow of fluids and nutrients from the cell in a process known as the "sodium pump." Sodium is also involved in the transport of carbon dioxide and amino acids across the cell membrane and intestinal wall. Because sodium causes high water retention, it saves the body from total dehydration—particularly in arid environments.

However, because of sodium's ability to pick up water, a large intake of it can lead to high blood pressure—at least partially so because there are some researchers who think that there should at the same time exist low levels of other minerals for this to happen. Minerals such as magnesium, potassium and calcium, when they exist in higher amounts, tend to neutralize the hypertensive effect of sodium.

Because American food is rich in sodium and the salt shaker is omnipresent, one should have very little concern with sodium deficiency. The concern most people have is of overindulgence. Besides the salt shaker that you find close at hand in every restaurant and at every dining table, there are many hidden sources of sodium. These can be cured meats, cheese, canned soups and vegetables, luncheon meats, etc.

In very rare instances, such as starvation, sodium malabsorption and diarrhea, deficiency may occur. The symptoms associated with sodium deficiency are loss of concentration, impaired carbohydrate metabolism, muscle weakness, dehydration and collapse of blood vessels.

The toxicity correlated with high sodium intake is the increase in blood pressure and excessive accumulation (edema) of fluid that can lead to swelling in ankles and feet, as well as buildup of fluid within the chest cavity and other tissues around the body.

Food Sources and RDA Requirements

The estimated RDA ranges from 120 mg for infants under six months to 500 mg for teenagers and adults-and on the average, roughly 280 mg for children over one year but younger than ten.

Food sources vary from various canned and frozen foods (soups, ice cream, olives, sauerkraut, ketchup, etc.) to eggs, meats, shellfish, carrots, beets, dried beef and bacon. There are other hidden sources like baking powders, soy sauces, monosodium glutamate (MSG) and several others that are used as preservatives, such as sodium sulfate, sodium nitrate and nitrite.

Absorption Suppressors: None known.

Absorption Facilitators: None known.

Chapter 6
Trace Elements

Chromium

One of the many amazing things about life and biochemical processes is how imperceptibly small things can contribute to health and well-being when available or become detrimental to health and life itself when absent. The mineral chromium is perhaps one example of this. This mineral is one of the micronutrients. That means the amount of chromium used by the body daily is so small (less than a pinch) that you think it should make no difference whether or not you have this mineral at all.

I have news for you. Without chromium, life could literally come to a clanking and sluggishly grinding halt. This shiny mineral's number one job is to help insulin bring glucose to your cells. As has been discovered, without chromium, blood sugar can never enter the cells. Glucose is very important as a fuel and for many biological processes. Your brain cells are entirely dependent (save for a few exceptions) on glucose for fuel, and they need chromium just as much as insulin to absorb and metabolize their fuel.

So what does the absence of chromium mean to you? Well, the first sign is that you start to feel lethargic and fatigued. If uncorrected, this can lead to depression, hypoglycemia and even diabetes. Glucose tolerance is the term used to describe your body's ability to process and metabolize sugar. Many adults in this country have very low glucose tolerance—some even being diabetic or borderline diabetic.

This is even more common in the older generation, because as one gets older, one's ability to absorb and metabolize nutrients decreases. Although we cannot say that chromium deficiency leads to diabetes, there are many instances where diabetics[9] were helped by being treated with chromium supplements.

In other areas, chromium also facilitates the metabolism of fats and proteins as well as the synthesis of genes (RNA and DNA). Studies with both human and animal subjects have shown that chromium deficiency can contribute to the accumulation of fat in the blood vessels, which can lead to atherosclerosis and other circulatory disorders.

---

9 Particularly those diabetics who are insulin-dependent.

Other conditions associated with low levels of chromium in the blood are high cholesterol and high blood pressure. In animal studies, these conditions were treated with chromium supplements.

In one study, when rats were given a low-chromium diet, their growth was stunted and they died sooner than average rats. Those that were given extra supplements of chromium, however, lived considerably longer, grew better and were healthier. All these studies indicate that chromium is indeed vital to health and longevity.

There are a variety of inorganic chromium supplements. But the one that is known to be highly absorbable is chromium picolinate. Picolinate is an organic molecule that acts as a carrier or transporter of chromium ions across the intestinal wall. In addition to increasing sugar metabolism (particularly important with hypoglycemics and diabetics, as well as the elderly), chromium picolinate is found to reduce fat and cholesterol levels in the blood. Because of its ability to mobilize and metabolize fats, chromium picolinate may be an excellent supplement to those who wish to lose weight.

Food Sources and RDA Requirements

Brewer's yeast, meat, poultry, shellfish, corn oil and whole grain cereals are good sources of chromium.

The RDA for this nutrient has not been formulated. The National Research Council (NRC) has yet to devise a method that quantifies the "active" chromium in food.

Nonetheless, based on research findings, anywhere from 50 to 200 mcg/day has been suggested by the NRC. Some nutritionists have recommended as high as 300 mcg/day. Because there is no known chromium toxicity, even higher amounts would be tolerable.

Absorption Suppressors: None known.

Absorption Facilitators: None known.

Copper

As you read and learn more about the various minerals mentioned in this book, you come to realize how much a part of the earth we are and how much the content of the earth's crust is a part of us. Copper is one more earthware that contributes to our health and well-being. It's not one of the most studied minerals, but what is known about it so far is pretty impressive.

Unlike calcium, iron or phosphorus, when you think of copper's benefit to health, you probably draw a blank. Perhaps the most you have heard about it is its role in traditional folklore, where arthritic people wore copper bracelets to alleviate their pain. As you can see below, copper actually does help in relieving arthritis.

Besides relieving arthritis, copper has many benefits, one of which is the production of energy from the food you eat. Copper is part of many enzyme systems that are involved in this process. Indirectly, copper is involved in the absorption and distribution of oxygen around your body. Considering life can cease within minutes without oxygen, this mineral is important to your health and well-being. Let's see how copper works in this area.

The hemoglobin in the red blood cells is what carries oxygen to all the tissues of the body. Iron, which gives blood its characteristic color, is very important for the formation of hemoglobin, and copper is largely responsible for the absorption of iron from the intestine. Without iron, the oxygen conveyor system can be quite weak and fragile. Incidentally, copper also combines with plasma protein to form ceruloplasmins. It's believed that ceruloplasmins protect hemoglobin and the red blood cells from free radical damage.

One of the most potent antioxidant enzymes is superoxide dismutase (SOD). Copper is also an integral part of this enzyme, which protects us from the savagely dangerous singlet oxygen free radicals. Free radicals are known to be one of the major causes of cancer and aging. In this connection, you may say that copper has an indirect (as part of SOD) anticancer role.

From both human and animal studies, copper has been found to lower the blood serum cholesterol while raising the HDL cholesterol. Regarding osteoarthritis, copper helps to relieve pain by reducing tissue swelling. The pain-relieving effect of copper bracelets on certain types of arthritis was experimentally verified by a double-blind[10] study. The researchers in this experiment discovered that body perspiration can dissolve tiny amounts of elemental copper and cause it to seep into the skin, where it can have healing effects on the affected tissues.

---

10   A situation where neither the experimenter nor the patient knows what treatment is being administered in the study.

Copper is also good for your skin and hair. It is involved in the formation and development of the fibrous proteins, such as collagen and elastin, found throughout your body but largely concentrated in the skin. The production of your natural sunscreen (melanin), as well as water, during energy-producing reactions in the cells also depends on the availability of copper in your body.

The amino acid tyrosine is a key nutrient for the formation of melanin, and copper facilitates its use in the synthesis of the pigment. The absence of the mineral in the body leads to skin and hair discolorations. How sharply discerning are your taste buds? Well, copper can help them work better, too.

Some of the other deficiency symptoms (although rare in humans) seen in animal studies include increases in blood cholesterol, anemia, malfunctioning of the nervous system, weakening of the blood vessels and poor development of the skeletal tissues. Some of the deficiency observed in humans involves infants. For example, infants who were fed only cow's milk had a copper deficiency. The expressed symptoms were malformation of the bones and hair follicles (causing hair to grow rough, twisted and kinked), and disorders that afflicted the circulatory and nervous systems.

Food Sources and RDA Requirements

Perhaps one of the reasons there are no widespread deficiencies of copper, although subclinical or marginal ones may occur, is because there are many common food sources of the mineral. These are all meats, almost all sea foods, whole grains, nuts, legumes, chocolate and mushrooms. If you live in an area where there is hard water or use copperware in your cooking, chances are you get a certain amount of copper from these sources as well. Copper pots, however, are deadly in interaction with Vitamin C and E and folic acid.

Be aware that there is a certain amount of toxicity associated with excessive intake of copper. Some of the symptoms of this effect are mental and sleep disorders and increased blood pressure. Those who cannot metabolize copper (Wilson's disease) can suffer from jaundice and cirrhosis of the liver (a result of free copper deposition in the liver.)

The adult RDA for copper ranges from 2 to 3 mg/day. Some nutritionists think this is less than half of what it should be. For infants up to 12 months old the RDA amounts ranges from 0.4 to 0.7 mg/day.

Absorption Suppressors: Excessive amounts of zinc, vitamins C and E and Folic acid.

Absorption Facilitators: Iron, cobalt.

Toxicity: Excessive intake of copper

Iodine

So far as we know, this is perhaps one of the few minerals that has limited but very important functions in the body. Iodine's primary function is in keeping the thyroid gland healthy. Thyroxine and triiodotyrosine, the two hormones produced by the thyroid gland, depend on iodine for their formation. These hormones regulate the body's energy-producing processes. For instance, thyroxine's major role in the body is maintaining a satisfactory rate at which the tissues convert food into energy. The significance of this is great.

First, when you have an efficient metabolism it means your cells are using more fuel and oxygen and you will have less fat storage in the body. This will also influence the synthesis of proteins and hormones as well as many other biochemical compounds that have a direct effect on the replication of cells, development, growth and health of the individual.

Second, cretinism is an iodine deficiency disease that afflicts in areas of the world where there is insufficient iodine in their diet. The characteristics symptoms of the diseases are mental retardation and poor, dwarfed muscular and skeletal development. The skin also becomes dry, rough and coarse with iodine deficiency. Cretinism is normally a congenital condition caused by a lack of iodine in the mother's diet. Unless an infant is treated with iodine supplement right after birth, the damage will be permanent and irreversible.

Third, in adults, goiter is the most common condition that results from iodine deficiency. Although now rare in this country, it affects over 200 million people world-wide. The classic symptom of goiter is an enlargement and protrusion of the thyroid gland (because it's trying to compensate for the absence of iodine). Goiter is an often painless, but nonetheless unattractive appendage. If caught early, goiter can be treated with iodine supplementation.

Be aware, however, that the lack of iodine may not be the sole reason for goiter or cretinism. Other factors such as a lack or malfunction of the enzyme responsible for the synthesis of the thyroid hormone, food and chemical goitrogens (agents that induce goiter) such as found in turnips, peanuts, cabbage, spinach, strawberries, radishes and rutabagas, can sometimes be the cause.

Food Sources and RDA Requirements

Sea foods such as fish and seaweeds (kelp) and plants and vegetables that grow in an iodine-rich soil are your best sources for this mineral. When buying table salt at the store, you can choose either iodized salt or plain salt. If you buy iodized salt or use a small amount of iodized salt, you might consider using iodine supplements.

The RDA for iodine is from 40 to 50 mcg for infants under one year old, 70 to 120 mcg for those between one and ten, and 150 mcg for teenagers and adults. Pregnant and lactating women require 175 and 200 mcg, respectively.

There is no known iodine toxicity from normal foods. As supplements you can take up to 1000 mcg/day without fear of toxicity. The thyroid gland has a built-in mechanism by which it maintains normal production of the hormones even in the presence of excess iodine. Extremely high doses, 10 to 20 times the above figures, can lead to simple skin rashes, abnormal breathing, headache and iodide goiterism.

Absorption Suppressors: None.

Absorption Facilitators: None.

Iron

As we have seen so far, many vitamins and minerals are needed to maintain human body's health and keep it properly functioning. It seems the more you learn about the benefits of one vitamin or mineral, the more important or beneficial that vitamin or mineral appears to be compared to any you have studied or read about so far.

When you read about the benefits of iron to your health, it will seem to you that this must be the most important of all the micronutrients you have studied thus far. In reality, one essential nutrient can't be more important than any other, because in the long run the body can be severely affected by the lack of any one of nutrients.

Iron is one of those minerals (or nutrients) you would think is so important you couldn't live without it. That seems a valid perception because the ability of oxygen (the breath of life) to the various tissues in the body is dependent on iron.

The hemoglobin in the red blood cells is a four-part protein molecule that contains four atoms of iron. The iron atoms combine with oxygen when you breathe air. Without iron, there is no oxygen for the tissue cells to burn the fuel and provide you with energy. In effect, there's no life. You can live without food for up to five weeks but only a few minutes without oxygen. In this regard, iron is perhaps the most essential of all the nutrients.

The characteristic symptoms of iron deficiency anemia range from weakness, fatigue and pale complexion to headache, irritability, forced breathing during exertion and cracks at the corner of the mouth. Some of the other conditions arising from iron deficiency are apathy, listlessness and loss of appetite for the normal food. Strangely, those who suffer from a severe lack of iron may have a craving for non-nutritional foods (pica) such as grass, clay, stones, ice or clothing. Children who are deficient in iron will have difficulty in concentrating, reading and solving problems. They also tend to be cranky and have little interest in activities.

Iron is important for the conversion of tyrosine to dopamine, one of the brain chemicals necessary for thought processes. Thus, iron not only brings oxygen to the brain but also helps the brain to work better.

How Does Iron Deficiency Come About?

After the epithelial cells of the intestinal tract, red blood cells have the highest turnover rate in the body. While the epithelial cells are replaced every three or four days, red blood cells can live up to three or four months. Every second, there are about 4 million births and roughly the same number of deaths of the red blood cells. Because these cells are in a fluid medium, they also tend to be lost quite easily through bleeding or menstruation. During its lifetime, a red blood cell makes roughly 75,000 trips between the tissues and the lungs.

Red blood cells are made up largely of hemoglobin—each cell containing approximately 300 million of these globular substances, each of which comprises four iron atoms. Given that the body has all the other nutrients necessary for the synthesis of the hemoglobin protein, iron will therefore be the only limiting factor for the formation and maturation of red cells in the bone marrow.

Although nearly 90% of all the iron from dead cells is reused, the other 10%, and that which gets lost through bleeding or menstruation, will have to be replaced through the diet or supplements. Incidentally, a small percentage of iron is also lost through sweat, urine, dead skin, hair and nails.

To make matters worse, the iron you get from ordinary food sources such as vegetables, beans, cereals and fruits is the least absorbed. Reportedly, only 2% to 10% of the iron in these foods gets metabolized by the body. Because of this, and the aforementioned problems, iron is one of the most commonly deficient nutrients in the human body. Yet iron is vital to life.

Iron deficiency is indeed prevalent in this country. Those who are most frequently affected are women of child-bearing age, teenagers, children, some infants, the elderly and certain economically disadvantaged people. Let's look at each group individually.

Teenage girls and premenopausal women suffer the most from iron deficiency because they lose much iron during the menstrual cycle. Some of these people, particularly the teenagers, are finicky eaters and don't get well-balanced meals. Because pregnant women produce a large volume of blood and share their iron with the fetus, women who bear children often have a problem with iron deficiency anemia. Lactating women can lose as much as three grams of iron a day.

It has been found that both men and women runners, as well as other athletes, have problems with a low level of iron in their blood, in some cases, as many as 50% of them were found to be borderline anemic.

After they are born, infants have just enough iron to last them a few months, and unless they are fed iron-rich nutrients they, too, are vulnerable to iron- deficiency anemia. Getting a sufficient amount of iron is particularly important to infants and children because the proper development of their bodies and brains depend on the availability of sufficient oxygen to their tissues. Children who have iron deficiency have difficulty concentrating, memorizing, reading and solving problems.

While economically disadvantaged people have iron deficiencies from not getting well-balanced meals, the majority of the elderly suffer from this malady largely because of insufficient absorption. As mentioned above, iron is one of the most poorly absorbed nutrients. To make matters worse, the elderly will have even less of it because of a lowered absorption rate. The elderly also tend to suffer more frequently from internal bleeding, such as caused by ulcers, and external bleeding, such as caused by hemorrhoids, increasing the loss of iron.

The absorption of iron in the digestive tract is also limited by such interfering factors as calcium, phosphates, zinc and plant-based organic substances, such as phytates, and oxalates found in cereal husk. Tannic acid (found in tea), egg yolk and aspirin are also found to be common antagonists to iron absorption. On the other hand, Vitamin C and chelating agents, such as amino acids and other organic compounds, increase the absorption and utilization of iron.

Finally, bear in mind that in addition to the formation of red blood cells, iron is used for other functions in the body. Roughly 25% of the total iron found in the body is used in enzyme synthesis and as part of organic molecules that are closely involved in the production of energy. Another 5% is found in myoglobin, a protein-iron complex used as a reservoir of oxygen in the liver and muscle cells. This is nature's backup arrangement that helps you weather any temporary short-age of oxygen supply.

In addition, iron helps strengthen the immune cells. The deleterious effects of toxic metals (such as cadmium, lead and mercury) are minimized when you have a high intake of iron. The syntheses of large proteins like collagen and other tissue fibers are facilitated by iron-rich enzymes. Iron is also important for absorption and utilization of all the B vitamins.

Looking at it from the aesthetic point of view, iron enhances your skin, teeth and nails. It is important for the formation of healthy bones and tissues. Iron helps you to cope better during times of mental or physical stress.

Food Sources and RDA Requirements

Pregnant women with a need for 30 mg of iron have the highest RDA requirements. Then come lactating women and females from 11 to 50 years old, with 15 mg. The requirement for children up to ten years old and for adult males above 19 years of age is 10 mg. Teenage boys need 12 mg.

Although adult males reportedly lose about 1 mg of iron a day from their total body reserve of 1,000 mg, females, who often have much less (200 to 400 mg), lose up to roughly 2.5 mg of iron a day. This is why the requirement for women is much higher. Even then, as it has already been mentioned, women have the worst time with iron deficiency.

At one point or another, between 25% and 50% of menstruating women and up to 60% of pregnant women are deficient in iron. According to one government survey,as many as 35% of infants were found to be deficient in iron. In another survey, 30% of the infants born to economically disadvantaged families were found to be anemic, while another 25% were shown to be deficient in iron.

It seems, therefore, that considering the low absorption and the wide prevalence of iron deficiency in this country we need to consume considerably higher than the RDA amounts to meet just the RDA figures for iron. It is reported that a person consuming a well-balanced meal can get about 6 mg per 1,000 calories consumed.

For men who consume up to 2,500 calories a day, meeting the RDA seems to be no problem. What is not accounted for, however, is how much of that 6 to 15 grams is actually being absorbed. Women who consume less (1,700 to 2,000 calories) get even less iron. This means both men and women can benefit by including nutritionally dense foods like the Four Pillars in their daily meals.

Some of the excellent food sources are liver, kidney heart, red meat, eggs, fish and clams. In addition, wheat germ, oysters, nuts, molasses, leafy green vegetables, beans, poultry, oatmeal and dried fruits are good sources of iron.

As we said earlier, the problem is with absorption. In general, the iron you get from meat sources is better absorbed than the iron you get from non-meat sources. Still, as a margin of safety, you might want to include iron supplements.

You should have very little concern about iron toxicity. In very rare situations, excessive iron could build up in the soft tissues, such as the liver and spleen, to cause some complications. This condition known as hemochromatosis, results mainly from excessive deposition of iron in the aforesaid tissues. Alcoholics and people with chronic liver problems are sometimes predisposed to the condition.

Absorption Suppressors: Excessive zinc, coffee, phosphates, phytates, oxalates and tannic acid.

Absorption Facilitators: Folic acid, copper, cobalt, manganese, Vitamin C and Vitamin B12.

Molybdenum

This tongue twister is relatively new to the human dietary scene, although it has long been known to be essential for plant growth and development. It is often added to steel and iron to give them hardness and strength, and as a food supplement, it may do just about the same for you.

In legumes, molybdenum is one of the two key minerals (the other is cobalt) used to catalyze the fixation of nitrogen. Its benefit for human health has gradually been establishing solid roots. Some of these involve the metabolism of iron (important in the production and growth of red blood cells), the prevention of certain cancers and even the health and appearance of your teeth. Regarding molybdenum and cancer, here's an interesting story.

In one Chinese province, the incidence of esophagus and stomach cancers was found to be the highest in the world. It was later discovered that such disproportionate rates of death from these cancers had something to do with a lack of molybdenum in the soil. By adding molybdenum to the soil, scientists were able to reduce deaths associated with the cancers.

In connection to its importance to teeth, studies have shown that molybdenum helps minimize the occurrence of dental cavities, possibly by promoting the retention of fluoride in the teeth.

Molybdenum has been found useful in removing certain food preservatives that accumulate in our bodies and become toxic. The sulfites are common additives used by the wine, restaurant and food-processing industries. Perhaps the most common food products containing sulfites are the salad accoutrements (dressings, etc.) and processed foods (bread, cakes, etc.). Often the symptoms resulting from sulfite buildup are diarrhea, nausea, asthmatic disorders and, in extreme instances, loss of consciousness and death. Molybdenum activates sulfite oxidase—the enzyme that destroys sulfite food additives.

The formation of urine, as well as the removal of toxic metabolic byproducts like aldehydes, is also aided by molybdenum.

Food Sources and RDA Requirements

Molybdenum is most commonly found in leafy vegetables, whole grains (barley, wheat, oats), legumes (beans, soybeans, lentils) and sunflower seeds. Please remember that the amount of molybdenum in these foods depends on the soil content of the mineral where they were grown and how much they have been spared by food-processing companies. Because of the great variety of fruits, vegetables and herbs in the Four Pillars drinks, chances are you get a good amount of molybdenum in your daily nutrition.

The estimated RDA ranges from 15 mcg for infants to 75 mcg for young children (up to age six). For older children and adults, it ranges from 75 mcg to 250 mcg, respectively. There has not been molybdenum toxicity reported in humans. In animals, however, growth retardation, weight loss, diarrhea and muscle wasting have been observed.

Absorption Suppressors: None known.

Absorption Facilitators: None known.

Selenium

Perhaps there is no better nutrient than selenium that can illustrate the relationship between the absence of a well-balanced diet and the incidence of major diseases such as cancer and heart disease. This element, which for a long time had been considered toxic for human consumption, has in recent years been elevated to an "essential nutrient" status. Now, for the first time, we have the RDA values for selenium.

Selenium's importance, for both human and animal health, is so great that in the areas of the world where there is little selenium in the soil, diseases like cancer, muscular dystrophy, heart disease and several other degenerative conditions prevail.

From the depths of mainland China to the far reaches of Turkey and Finland to the heartlands of America, scientists have found uncanny correlations between the occurrence of heart disease, cancer and other afflictions and low levels of selenium in the soil.

One disease stemming from a selenium-poor region in Turkey, where the peasants suffered and died from weak and scarred hearts, is called Keshan's disease. It was later discovered that it afflicted children in China as well. The Finns have the worst incidence of heart disease. This is correlated quite well with their low level of selenium intake compared with other nations. To bring this home, similar heart problems are seen in the "stroke belt" of Georgia and the Carolinas, as well as in Ohio, Vermont, Texas, New York and Indiana.

For a long time, this geographically specific occurrence of cardiovascular disease and cancer was a mystery to scientists. It was only in the past three decades or so they discovered a connection between the low level of selenium in the soil and the frequency of heart disease in these specific areas. With this discovery came the resolution: in China, for example, Keshan's disease has now been virtually eliminated through the use of selenium supplementation.

Figure 6.1 shows the distribution of selenium in American soils.

Depending on where you live, it will be important for you to have access to foods that are grown in selenium-rich soils or to take supplements as a protective measure.

Selenium's value to human health lies in its ability to fight free radicals and retard the process of aging. Selenium can do this as part of the enzyme glutathione peroxidase, or in conjunction with vitamin E. Of course, as a team these two nutrients are very powerful in protecting the body from free-radical damage. The parts of the body that ate susceptible to free radicals, particularly those produced from the oxidation of fats, are the cell membranes and the contents inside the cells, like the DNA and RNA, mitochondria and other organelles.

Selenium is found throughout the body, but the organs that seem to have the greatest concentration ate the liver, kidney, heart, testicles, spleen and pancreas.

Besides its ability to help prevent cancer and heart disease and in moving toxic metals[11] (i.e., cadmium, mercury, lead, aluminum) out of the system, selenium is found to reduce problems associated with dandruff and acne and keeps the skin elastic and youthful.

---

11   Some of the physical symptoms of these metals are irritability depression, mental retardation, fatigue and headaches.

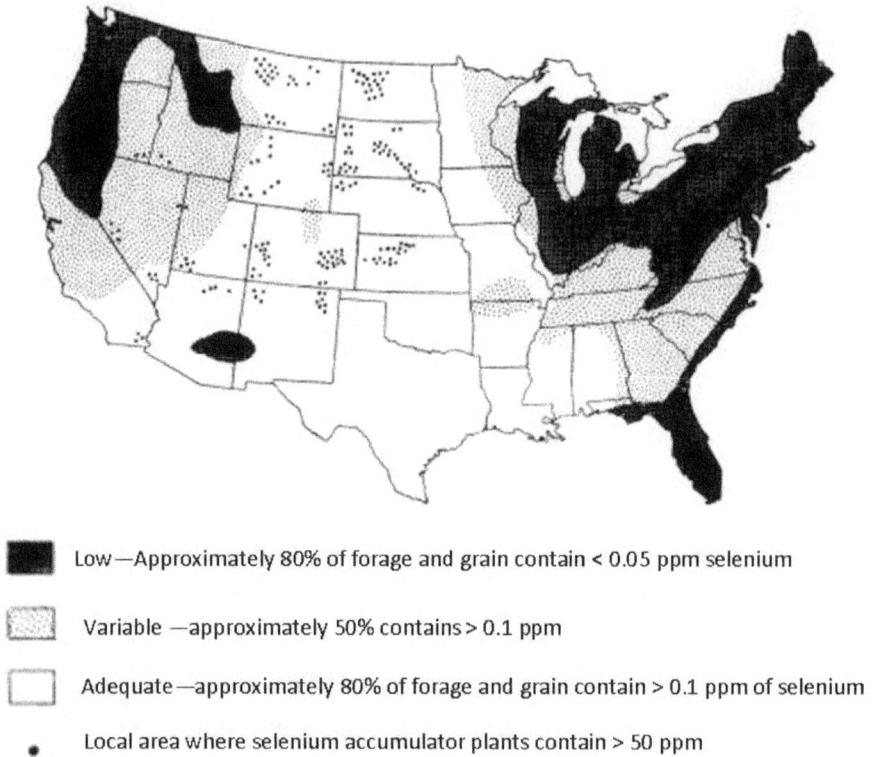

Low—Approximately 80% of forage and grain contain < 0.05 ppm selenium

Variable —approximately 50% contains > 0.1 ppm

Adequate—approximately 80% of forage and grain contain > 0.1 ppm of selenium

•   Local area where selenium accumulator plants contain > 50 ppm

Source: Data from USDA Technical Bulletin No. 758 (1967)

Figure 6.1 Geographical distribution of selenium in the U.S.

Food Sources and RDA Requirements

Food sources of selenium range from whole grain foods (wheat, barley, rye) to fish (tuna, herring, shellfish) and organ foods (kidney and liver). To a limited extent, green vegetables, brewer's yeast, asparagus, tomatoes and peanuts may also contain selenium. Bear in mind, though, that all these depend on the selenium richness of the soil in which the foods are grown.

The current RDA requirements for selenium range from 10 micrograms for infants to 75 mcg for lactating women. Many researchers feel that these values are far below what they should be for the body to have optimal protection from the myriad of substances that attack the tissues every second. From their research, many scientists believe that we need to have as many as 250 to 350 mcg of the mineral daily.

In those areas of the country where the incidence of cancer and heart diseases is less frequent, the average daily dietary intake of selenium was reported to be over 100 mcg. Selenium is absorbed at over 90%.

Absorption Suppressors: None.

Absorption Facilitators: Vitamin E.

Manganese

Manganese is one of the most prevalent micronutrients in nature, yet the body tissues use very little of it. Although it is found to be essential and has many important functions in the body, the Food and Nutrition Board of the National Research Council (NRC) has not made manganese a nutritional requirement for a long time. This was primarily because there has not been, according to the NRC, "a practical way for assessing manganese status" and because of the abundance of manganese in food sources.

Manganese is involved in many different biochemical processes. These include its role in the synthesis of mucopolysaccharides—a group of complex carbohydrates used as structural components off tendons, bones, cartilages and ligaments. As a cofactor of many enzyme systems, manganese is also involved the synthesis of proteins, collagen fibers, fatty acids and cholesterol. The proper functioning of mitochondria is aided by the presence of manganese.

The digestion of protein and the formation of urea (a byproduct of protein breakdown excreted in the urine) are facilitated by manganese. The synthesis of thyroxine, the key hormone made by the thyroid gland used to stimulate the production of energy in the body, is influenced by manganese. This versatile mineral is involved in reducing the symptoms associated with diabetes, convulsions and epileptic seizures, as well as those in schizophrenia. Manganese facilitates blood clotting and insulin utilization. The efficacy of this mineral with all these conditions was observed in both human and animal studies.

Manganese plays a role in keeping the immune system healthy and in reducing the effect of certain free radicals. Superoxide dismutase (SOD) is a key antioxidant responsible for neutralizing the singlet oxygen free radicals (see Appendix A). Manganese is one of the minerals that make up SOD. Without manganese, the enzyme would not be formed and the free radicals could have a field day in your body and immune system.

Although there are no outright deficiency symptoms associated with manganese in humans, in animals a variety of conditions have been observed. These range from skeletal deformities, growth retardation and poor glucose tolerance to neuro-muscular disturbances that resulted in epileptic seizures and convulsions. Animals that were fed a manganese deficient diet had offspring that were poorly developed.

Like iron, manganese is responsible for the production of dopamine from tyrosine. This chemical is important for the proper functioning of your brain. It's involved in thought processes, emotions and muscular control. This is why manganese supplementation seems to help children who have poor muscular coordination and learning and speech problems.

Food Sources and RDA Requirements

As mentioned, there is no RDA requirement for manganese primarily because it has not been fully studied. However, there are amounts that have been suggested as enough for the proper functioning of the body. The RDAs range from 0.3 to 1.0 mg for infants to 1.0 to 2.0 mg for children from one to ten years old. Teenagers and adults can use from 2.0 to 5.0 mg of the mineral per day.

There is very little toxicity associated with manganese except to those who work in industrial and mining environments. In these cases, excessive amounts of the mineral can collect in the lungs and other tissues in the body where it can cause anorexia, cramps in the legs, headaches, apathy and even impotence. In an advanced situation, more sever neuromuscular conditions such as muscle tremor, rigidity and a loss of spontaneous movement can occur. In some cases, the afflicted cannot modulate their voices or show facial expressions.

The best natural sources of manganese are organ meats, nuts, whole grains, peas and beans, beets and egg yolks. Leafy vegetables, seaweed, oatmeal, avocados and dry fruits also have a significant amount of manganese.

Absorption Suppressors: Excessive intake of phosphorus and calcium and phytates.

Absorption facilitator: Vitamins B1 and E.

Zinc

Zinc's name may start with the last letter of the alphabet, but what it can do for health is absolutely numero uno. There are roughly 2 to 3 grams of zinc in a human body, but those areas that have the highest concentrations include the eyes, liver, kidney, bones, muscles, hair and the male reproductive organs (prostate and seminal fluid). Zinc is a remarkable mineral that has many important functions in the body.

For starters, zinc works as a cofactor in at least 40 enzyme systems in humans (as many as 59 have been reported, including those in animals). All these enzymes have very specific functions and without zinc many of the biological processes would be in a serious trouble. For example, the synthesis of DNA and RNA—two substances critical for the growth and replication of the cells—is dependent on enzymes that use zinc.

Several other enzymes that help digest food in the stomach and small intestine and those that break down sugar and fat molecules in the cells are also dependent on zinc. Alcohol dehydrogenase breaks down and detoxifies alcohol (including methanol and retinol). This enzyme is necessary because alcohol will become toxic when allowed to accumulate in the liver and other tissues. This enzyme contains zinc.

The breakdown, or removal, of carbon dioxide from the cells and body fluids is also accomplished by a zinc-dependent enzyme. Imagine what these two substances would do to the body if allowed to collect—a very dangerous and explosive situation would ensue.

From a less technical point of view, here are some of the things zinc can do for you. Let's start with the skin, hair and nails. The basal layer of the epidermis, the papilla of the hair and the matrix of the nails are among the fastest reproducing tissues of the body. Since Zinc is very important for the replication, growth and repair of the cells, the health and appearance of your skin, hair and nails will depend as much on the level of zinc in these tissues as on the level of other essential nutrients.

To cite another example, how fast and how well a wound can heal is greatly influenced by the amount of zinc present in your body. In one study, surgical patients who were given zinc supplements healed on the average twice as fast as those who were not supplemented. In another study, zinc sulfate was used to dramatically reduce scars left from chemical treatment of acne.

Acrodermatitis enteropathica is a congenital and often fatal disorder affecting the hands, feet, mouth, scalp and anal areas of infants. The skin in these areas is characterized by red and ulcerated rashes and hair loss. Acrodermatitis is caused by the body's inability to absorb zinc. Sometimes similar symptoms can result when an infant is switched from breast-feeding to formula that maybe lacking zinc. For years, this disease was a mystery. Now doctors can successfully treat individuals who suffer from acrodermatitis with zinc supplements.

Another area where the absence of zinc has a profound impact is on the reproductive system of both sexes and on the subsequent offspring. It was mentioned earlier that the reproductive organs are some of the areas where zinc is found in high concentration. Since zinc is very important for replication of strong and healthy cells, and since sperm cells are some of the fastest producing cells, the availability of a sufficient amount the mineral will determine the proliferation, maturity and fertility of the sperm cells. In this case, zinc deficiency can lead to a retardation of sexual development in teenagers and young adolescents and perhaps even in impotence or sexual dysfunction in adult men.

Zinc deficiency in a pregnant woman could have many complications, including miscarriage. For the baby, it could lead to mental retardation or physical deformity. In one animal study, zinc-deficient female rats showed nearly a 100% incidence of birth defects. These varied from severe complications with the nervous system of their offspring to physical deformities, such as clubbed feet and cleft palates.

Some of the other manifestations of zinc deficiencies are loss of appetite, taste and smell. There may be complications in the eyes that lead to color blindness, inflammation of optic nerves and the formation of cataracts. Zinc seems to be critical for the activation and proper function of vitamin A—the nutrient that is often associated with the eyes. Zinc deficiencies elsewhere in the body also seem to lower the body's stress response and affect its ability to fight infections or cope with toxic foreign elements such as alcohol, heavy metals and air pollution.

Zinc is truly a remarkable mineral that has beneficial effects on blood circulation, rheumatoid arthritis and sickle cell anemia. The health and proper functioning of the prostate gland and of the skeletal, nervous and immune systems are aided by the sufficient availability of zinc in the body.

Millions of germs, bacteria, parasites and viruses seek entry into the body every day. Within the body, certain cells may tend to become cancerous, and toxins may build in tissues to threaten the health and well-being of an individual. These elements, to a large degree, are put in check or neutralized by body's own defense forces.

Although most of the body's defenses are born in the bone marrow, they reach mature elsewhere in the body. For instance, the B-cells, which produce antibodies, develop in the thymus gland, the spleen, lymph nodes and the intestinal wall. T-cells develop in the thymus gland, and after maturity they migrate into other locations such as the spleen, lymph nodes, blood and liver, where they are needed to deal with any potential foreign agents. It seems zinc is intimately involved in the proliferation and maturation of all these cells, as well as in the health of the organs and tissues that produce them.

Both animal and human studies have shown that the immune system is one of the first areas to be affected by zinc deficiency. People who took zinc supplements had fewer infections. Those who had an infection such as the common cold or were recovering from surgery and took zinc supplements regained their health faster than those who were not taking supplements. AIDS is probably the worst communicable disease of the twentieth century. Researchers have found that those who succumbed to the disease were sometimes found to have a low serum level of zinc.

Food Sources and RDA Requirements

Zinc is one of those minerals that does not store well in the body. If you are sick, recovering from surgery or undergoing mental or physical stress, some of the zinc stored in your body can be used up. Moreover, this mineral is easily lost from the body through sweat and in the feces. In a hot climate or during strenuous exercise where there may be excess sweating, the loss of up to 3 mg/day is reportedly common. This means that considering its multipurpose function and your body's inability to store it, you may need a regular intake of the mineral to keep your body healthy and strong.

The RDA for zinc ranges from 2 to 5 mg for infants and up to 30 mg for pregnant women. Children from 1 to 10 years old need 10 mg, while females and males above 10 years old require 12 and 15 mg, respectively. The recommended intake for lactating women is 15 mg.

The best food sources are meats, poultry, wheat germ, brewer's yeast, eggs, pumpkin seeds, liver, legumes, nonfat dry milk, whole grains, herring and oysters. Speaking of oysters, perhaps now you know why they are erroneously considered aphrodisiacs. Other foods such as vegetables, fruits, potatoes, onions, carrots and nuts may also have zinc, albeit in low levels.

The levels of zinc in various plants vary depending on the mineral content of soil they were grown in. Most of the farmlands in this country have been depleted a long time, and as a result not many people get the RDA amounts of zinc. Moreover, processed foods, particularly grains, can lose up to 80% of their zinc.

There are also absorption problems you have to be concerned with. It's reported that zinc uptake by the intestinal walls could vary from 20% to 80%.It all depends on the food sources and factors that might interfere with its absorption. For example, the zinc in meats is better absorbed than that in cereals. Phytates in cereal fibers can interfere with absorption. Drugs such as diuretics and oral contraceptives can inhibit zinc absorption. High intakes of alcohol and calcium are some the other culprits. On the other hand, vitamin A, copper and phosphorus are good absorption facilitators.

Zinc is a relatively nontoxic mineral. When up to 150 mg/day of zinc was given to individuals for a certain period, no toxicity was observed. It seems that the body has a way of monitoring zinc intake—stepping up its absorption of the mineral when it's low and eliminating it when there is more than enough. A very large dose, say 300 mg at one shot, can cause vomiting.

Absorption Suppressors: Phytates, diuretics, oral contraceptives, high intakes of alcohol and calcium.

Absorption facilitators: Vitamin A, copper and phosphorus.

Chapter 7
Acid/Alkaline Foods

There is a buzz around the Internet about acid- and alkaline-forming foods. Various web sites show categories of foods, classified as alkaline- and acidic-forming when consumed by humans. The story is based on the assumption that the body's acid-base balance has to be maintained between its normal ranges, between pH of 7.35 to 7.45. If we choose and consume the right food we are supposed to maintain those homeostatic ranges. The pH is the measure of the acidity or alkalinity levels of a fluid. In the acid-base scale, zero is most acid, 14 is most alkaline. Seven is neutral. The above pH range of the human body indicates that it works in a slightly alkaline environment. Anything that throws this balance off—like stress, eating foods that are acid-forming (animal products, grains and processed food), toxic build up—can compromise a person's day-to-day life as well as his/her long-term health. If the range shifts by a few degrees either way, the person's life can be in jeopardy.

It's believed that the body, in its propensity to keep itself on an even keel, mobilizes alkaline forming minerals such as calcium, magnesium and phosphorus from the bones and elsewhere if it does not find them from the food the person eats. A chronic problem of this kind is supposed to lead to osteoporosis and osteomalacia and other diseases. Therefore, it's recommended that to minimize this problem and promote good health, we need to consume foods that are rich in minerals. This means largely vegetables and most fruits.

Purely from a scientific point of view, there has not been a controlled, double-blind study to corroborate the claim. The clinical trials have not been conclusive. I don't buy the theory entirely, because just by eating alkaline-based foods, people can keep their body alkaline and less so (i.e., the normal range) if you consume acid-forming foods. The system naturally regulates its pH level. We cannot monkey with it by simply eating one type of food or another. Nature is a lot wiser and more capable of doing its thing without our interference. Yes, in the extreme situation, the body's pH can drop. For example, if someone is diabetic, severely starved, or on a carbohydrate-restricted diet, the liver converts fatty acids into ketones to fill the body's energy demands.

In a diabetic, the build- up of ketones and un-metabolized sugar can make the blood acidic, thus lowering the pH and posing a threat to the person's life. This could happen with a starving person as well. In normal circumstances the body regulates its acid-base balance without our interference. The body can, indeed, lose minerals from the bones if the blood level is low. Minerals such as calcium and magnesium are critical for muscular contraction and for maintaining the heart's natural rhythm. In this instance, maintaining life is more important than having strong bones. The body starts to break down the minerals from the bones and make them available for these tissues.

As we discussed earlier, minerals are vital to life. If you're a believer in the acid/alkaline value of foods, the fruits and vegetables configured in the Four Pillars drinks can be excellent sources. Here are some examples.

Alkaline Food Chart

ALFALFA	COLLARD GREENS	LETTUCE	SEA VEGGIES (SEAWEED)
ARTICHOKES	COMFREY	MUSHROOMS	SORREL
ARUGULA	CUCUMBER	MUSTARD GREENS	SOY SPROUTS
BARLEY GRASS	DANDELION GREENS	NIGHTSHADE VEGGIES	SPINACH, GREEN
BEET GREENS	EGGPLANT	OKRA	SPIRULINA
BEETS	ENDIVE	ONIONS	SPROUTS
BROCCOLI	GARLIC	PARSNIPS	SWEET POTATOES
BRUSSELS SPROUTS	GINGERROOT	PEAS	TOMATO
CABBAGE	GREEN BEANS	PEPPERS (BELL)	TURNIPS
CARROT	GREEN PEAS	PEPPERS (FRESH, HOT)	WATERCRESS
CAULIFLOWER	HORSERADISH	PUMPKIN	WHEAT GRASS
CELERY	KALE	RADISHES	WILD GREENS
CHARD GREENS	KOHLRABI	RHUBARB	YAMS
CHLORELLA	LEEKS	RUTABAGA	ZUCCHINI

courtesy of H2Oalkalizer.com

Pillar Three

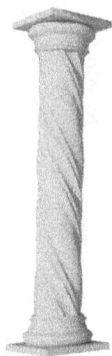

Dietary Fiber

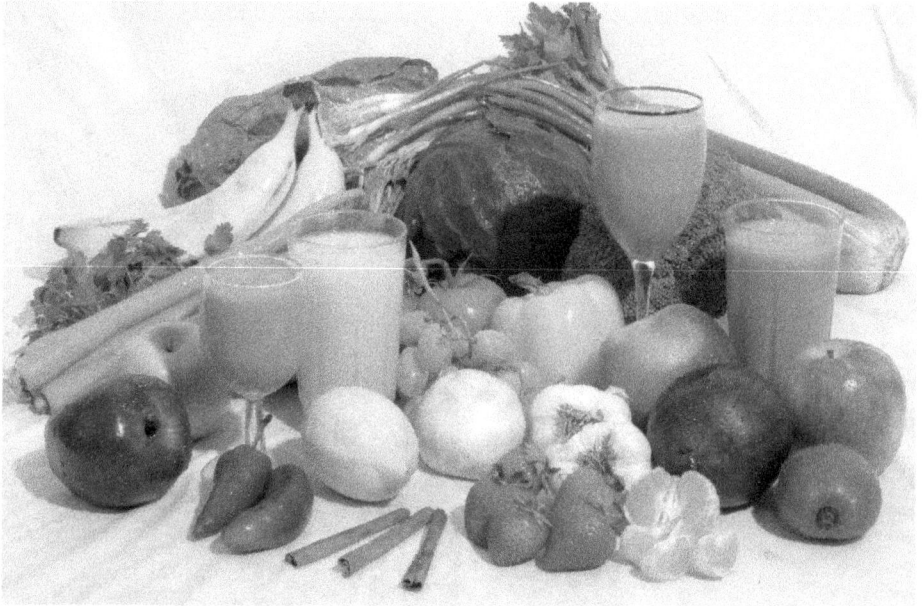

Figure 8.1 Fiber rich fruits and vegetables

Chapter 8
Dietary Fiber

Fibers are indigestible substances that have no nutritive significance whatsoever. Because of this, for a long time fibers have been some of the least understood and most unsung heroes of the nutrition world. Only recently, scientists have come to recognize the importance of these inert, stringy substances in our diet. As you can see below, fibers do play a crucial role in our health.

Fibers come from many different sources, and depending on their origin, they have different functions and classifications. The so-called water-soluble fibers include the ones in apples, squash, potatoes and all the citrus fruits. These are the pectin family. The gums, which are in oat bran, lentils, guar gum, peas and beans, are also water soluble. These and pectin are great at absorbing fats, cholesterol and bile acids (involved in fat processing) in our stomach and intestinal tract. Because these fibers expand as they absorb water, they can quickly give you a sense of fullness. For those who want to lose or control weight, fibrous foods can help suppress the temptation to overindulge.

The insoluble fibers are also divided into two major groups. The lignins are in green beans, broccoli stalks, celery, popcorn hulls, eggplant and cereals. The cellulose and hemicellulose consist of beans, Brussels sprouts, wheat flour and carrots. The insoluble fibers function as vacuum cleaners in your intestinal tract. They suck up toxic chemicals, fats, cholesterol and heavy metals, such as cadmium, lead, mercury and aluminum. Because of their fibrous consistency, these substances move relatively fast through the alimentary canal, which, as explained below, is a great benefit to your health.

The advantages of these fibers' short transit time in the gastrointestinal tract and their toxin-gathering ability can be explained by the difference in the health of those people who consume a lot of fiber and those who don't. For example, in those countries, such as the U.S., in which people consume a significant amount of processed foods (and too little fiber), the incidence of cancer, obesity and heart disease is very common. By contrast, in those countries, such as Japan and many African countries, in which the people eat fiber-rich foods, the aforementioned health hazards are much less common.

The Importance of Fibers for Your Health

Constipation When one thinks of fibers one often associates their benefit with minimizing constipation-abnormally difficult and irregular bowel movements. Because of the highly refined and processed foods people consume in this country, constipation is a frequent problem-particularly among older adults. This, in itself, is not a life-threatening situation. As food stays longer in the intestinal tract, however, it could lead to potential health hazards. These include cancer of the colon, hiatus hernia, diverticulosis (the ballooning of intestinal membrane due to hard feces accumulation), appendicitis, hemorrhoids, irritable bowel syndrome and other maladies.

To give you an idea of the prevalence and significance of some of these health problems, colon and rectal cancers, for example, are the second (after lung cancer) most common cancers in the U.S. Each year there are over 60,000 deaths from these two cancers. Scientists attribute these mortalities to the fat- and protein-rich and low-fiber foods people consume in this country. In one study, for instance, people who had low-fiber diets had four times the incidence of colon cancer as those who ate fiber-rich foods. Similarly, diverticulosis is a common health problem among the older generation. According to one report, 30% of Americans over 60 years old suffer from diverticulosis-a condition that can lead to internal bleeding, pain and distress.' Irritable bowel syndrome, which can lead to diarrhea, flatulence, cramps and spasms, is also a frequent problem among millions of Americans.

Heart Disease Fiber can play a very important role in keeping your circulatory system trouble-free. Since nearly all heart disease is caused by an excessive presence of artery-clogging fat in the bloodstream, a high-fiber diet serves as a purging device to your cardiovascular system. Fiber does this by absorbing fat and cholesterol from your stomach and small intestine and eliminating them along with other waste before it has a chance to get absorbed by the bloodstream.

The fibers that are highly effective in absorbing fat are the pectin and the gum family mentioned above. In a Stanford University study, when patients were given a concentrated level of guar gum with their meals, they showed a reduced level of the LDL cholesterol while at the same time showing an increase in their HDL level (the good cholesterol)[2] Similar results were also shown with locust bean gum, oat bran and pectin (from apples, pears and potatoes).

Blood Pressure Fiber is also known to minimize high blood pressure (hypertension). Normal blood pressure is created when the heart pumps blood through the arteries. The accumulation of cholesterol and fats in the arterial walls can, however, impede the blood flow, thus forcing the heart to pump harder. The constriction of blood vessels due to hardening of the arteries can lead to a similar situation.

In addition to these culprits, hypertension can result from smoking cigarettes and excessive consumption of stimulants like coffee or tea, drug use and high sodium intake. One of the best and most natural ways to deal with this problem is to include a fair amount of fiber in your diet. By absorbing fat and cholesterol in the digestive tract, fiber can reduce the occurrence of high blood pressure. Hypertension is sometimes age-related. For this and the above reasons, it is important that you increase your fiber intake as you get older.

Environmental Pollution Through the food and water we consume, our bodies are constantly exposed to toxins and some of the cancer-causing agents like food additives and heavy metals, such as cadmium, mercury and lead. When you have a high amount of fiber in your diet, these toxins and pollutants will have a smaller chance of getting into the bloodstream. They will be sucked up and carried out of your digestive tract.

Blood Sugar The consumption of sweets and processed foods can cause havoc in one's body. Since these foods are easily digestible, they are absorbed into the bloodstream quickly. This leads to an elevated blood sugar level, which triggers the secretion of a large amount of insulin to help burn off the excess sugar. As a result, a person could experience unpleasant mood swings-including depression, irritability, etc.

When your food is rich in fiber, however, you experience fewer problems. The fiber, by trapping the sweets longer and releasing them gradually, can provide a more even sugar level in the blood. For some diabetics, this can be a realistic and welcome alternative to insulin injection or the use of antidiabetic drugs. In addition to their cholesterol-lowering effect, gaur gum, xanthan gum, oat bran, pectin and locust bean gum are known, important sugar-trapping agents in the digestive tract.

Xanthan gum, by itself, was found to help diabetics and weight watchers.

Weight Loss The other area in which fiber has found popularity is in weight control. One of the most frequent problems encountered by people who try to lose weight is their inability to suppress or contain their craving for food. As a result, no matter what they do to deal with this problem, they end up frustrated, depressed and angry at themselves.

Several experiments have shown that fibers can be effectively used as natural suppressants of hunger and consequently aid in losing or controlling weight. Fibers do this in three ways.

One, when a soluble fiber, like guar gum absorbs water in the stomach, it swells and turns into a viscous gel. This gives the individual who is trying to lose weight a sense of fullness. This sense of satiation will help the person to eat less. The same thing can be experienced with those fibers that are not water soluble. With these types, you might need to consume larger quantities to get the same effect.

Two, because fibers have a capacity for absorbing things in the stomach, fewer of the fattening food products, such as sweets, proteins and fats, have a chance to get absorbed in the bloodstream. This is consistent with what was stated earlier regarding the blood sugar stabilizing effect of fibers. When the sugar level in your body is stable, you feel less hungry.

Three, because fiber-rich foods take longer to chew and digest, people often eat less of them. When combine this with the other two factors, you end up eating much less and ultimately lose weight.

In summary, considering that both cardiovascular diseases and colorectal cancers are some of the major killers in this country, eating plenty of fibers and less fat and protein-rich foods will help you live longer. Losing weight is one of the major concerns people have in this country. When you give your body fiber-rich foods or supplements, you can effectively (along with other weight-reduction measures) deal with this problem as well. Constipation, high blood pressure, diabetes and environmental toxins are the other health problems that affect most of us at one time or another. By increasing our fiber intakes, we may be able to keep many of these health hazards at bay. It is reported that the average American consumes only 11 to 13 grams of fiber a day. According to the National Cancer Institute, our intake should be somewhere in the range of 20 to 30 grams a day.

The Dietary Fibers in The Four Pillars

Take a good inventory of what you eat every day and see if you get all the different fibers in your meals. Chances are you probably don't get even one type of the dietary fibers in sufficient quantities daily let alone the four different fiber groups—the pectins, the gums, hemicellulos and lignins that are found in the Four Pillars drink.

If you eat out, take a look at the menus of the restaurants—from fast foods to five-star establishments, you will see that they are mostly meats, white breads, pasta and maybe one or two or three vegetables. Even in oriental restaurants where greens are commonplace in most dishes, the variety is not large enough to get all different fibers you find in the Four Pillars drinks.

Consuming the "balance diet" every day is a dream for most people. For many the little mounds of salad or mixed vegetables they eat with their rice and meats are the sources of their balanced diet—not the nutritionally dense foods like The Four Pillars which contain a great variety of vitamins, minerals, phytonutrients and fiber.

Talking directly, you probably are too busy to prepare even your normal meals—the two or three dishes—let alone configure a meal from fifteen to twenty different fruits and vegetables. But, if you plan and dedicate two to three hours once a week to making these drinks, you will find that consuming the truly balanced diet will no longer be a dream. It will be an everyday reality for you. You'll feel great and this practice will surely improve the quality of your physical appearance and long-term health.

"Every time you
  eat or drink,
you are either
  feeding disease
or
fighting it."

~ Heather Morgan, MS, NLC

Pillar Four

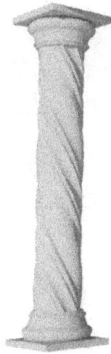

Phytonutrients

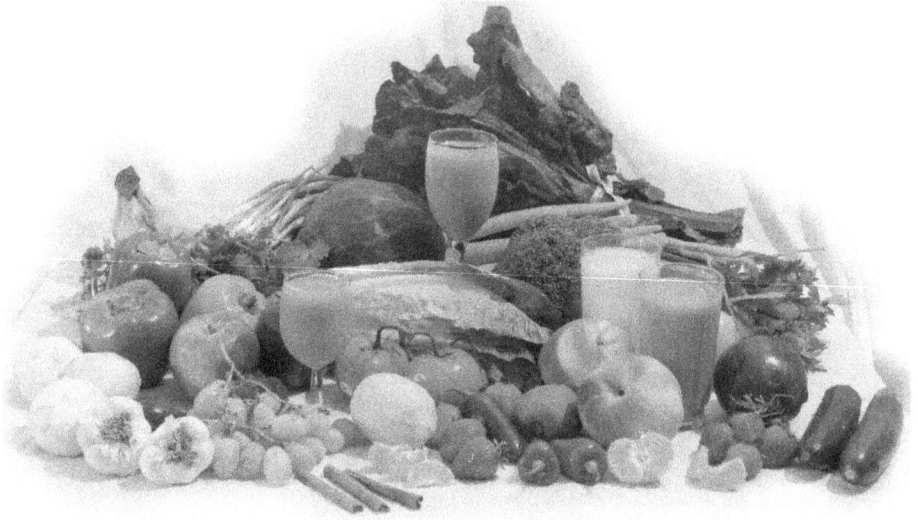

Figure 9.1 Fruits and vegetables rich in phytonutrients

CHAPTER 9
Phytonutrients

We've heard it from our mothers, nutritionists and some doctors about the importance of consuming vegetables and fruits daily. We are also cognizant of Hippocrates famous dictum: make food thy medicine and thy medicine thy food. We even find references in the Bible about the significance of vegetables in our health and appearance. During the reign of Nebuchadnezzar (about 6th century B.C.), Daniel along with other young men was recruited to be trained and eventually enter the king's service. When he began his training, one thing was not quite right to Daniel: the food and drink being consumed at the royal court. Daniel said to the chief official that he would not defile himself by indulging on the royal food and wine.

When the official, for fear of punishment, demanded that Daniel comply with the existing dietary practice, Daniel challenged him by asking the guard whom the chief official had appointed over him and his colleagues to instead feed them vegetables and water for ten days and compare their appearance with those who consumed the royal food and wine. The guard agreed to do so, and after the ten days, Daniel and his colleagues indeed "looked healthier and better nourished than any of the young men who ate the royal food." From then on, the guard took away the royal food and gave the men vegetables and water for their meals.

From early on we have been indoctrinated about the benefits of fruits and vegetables, but until recently, neither we nor our educators knew about the real benefits of these groups of foods. Even nutritionists, when they recommended that we eat a balanced diet, often did so that we would obtain enough vitamins, minerals, carbohydrates and proteins for sufficient energy and to adequately build and repair tissues. Beyond these basic but important functions, to most of us, the idea of eating a balanced diet as a way to prevent disease, enhance one's memory, improve one's appearance or increase one's life span has never been a consideration.

Now thanks to the advancement of science, we are discovering that grains, fruits and vegetables are a storehouse of substances that hold the key for our day-today well-being as well as for long-term health. These substances are called phytochemicals and are found locked in the green, red, yellow, orange or blue of the fruits and vegetables we consume daily. In fact, it's these substances that give flowers, autumn leaves, and various fruits and vegetables their distinct colors. See chart for the different categories of these color groups.

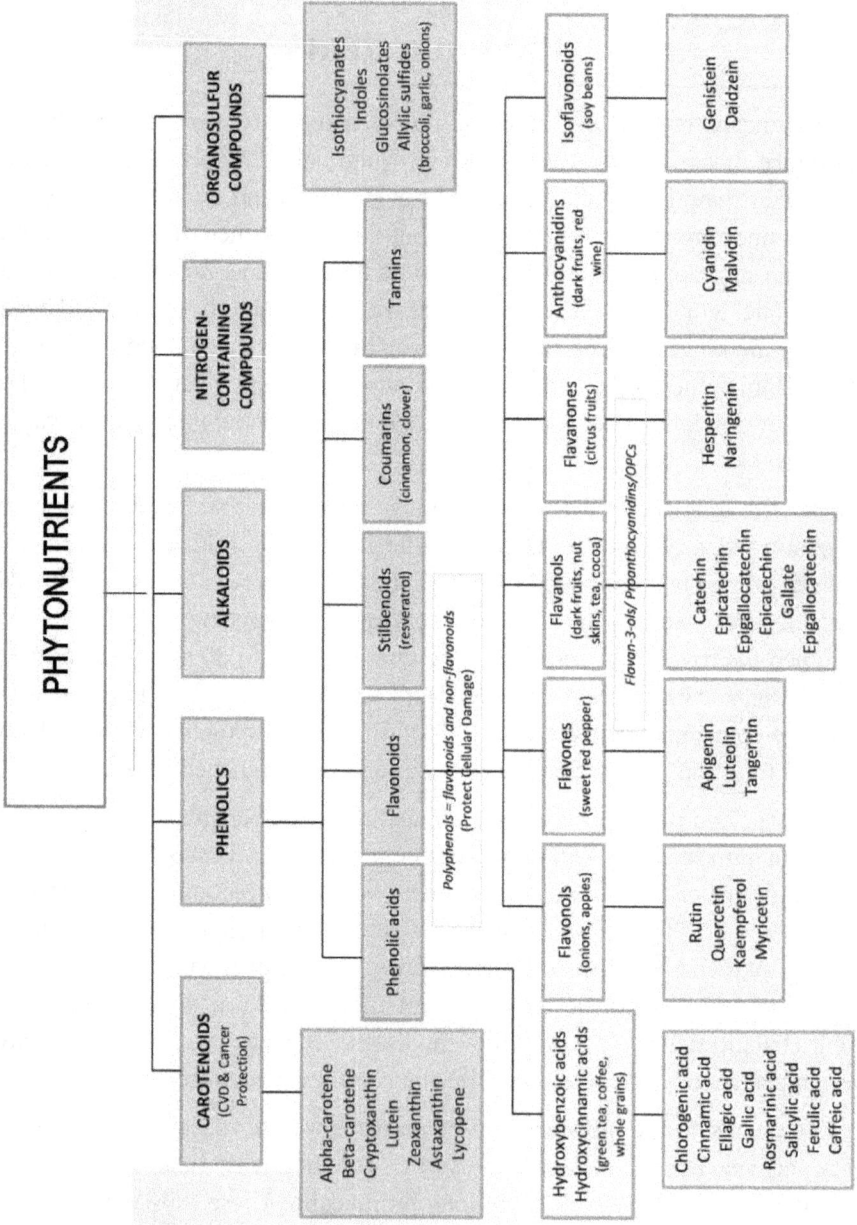

Figure 6.1 The five phytonutrients groups and their associated derivative compounds

Also called "phytochemicals," "designer foods," "medicinal foods," "neutra-ceutical foods," "physiologically functional foods" and "pharma foods," phyto-chemicals are not nutrients, at least so far as we know, but are organic compounds that have a tremendous influence in the biochemical and physiological processes that take place in our bodies. We will talk about the specific compounds and their functions in our bodies later, but for now let me give you some general comments.

One, as mentioned, phytochemicals are not nutrients and are not converted into tissues or used up as fuel by the body. There are no known deficiency symp-toms associated with them if we stop taking them, although, as you'll see later, opportunistic disease may take over in their absence. From research that has been conducted around the world, phytochemicals play crucial roles in our bodies. These range from minimizing the incidence of cancer and heart diseases to improving with conditions that come with aging, such as arthritis, inflammation of the joints and loss of memory and concentration, to the slowing of the aging of the body itself.

Two, although potentially there can be found millions of phytochemicals in plants, the ones that are known so far number only several thousands. James Duke in his book, Handbook of Phytochemical Constituents of GRAS Herbs and Other Economic Plants, has cataloged 3,000 phytochemicals extracted from 1,000 plants. Depending on the effect they have on the body, these compounds can be either GRAF (generally regarded as food), GRAS (generally regarded as safe) or GRAP (generally regarded as poisons or medicinal.)

Three, phytochemicals are found scattered throughout the plant kingdom. But some plants, fruits or vegetables may have a higher concentration of one kind of phytochemical than another. This variation in the phytochemical constituents of plants is the reason for the recommendation to consume a wide variety of fruits and vegetables, which you can now consume as a Four Pillars drink.

Four, the phytochemicals discovered so far function by serving as antioxidants, helpers of other antioxidants (such as vitamins A, C and E) and by blocking or interfering with processes that lead to disease conditions in our bodies. All these happen at a biochemical and physiological level, and hence the impact they have on our health can be profound.

Finally, phytochemicals are not always single compounds. There can be many variations of the same compound[12] or substance, and for this reason, it's often suggested that we eat whole foods as opposed to relying on supplements that contain only the active principle of these compounds. Of course, supplements when available and are of good formulation can sometimes serve as nice stand-ins for some of these phytochemicals found in these foods.

Phytochemical samplers: their food sources and benefits

To understand and appreciate the importance of phytochemicals, we need to begin with the amazing world of cellular operations. It's what happens in the cells that determine who we are as humans: young, middle-aged, old, sick or healthy. As you know, the cell is the fundamental unit that when duplicated (sort of) 60 trillion times forms the human body.

Hence, if we understand what goes on in a cell, we can pretty much understand what goes on in the rest of the human body. To illustrate this point and how phyto-chemicals play a role in our health, wellness and longevity we'll need to understand what an ordinary day is like in the life of a cell.

An ordinary day in the life of a cell, assuming you have properly nourished it, involves the conversion of food molecules into energy, body tissues or thousands of other substances that take part in the operation of the cell and the rest of the body. During these processes, there can also be many agents that interfere with or hinder the normal operations of the cell, including threatening its very existence.

Hence, part of a cell's daily task is housekeeping or maintaining order so that it can function continuously and comfortably. But how does the cell manage its house maintenance job, and what specifically are the agents that can damage the cell or disrupt its operation? How does the food we eat, particularly fruits and vegetables give us protection against those substances or agents that threaten the life of the cell and the rest of the human body? Let's answer each of these questions.

Some of the agents or substances that can be deleterious to the cell can come along with the water, air and food we consume. Considering the level of pollution in our environment, the different chemicals that are added to foods as preserva-tives, coloring or bulking agents and fruits and vegetables that are often treated with pesticides, herbicides and other chemicals, it comes as no surprise that bodies are at constant threat from these various elements. Internally, just the normal metabolism (the process of food utilization by the body) and everyday stress can

---

12   For example, beta carotene comes in six different versions. Similarly, Vitamin E has six forms. So, eating foods that contain all these different forms of the vitamins is now believed to have greater benefits than just one or two of the active components.

also produce substances that can be toxic or damaging to the body. Many these, as discussed in Appendix A are free radicals.

Scientists have discovered that free radicals and many of the extraneous substances that we get from outside sources can lead to degenerative diseases such as cancer, cardiovascular diseases, diabetes, Alzheimer's, and other illnesses that afflict us in this country.

Fruits, vegetables, grains, nuts and seeds can give us protection because they contain phytochemicals that interfere with or block certain processes that may lead to diseases. They do this either by serving as antioxidants to free radicals, by inhibiting certain enzymes that facilitate the formation of diseases such as cancer or by whisking out of the cell those chemicals or substances that are going to be deleterious to our body. Almost all of these substances, as you'll see below, are found in the dark green, yellow, red, orange or blue variety of the vegetables and fruits. Let's see what these foods are, what substances they contain and how they function in our bodies.

Berries, citrus fruits, cherries, grapes and grape seeds. This group of vegetables is a great source of a class of water-soluble phytochemicals called phenols, of which phenolic acids, flavonoids, stilbenoids, coumarins, and tannins are members. Of these group flavonoids are the most studied. Important contributors to the vivid colors we see in fruits, vegetables and flowers, in your body, these compounds may likewise bring you vibrant health, good looks and longevity. Let's see how and why.

One, flavonoids (aka bioflavonoids) are sometimes referred to as vitamin P. They serve as helpers of Vitamin C and as important contributors to the health, function and integrity of the capillaries (the smallest of blood vessels). Because it's these tiny tubes that ultimately deliver nutrients and oxygen to all the cells of the body, you can see the significance of these phytonutrients to the health and appearance of your body. This can range from the smoothness and elasticity of your skin to improved circulation, greater resistance to bruising to enhanced memory and visual acuity. In fact, the "P" in the vitamin name stands for permeability factor, because, bioflavonoids enhance the transference of nutrients across the blood vessels to the various cells in the body.

Two, as co-workers of vitamin C, flavonoids contribute to the health and function of the body wherever Vitamin C is involved. This benefit varies from the neutralization of free radicals to building and strengthening of the collagen matrix of your skin, gums and bones to helping alleviate cold and flu symptoms. Those who suffer from asthma, allergies, arthritis and bursitis may also benefit from bioflavonoids.

Three, because they can function as antioxidants and also help recycle vitamin at may have been destroyed by free radicals, bioflavonoids may help protect body against cancer, heart diseases, reduced memory and other degenerative conditions.

There are reportedly over 20,000 bioflavonoids registered in Chemical Abstracts, but a few well-studied ones that you may want to be familiar with include hesperidin, rutin, quercetin, pycnagenol and catechin. Hence, for example, catechin helps reduce histamine release and hence helps with those people who have allergic reactions; quercetin can help with inflammatory responses such as those experienced by people who have arthritis or suffer from injury, bursitis and asthma, and rutin is important in maintaining the health and integrity of the capillaries, veins and arteries.

But bear in mind that for maximum benefit, it's import to have all the bioflavonoids together instead of the individual compounds. This means that as much as possible you need to consume whole foods instead of relying on supplements. Again, supplements can sometimes be good concentrated sources of some of the compounds as well serve as stand-ins for some nutritional inequities.

Finally, remember that there are many other sources of bioflavonoids, including buckwheat, rose hips, apricots, black currants, plums and papayas. Broccoli, yams, cucumbers, green pepper, tomatoes, red and yellow onions and apples also contain a fair amount of these phytochemicals.

Broccoli. This dark green vegetable is a storehouse of many nutrients including of course, phytochemicals. One of the most known anticancer vegetables, broccoli contains a well-studied, antitumor compound called sulforaphane. The power of this phytochemical comes from its ability to promote the formation and function of a group of enzymes called phase I1 enzymes. These enzymes are responsible for processing and removing carcinogenic substances from our cells.

In one study, rats were divided into two groups. Twenty-five of them were a cancer-causing compound called DMBA, 29 of them were given both DMBA and high or low doses of sulforaphane. Of those that received just the DMBA, 68% got breast cancer. However, of those that took the low dosage and the compound, only 35% got tumors. Of those that took higher doses along with the compound, only 26% got cancer. Although study has not been done on humans, the addition of sulforaphane to human cells grown in petri dishes showed an increased synthesis of the anticancer or phase I1 enzymes. Brussels sprouts, cauliflower, collard greens and kale are other vegetables that contain sulforaphane.

Cabbage. Like broccoli, this vegetable contains many nutrients and exciting phytochemicals that have been found to possess a number of benefits for the body. Some of these compounds are called isothiocyanates and indoles. Isothiocyanates function by inhibiting the production and activity of the "bad" group of proteins called phase I enzymes. These enzymes have a special knack of converting the benign, even beneficial compounds into carcinogens. Isothiocyanates simply snarl the enzyme, thereby minimizing the formation of cancer-causing compounds in the body.

Isothiocyanates reportedly can also increase the activity of the phase II enzymes mentioned above, thus giving the compounds dual roles. In doing so, this crinkly coleslaw- and sauerkraut-maker can prevent esophageal, stomach, colon, liver and lung cancers. Also found in watercress, in one animal study, isothiocyanates reduced the risk of developing lung cancer by half when the animals were exposed to carcinogenic chemicals such as those found in cigarette smoke.

Breast and prostate cancers are believed to be a result of higher production of harmful versions of the estrogen and testosterone sex hormones. The indoles in cabbage and other cruciferous vegetables (such as broccoli, cauliflower, turnips, Brussels sprouts) promote the activity of the enzymes that break down these harmful substances and thus minimize the incidence of the gender-related cancers.

Celery. This fibrous, rib-like green has not attained the status or respect of the other vegetables like broccoli, cabbage and cauliflower. Yes, you have heard about its importance as a fiber source and as an ingredient in certain soups, chicken and other meat dishes, but celery contains phytochemicals that can be of a benefit to you. One of these phytonutrients is 3-n-butyl phthalid. This compound functions as a calming or sedative agent to the nervous system and also has a capacity to reduce blood pressure, through regulation of hormones that induce the condition.

For its healthful benefits, always consume fresh celery and avoid or discard any old or wilted celery that is more than 3 weeks old. This is because cancer-causing substances called furocumarins, found only in tiny amounts in the fresh celery, can significantly increase as the stored celery ages.

Onions, garlic and peppers. These three vegetables contain specific compounds or plant chemicals that make them such important dietary components. Onions, are rich in bioflavonoids and reportedly contain as many as 50 of these and other phytonutrients. Allylic sulfides (sulfur-containing compounds) are the predominant ones, and these compounds serve as cancer fighters in the body. For instance, researchers in China have shown that high onion consumption was attributable to a 40% reduction in the incidence of stomach cancer in one region of that country.

Garlic contains, among many compounds, a phytochemical known as diallylsulphide. It is this substance and others in this smelly, bulbous clove that block carcinogens from getting into the cells and inhibit those cells that have become malignant from growing further. The garlic compounds are also known to reduce cholesterol and blood pressure, improve circulation and strengthen the immune system.

Red pepper has similar benefits. The capsaicin compound, which gives peppers their hot characteristics, may help kill bacteria, neutralize the carcinogen chemicals such as nitrosamines and reduce the bad cholesterol and triglyceride levels in the body This substance is also known to relieve muscular pain and elevate moods by releasing brain chemicals called endorphins.

Soybeans. For a long time, scientists couldn't figure out why there is less incidence of cancers including breast cancer, in Japan and other Oriental countries than in the West. Now the mystery seems to have been solved: it's because of the phytonutrients found in soy called genistein, daidzein and saponins. These compounds are effective in preventing the early development and spread of cancerous cells by blocking their food supply line.

When cancer cells grow and migrate to other parts of the body, they need new capillaries to bring them food. Genistein block the formation of the tiny blood vessels. For women, because genistein is similar to estradiol, one of the estrogen hormones, a known breast cancer promoter, the phytochemical blocks the formation of cancer by blocking the cell receptors in the mechanism of cancer initiation and formation. Saponins block cholesterol-absorbing sites in the intestine and hence help reduce cholesterol levels in the body To obtain the beneficial effect of these compounds consume more soybeans and soy products such as to&, soy milk, tempeh and tamari.

Teas. The most common active constituents of the humble green and black teas are tannins, catechins and theobromine. While theobromine acts as a central nervous system stimulant, the tannins and catechins primarily function as antioxidants in the body.

In terms of their overall effectiveness, the green teas, which are less processed than the black teas, may be more beneficial. In fact, this point has been postulated as the reason why there is a lower incidence of cancer and heart disease in a certain section of Japan where a large quantity of green tea is consumed than in those areas where less of it is consumed. In one animal study, catechins in green tea were shown to lower cholesterol and blood pressure and inhibit esophageal and gastrointestinal cancers. Catechins may also strengthen the immune system.

Besides serving as an antioxidant, tannic acid can help fight tooth decay. This phytochemical is lethal to the plaque-forming bacteria. In one experiment, when tannic extracts were added to saliva-coated tooth enamel, 85% of the cavity-forming bacteria were destroyed.

Tomatoes. Carotenoids are a group of related compounds that have remarkable benefits to the human body. Found in almost all the red, yellow, orange and green vegetables, carotenoids are associated with the reduction of all types of cancers.

Carotenoids work as antioxidants, protecting the cells against the damaging effect of free radicals. If these marauding chemicals are not put in check, they can shatter the DNA molecule in your cells and the protein matrix in your skin and other tissues in your body. When the DNA is damaged the cell loses control of its own growth and division, and becomes cancerous. A diet low in antioxidants may increase your cancer risk and heart disease.

The carotenoids are found in the red, orange and yellow and dark green of the fruit, vegetable and flowers. These include the alpha and beta carotene, lycopene, lutein and zeaxanthine, representatives of the more than 600 similar compounds found in these foods.

The alpha and beta carotene are known as the pro-Vitamin A because when processed in the liver, provide the biologically active form of Vitamin A, which as described earlier, is important for the health and proper functioning of the body.

Here are a few examples what the carotenoids can do for you. They support and enhance the function of the immune system, thus reducing viral infections and your chance of catching colds and flus and your cells from becoming cancerous. They do this by making your natural antibodies respond efficiently to antigens, invading molecules from outside or modified and harmful substances from within the body. They support the production of "Natural Killer Cells", a type of white blood cells which have the ability to recognize and destroy cancer cells.

As we mentioned in the Vitamin chapters, Vitamin A along with the rest of the carotenoid members keep the linings of your digestive tract—from the mouth to the intestines and the respiratory pathways—from nose to sinuses to trachea and lungs—healthy and properly functioning. These linings are primary target to food, fluid and air-borne bacteria and viruses.

The carotenoids also are important for the formation, growth and cohesiveness of your cells. When these normal processes are disrupted there is a greater risk that they will turn cancerous. These compounds are important for good night vision, the health of the reproductive organs and for the formation of strong bones.

Lycopene, the other well-studied carotenoid, found largely in tomatoes, is an important protector of the cell membrane and LDL cholesterol and triglycerides in the blood from free radical attack. This means this compound can help reduce the risk of heart diseases, cancer, cataract formation and other degenerative conditions. For example, researchers in North Italy found that people who ate more servings of raw tomatoes every week, had a 60% less chance of developing cancer of the stomach, colon and rectum than those who consumed fewer servings of the vegetable.

And unlike most vitamins, lycopene reportedly survives cooking and processing, so you are more likely to find lycopene in pasta sauce, ketchup, tomato juice and pizza. Other sources of lycopene are pink and red grape fruit, watermelon, guava and sweet red peppers.

P-coumaric and chlorogenic acids are some of the other compounds found in tomatoes. They too are effective in fighting the formation of cancer-causing substances in the body. Also found in pineapple, green pepper, strawberries and carrots, p-coumaric and chlorogenic acids are powerful in disabling the formation of carcinogenic substances called nitrosamines. These noxious compounds are formed when nitrates often used as food preservatives and the proteins from our diet interact in the digestive tract.

All the red, yellow, orange and dark green fruits, vegetables and herbs are rich in carotenoids. They contain the alpha and beta carotene, lutein, lycopene and zeaxanthine—just to name a few. When these foods are blended together and consumed, they become the four pillars on which your health, wellness and longevity stand.

In summary, as you can see from the above examples, mothers were indeed right for demanding that we eat our vegetables when we were little. Daniel of the Bible and Hippocrates were astute observers about the benefit of foods, particularly those of plant or vegetable origin. To be the beneficiaries of their advice, we need to regularly consume our vegetables, fruits, grains and seeds. These foods may help fend off cancers, keep our blood vessels clean and our minds sharp, improve the appearance of our skin and provide us with a vibrant and dynamic health to the very end.

For a list of various colored fruits and vegetables, their phytonutrient content and benefit to human health, please go to Part IV, The Four Pillars Recipes.

The healing comes from nature
and not from the physician.

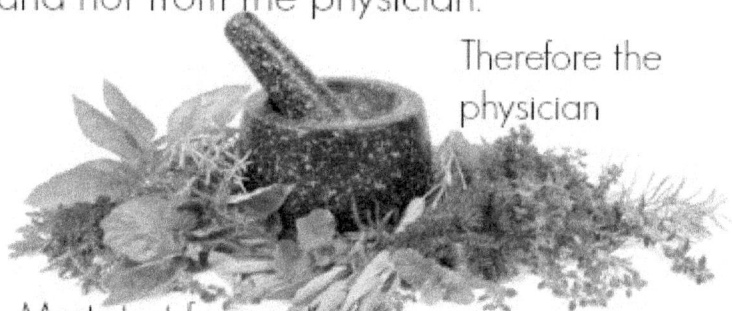

Therefore the
physician

Must start from nature
with an open mind

~ Paracelsus ~

PART III
The World of Herbs and Spices

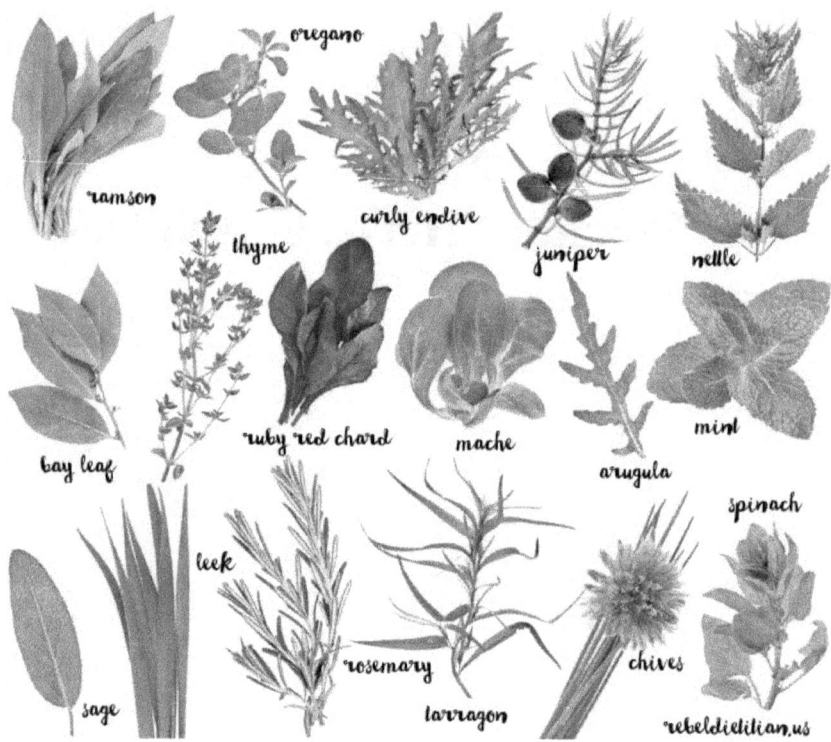

ramson
oregano
curly endive
juniper
nettle
thyme
bay leaf
ruby red chard
mache
mint
arugula
leek
spinach
sage
rosemary
tarragon
chives
rebeldietitian.us

The World of Herbs

CHAPTER 10
The World of Herbs

To most Americans, and for that matter most people in the western world, herbs or the use of herbs has been as alien as the use of vitamin and mineral supplements have been. In fact, if you randomly ask people in this country about the value of herbs to the human body, most of them will probably draw a blank. Just as with vitamin and mineral supplements, though, the use and application of herbs in this country has been rapidly changing. This is so primarily because people are finding that the best way to care for the body is not through drugs or synthetic chemicals but rather through proper nutrition and other natural means, such as homeopathy, herbs and spices.

Some or all of these practices, as John Lust, author of *The Herb Book*, puts it, are in "harmony with life" as opposed to being against it, which often can be the case with the synthetic drugs.

What are Herbs?

The answer to this question can depend on how you perceive herbs. If you are tea drinker, you may be thinking of the different herbal teas now available in grocery stores. If you have a particular affinity for greens and spices, you may be thinking of the variety of fresh herbs or spices (parsley, sweet basil, etc.) that you can buy in the produce section of your supermarket. Gardeners and forest rangers may have their definition or perception of herbs. To them, herbs may mean those soft stalked plants or weeds that grow near the ground and die after they have flowered or completed their life cycle.

To herbalists, the term herb applies to those plants or parts of plants (such as roots, barks, leaves, flowers or seeds) that can be used to enhance, support and vitalize the human body. In this book only this last definition or interpretation will be used. Before, we discuss the many great attributes of herbs and their significance in our lives, let's first take a brief look at the historical background of these plants and their overall characteristics.

As you may well be aware, the use or application of herbs is not new. Herbs have been part of human societies for over 5,000 years. The oldest herbal book found in China dates back to 2700 B.C. This book documents some 365 plants and their beneficial properties. The Babylonians, Africans, Romans and Greeks as well as American Indians depended on herbs for all kinds of home remedies and treatments. In Europe, herb gardens were common at monasteries and in private homes in earlier centuries.

According to the World Health Organization, some 80% of the world's population still relies on traditional medicines and remedies. Aside from uses in witchcraft, prayer, sorcery and psychic healing, herbs and plant extracts account for a very significant part of those remedies. Practically all the medicines of earlier eras were obtained or derived from plants. Even now, the active ingredients in a quarter of the pharmaceutical drugs come from plants.

Regarding their overall characteristics, herbs require you to remember a few rules of thumb. One, the quality and potency of the herb will depend on where the herb was grown, when it was harvested (seasonally speaking), what part of the plant was used (leaves, flowers, roots or bark) and how the herb was dried, processed and packaged.

As to regional or geographical variations, herbs grown in mountainous areas can have certain specific qualities or properties compared to those grown in the lowlands; those herbs grown near water or in warmer climates can still have other qualities or properties. Quantitatively speaking, plants grown in fertile or nutrient-rich soils can have a higher concentration of the active ingredients than those grown in poor soils or harsher climatic conditions.

As mentioned, seasons can also affect the distribution and concentration of the active ingredient in the plant. This is to say that in spring the active constituent of the herb may be in the young leaves and buds, in the summer it may be in the fruits and flowers and in the fall and winter it may be in the roots and barks.

The quality of the herb can likewise vary depending on whether rootlets, twigs or leaves are used, or whether the herb has been adulterated with excipients of other plants. Sometimes age can be a factor, too. If the plant is old or too young, the quality and the quantity of the active ingredients may be low. As with vitamins and minerals, how the herbs are processed or extracted can determine the quality or potency of the herb. (For more information on this, see the reference given at the end of the book.) However, bear in mind that fresh herbs are often the most potent.

Two, with herbs you should not expect results on the first use or application. You have to give herbs time. Of course, there can always be an exception to this rule.

Herbs' Function in the body

The list of herbs or plants to aid and strengthen the function of the body is long growing. Of the some 250,000 plants discovered so far, less than 1% are currently used for a variety of health and wellness-enhancing purposes. Those plants employed for such purposes range from the tonics—herbs that improve the overall function of the body—to those herbs that enhance the functions of individual organs and tissues.

Thus, the tonics are generally for people who want or need energy and vitality. The herbs used for this purpose are seaweed (such as kelp), Irish moss, alfalfa, comfrey, dandelion leaves, burdock, parsley, goldenseal root, ginseng, milk thistle and others. The herbs used for specific tissues, organs or body states (such as appetite, fluid balance, constipation) are equally varied.

Unfortunately, neither space nor point of emphasis permits us to list all these herbs and their benefits to the body. For more information on the different herbs and plants used for a variety of purposes, refer to some of the herb books listed in bibliography or search the Internet. What you need to bear in mind, is that all herbs (including spices) vegetables as well as other plants can have some benefits to the human body. Knowing the specific attributes of each herb, spice or plant can make you appreciate or value these wonderful natural gifts.

In summary, regardless of how you perceive or use herbs—as condiments you add to your favorite dishes or as substances you infuse to tea or as trouble-some weeds in your yard or garden—from what we have said so far, herbs can have many important and healthful benefits indeed. You may also be one of those people who think of herbs as folklorish and therefore doubt their significance to the human body. Think again.

One, herbs have been used by many societies for thousands of years. This means, even though now we also have much scientific data that support their historical functions or benefits, even if we didn't, these plant extracts have been in experiment in many cultures much longer than drugs and vitamins and minerals have. They have a track record, a richer heritage than these substances.

Two, many of the drugs used today have their roots in plants, but from what we said earlier, the whole plant or herb can have greater benefit to the body than one or two components of the herb or plant. Most drugs contain just one active ingredient and can be tolerated by the body within limited ranges. Drugs are used to treat a disease or a symptom-as a quick fix or a mending device. Herbs, on the other hand, are used to support the function of an organ or the entire body.

Herbal Preparations and Application Methods

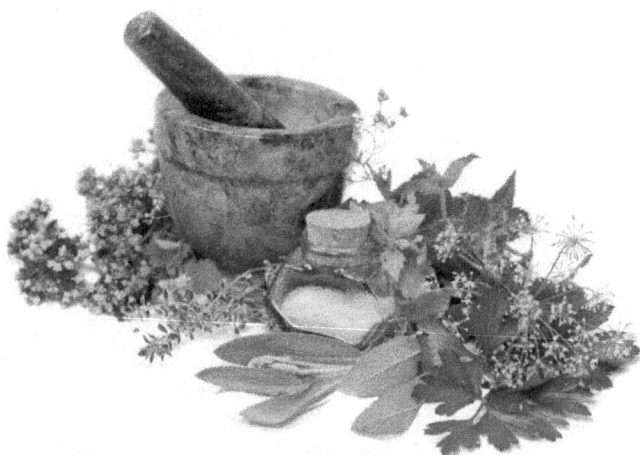

Depending on their applications, herbs can be prepared in several ways. The traditional method has been to make any one of the following preparations using the end product for a given application.

Infusion. This method of extraction involves steeping the plant part (such as leaves or flowers) in hot water, just as you would steep tea, for a certain period of time (10 to 20 minutes is usually enough) to let the active ingredients and other substances such as vitamins and minerals release into the water. The amount of liquid and plant part used will depend on the concentration of the active ingredient you are trying to attain—usually 1/2 to 1 ounce of the plant part is used per pint of water. After the necessary allotted time, strain the fluid and drink or use for whatever external applications the herb is recommended. In the event the infused end product is bitter, you may add honey or sugar to make it palatable.

Regardless of what you're using the herb for, remember not to expect a result from one application. You may need to continue to use it for a certain period of time. Employ a porcelain or nonmetallic pot or cup to make the infusion.

Decoction. This method of extraction is often for a plant's hard parts, such as the roots, bark or stems and in a situation where your goal is to remove the plant's active ingredients and mineral salts (instead of vitamins and volatile oils). Depending on the hardness of the raw material you work with, in this method of preparation, you simmer (not boil) the plant parts anywhere from 3 minutes to 30 minutes. The amount of water used can vary from a cup of water to a cup and a quarter, the latter amount being used when the herb is simmered for 30 minutes.

Tincture. For potent herbs and when the goal is to use a very concentrated form of the active ingredient, you use tincture as your technique of extraction. In this technique, you add 1 to 4 ounces of powdered herb into a 50% alcohol solution and let it sit for two weeks. You shake it once or twice a day for the duration of the extraction. After this time, you strain or press out to yield the tincture. Tinctures are good for herbs that have a bad taste, for herbs you want to use as an ointment or when the herb is to be used for a long period of time. The alcohol solution serves to preserve the extract.

Extraction. Liquid extracts are a form of tincture but more concentrated than tinctures. They are usually obtained by removing some of the alcohol using low temperature and a vacuum distillation technique. When you remove the fluid completely, you're left with a thick paste-like residue known as solid extract. This residue can be dried and granulated or powdered to be used for a variety of applications. As you can imagine, a solid extraction method can give you a highly concentrated form of the active ingredient. If necessary, this exact can be made into a pill. Solid extraction can give you a much longer shelf than any of the other forms of preparation.

Besides the methods of extraction described above, sometimes whole herbs can be dried and ground into a powder. At other times, honey or brown sugar can be added to a liquid containing the raw herb and boiled together until the right consistency is reached. Freshly cut herbs can also be pressed or processed through a juicer.

Freeze-drying is the other technique often used with herbs. In this process, you freeze the whole herb and then under a very low pressure and high vacuum remove the water (or rather the ice) naturally found in the herb by sublimation— the transformation of ice into vapor. Freeze-drying is probably better than any of the other techniques because there may be less degradation or loss of potency of the active constituents.

As indicated above, the extracted herb can be used for a variety of applications.

You can make salve or poultice—a thick paste prepared by mixing the extract with a carrier medium such as flour, corn meal, milk or water to be applied on a wound or cut. Sometimes, you may also use herbal preparations as laxatives, ointments and liniments as well as emetics.

From the above brief introduction on herbs, you might by now wonder how can one be assured of potency of an herbal product—particularly given the potential difference in the quality of the herbs used as well as in the processing or manufacturing technique. In other words, knowing that herbs are not regulated the way drugs or medicines are, how can you be assured that you're getting what the manufactures says you're getting on its label of an herbal product?

Quantification and Standardization of Herbal Extracts

It's true that in the past, since the active ingredients were not known, it was difficult to precisely know what is contained in an herbal concoction. Now, besides the following common practices, we also have many sophisticated techniques to identify and quantify an herbal active ingredient.

The usual method of quantifying an herbal extract is using concentration ratios. For instance, a 4:1 concentration means 1 part of the solid extract is derived from 4 parts of the crude herb. A tincture is usually given in 1:10 or 1:5 concentration ratio, while liquid extract is expressed as a 1:1 ratio. These ratios can also be expressed in terms of grams or ounces. Hence, one gram of 3:1 extract is derived from 3 grams of the starting raw or crude herb.

If you're interested in the weight of the active ingredient, concentration ratios are not very useful because they can contain, besides the active ingredient, hundreds of other compounds, many of which may not be useful. But in some cases, these extraneous compounds may help the principal substance function better in the body. Nevertheless, in the past, accurately assessing or quantifying the active principle in an herbal extract was difficult.

Now, however, because of new tools and techniques of measurement, it's very easy to determine the active ingredients and measure their amounts. The most common techniques used are high pressure liquid chromatography (HPLC) and thin layer chromatography (TLC). By using these analytical tools, we can determine the amount of active ingredient in an herbal preparation and express this value in terms of grams or ounces. In other words, with these new techniques, we no longer have to talk about crude extract weights or concentration ratios. We'll have a more precise and standardized method of assessing herbal extracts. Thus, for instance, allicin is one of the many beneficial compounds found in garlic. Using the tools and techniques just mentioned, we now can give the amount of this compound in grams or ounces. This method of disclosure will enable us to know precisely how much of the useful ingredient we're ingesting.

CHAPTER 11
Herbal Samplers

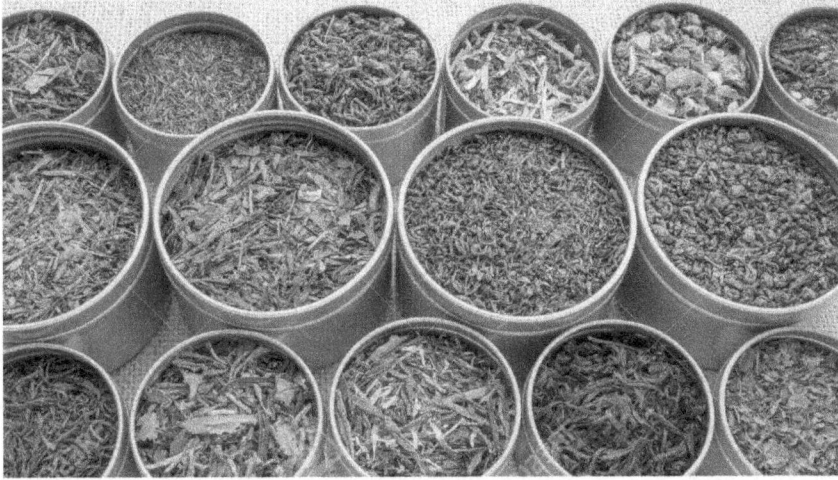

As we indicated in the previous chapter, the kinds of plants or herbal extracts that can contribute to human health are many and cannot be covered in just two or three chapters. However, the following information on some of the most prominent herbs, widely used spices and herbal teas may be of benefit to you.

Astragulus. Steeped in Chinese tradition as an immune stimulant and for a number of other purposes, astragulus is finding similar uses in Western societies.

Researchers here in the U.S. have confirmed these particular attributes of the herb. The active ingredients come from the root extract—usually prepared by decoction (simmering the root in water at low heat for a protracted time). Besides having a role as an immune stimulant (it helps increase the production of T-cells, the white blood cells of the body that attack foreign substances or invaders), astragulus may benefit the proper function of the heart and respiratory system. This herb also has adaptogen properties and thus helps prolong the function and life of the cells in the body by making them withstand extremes of physiological conditions.

The principal components of the herb include a polysaccharide known as astragalan B, a bioflavonoid and choline. Like most herbal products, the benefit of some of these active ingredients may not be immediate. For this reason, you may have to take the herb for several weeks before you see any significant effect. As we said earlier, there can always be an exception to this rule of thumb. Some people have reported seeing results within a few days of taking herbal products.

Baptisia Extract. This native American plant goes by various names, some of which are wild indigo, American indigo, horsefly weed and indigo broom. Baptisia is a multi-branched perennial plant that produces gray green leaves and yellow flowers.

The whole plant as well as the root bark can be used for many of this plant's beneficial properties. Although it has sometimes been used for a variety of external applications, it has also useful for many internal purposes. These include its use as a stimulant, emetic or purgative and to enhance the function of the immune system.

Bilberry. Also called huckleberry or blueberry, bilberry is a shrubby perennial plant that is found wild in parts of Northern United States and in the woods and forests of Europe. For more information about other berries, read the chapter on phytonutrients.

Now also cultivated, Bilberry has reddish bell-shaped flowers that turn into blue-black fruit on maturity.

The most important chemical components of bilberry are the bioflavonoids, particularly the anthocyanosides. As you can see below, anthocyanosides have been found to have beneficial properties in the body. These range from increasing the production of collagen and maintenance of its structural integrity to serving as antioxidants. Since collagen is the most abundant protein in the body and is the fabric that holds our skin, bones, blood vessels and other tissues and organs together, you can see that anything that helps with the health and function of collagen is also going to help with the overall health and structural integrity of the body.

More specifically, anthocyanosides maintain the health and function of the arteries, and capillaries, fortify the brain from toxic substances by strengthening the blood-brain barrier and by serving as antioxidant. In the circulatory system they help disperse clot-forming platelets thus minimizing heart attack and stroke.

Since they function as an antioxidant and promote the health of protein fibers, anthocyanosides can help prevent or treat glaucoma, reduce peripheral vision loss and improve night time visual acuity. Anthocyanosides are also known to help ease the effects of stress, improve memory, alleviate joint inflammation and enhance flexibility.

Because it helps lower blood sugar level and improve capillary fragility, the bill-berry extract can also be important for those who suffer from diabetes. Reportedly, anthocyanosides are also effective in reducing cholesterol and triglycerides in the blood.

There are many other benefits of anthocyanosides but, just from the above description alone, you can see that blue-black fruit, of bilberry is an important food. To take advantage of this important fruit make sure to include it in all your Four Pillars drinks.

Burdock. This wide and long-leaved plant is used primarily as a blood purifier, but herbalists have also used it for a variety of applications, ranging from its use for coughs, colds and sore throats to help in healing stomach ailments to neutralization and removal of poisons and waste matter from the body. The herb does this by acting as a diuretic and diaphoretic (as a substance that increases perspiration). The herb can also restore the liver, kidneys and gallbladder to their normal operations during illness. This property of the herb is what classifies it as an "alterative," meaning that it helps alter or restore the body during illness.

In the literature, even antibiotic, antifungal and antitumor benefits have been mentioned of the herb. When applied externally, burdock can also be used to treat scrofuloderma (tuberculosis of the skin) and venereal eruptions, and other skin conditions, including those that are cancerous. The seeds, roots and leaves can be used for many of the herb's beneficial properties.

Chicory. This scruffy European native is often cultivated and found in the wild. Now it's also grown in the United States. Chicory has bright, iridescent flowers and yellow root bark with white stalk that contains milky juice.

Chicory is a tonic herb but also has specific functions to organs and tissues of the body. It helps stimulate the production of bile in the liver as well as serve as a cleanser to the liver and the spleen. It may assist with nausea or stomach disorders and help heal skin that is affected by such things as insect bite, sunburn or rash.

This interesting herb is good for the kidneys as it decreases uric acid level (hence minimizing gallstones) from the body, increases urine flow and helps eliminate excessive mucus in the digestive tract. Chicory is often recommended with people who have jaundice and for those with spleen disorder.

Comfrey. Comfrey is one of those herbs whose use by humans goes far back in time. Ancient Greeks, Native Americans as well as other societies used comfrey to treat many internal and external bodily problems.

Externally, comfrey's power comes from is ability to heal wounds, bruises, sores, fractures, broken bones and insect bites. Burns, ulcers, sprains swellings and pimples can also be treated with comfrey. Allantoin, a compound found in comfrey is responsible for rapid cell proliferation and healing of any of these maladies. For this purpose, a poultice of the root or fresh leaves is applied over the affected surface to help it heal.

Internally, comfrey can be used to stop bleeding of gums and hemorrhaging, relieve congestion in the lungs and alleviate irritation and inflammation of the stomach, intestines, kidneys, urinary tract and the bladder. In short, any part of the body that is injured or bleeding can be helped by comfrey, so much so that comfrey is sometimes referred to as the knitter and healer herb.

Because of its high mucilage content (substances that swell without dissolving), comfrey root can also be an excellent demulcent—a liquid used to soothe inflamed surfaces and protect them from irritation. Additionally, in the digestive tract, comfrey promotes the production and secretion of pepsin, one of the enzymes that aid digest protein.

For any of the above applications you can make a decoction, infusion or tincture of the herb. Although the root is used for many of the comfrey's benefits, the leaves can also be used for a number of external treatments.

To make a decoction, simmer 6 teaspoons of ground comfrey root in 3 cups of water for 30 minutes, cool, strain and put in the refrigerate. Heat and take 2-3 teacups a day from this batch for any of the internal benefits mentioned above. To enhance taste, you may want to add six to eight spoons of honey to the initial batch.

Dong Quai. Dong quai is one of the most popular herbs in China and Japan and has been in use there since ancient times. It has primarily been used to help with the function of the female reproductive system, including its ability to maintain the proper amounts of the female hormones and regulate menses after child birth. Because it tends to cleanse and purify blood, dong quai is beneficial for the circulatory system. This herb also enhances the utilization of Vitamin E by the body.

Dunaliella Salina. As mentioned elsewhere in the book, beta-carotene, a Vitamin A is an important antioxidant that has many healthful properties. Beta-carotene is important for, among other things, healthy functioning of the immune system, the skin, the eyes and the mucous membranes. Dunaliella Salina happens to be one of the best sources of this important nutrient.

Echinacea. An indigene of North America, Echinacea has been used by both Native Americans and health-care professionals for many purposes. These range from elevating the production of immune cells to stimulating the generation of new tissues, particularly when applied externally on burns or wounds. Echinacea also has overall tonic properties that it enhances the function of the body as a whole. This great herb has many wonderful qualities, some of which have been documented by researchers both here and in Europe.

For starters, Echinacea can help boost the immune system, which is important for the health of the entire body. The herb does this by stimulating the production of T-cells (a type of white blood cell) and interferon (a group of protecting proteins) against viruses and bacteria. This amazing herb, which helps with the health of various tissues and glands, including the prostate gland is also an effective blood cleanser. Echinacea can help remove toxins from the body, enhance digestion and reduce the problem of gas in the digestive tract.

Echinacea has thick hairy leaves and large, pale purple flowers. It's the root, however, that has been used for a variety of its healthful benefits. A root extract usually contains a host of compounds, but the predominant ones are inulin[13], glucose, fructose, betaine, echinacin, and echinacoside.

Whether you use it for a specific purpose or to aid in the overall function of the body, Echinacea is one of those herbs that you can appreciate having as part of your daily good nutritional program.

Fennel. Fennel is one of the common herbs you find in the product aisle of your supermarket. It has a round light greenish bulb, stout stems and hair-like green leaves. A perennial plant, fennel can have very wide uses or applications in the body. It helps eliminate gas and aids with the proper function of the digestive tract. It helps relieve congestion in the chest and throat and assists with the production and flow of milk in nursing mothers.

---

13   a type of carbohydrate

Fennel seeds contain a special type of oil that also can help with weight loss and weight management. In addition, this interesting herb can also be an effective liver and gallbladder cleanser. Because of its ability to dissolve uric acid crystals, fennel may also help eliminate gout. Its high Vitamin A content can also help with night of time vision and prevent snow blindness. Fiber, antioxidant phytochemicals and iron are fennel's other assets.

Garcinia Cambogia. Garcinia cambogia, also known as brindall berries or mangosteen, is a fruit that customarily grows in India and Thailand. Its primary function in the body is to suppress the appetite so that you have less craving for food. This interesting herb also tends to increase the oxidation of fat (through thermo genesis) while slowing or limiting the conversion of carbohydrate into fat. In this instance, the body converts more glucose into glycogen and stores it in the liver muscles so that it can be used as fuel at times when you're low in energy. It's also reported that this herb may help with the health of the throat and the urinary tract.

The active ingredient in this herb is called hydroxycitric acid, and apparently it's this substance that blocks or inactivates the enzymes systems that are involved in fat synthesis and storage in the body. It is reported that 50% of the herb consists of hydroxycitric acid. This compound also blocks the formation of fatty tissues in the body, and with the proper exercise and nutritional program, such as the inclusion of metabolic enhancers such as chromium, L-carnitine and magnesium, one may be able to lose or maintain weight.

Ginkgo Biloba. So far as we currently know, no other life from earth has witnessed and survived the climatic and other vagaries of the world for 200 million years in its present form as ginkgo biloba. The average life span of the ginkgo tree may, however, range from only 1,000 to 3,000 years. Considering its antiquity, it is quite possible to think that dinosaurs may have once plucked its leaves or scratched their shoulders against the trunks of this giant tree. This amazing, tall and hardy tree once grew in many parts of the world, but now it's found only in China.

Although it bears fruit, only the leaves and the seeds are used by humans.

The ginkgo leaf extract has many chemical compounds, but the ones that have been extensively studied are the ginkgo-flavone glycosides, which you often see as 24% of the total compounds found in a ginkgo extract. The standardized ginkgo leaf extract (i.e., an extract that shows a 24% ginkgo-flavone glycosides content) has many important benefits to the human body.

Some of these include their serving as antioxidant or free radical scavengers and in enhancing the utilization of oxygen and glucose by brain cells. The specific antioxidant activity involves the neutralization of free radicals that attack lipids (fats) of cell membrane and other fats elsewhere in the body.

The brain cells, for instance, are largely made from unsaturated fatty acids; hence, ginkgo biloba extract may serve as an antioxidant for these cells and the rest of the nervous system. Because the ginkgo extract may serve to facilitate entry of glucose and oxygen into the cells, brain cells may get sufficient quantities of these important nutrients and hence are allowed to function better.

A ginkgo extract has also been found to enhance nerve impulse transmission due to the brain's improved synthesis and turnover of brain chemicals (or so-called neurotransmitters). It's reported that the circulatory system may also benefit by ginkgo extract, thus increasing blood flow to all tissues and organs of the body, which ultimately improve the health and nourishment of the body.

Like ginseng, ginkgo extracts have been used in China for thousands of years. And like ginseng (see below), its use in Western societies is relatively new. In Europe and Mexico, ginkgo extract is fairly popular and is being sold under various trade names: Tebonin (Europe and Mexico), Tanakan (France) and Rokan (Germany). As mentioned earlier, although there can be many different concentrations of the plant extract, the extract that contains 24% of the active ingredient (ginkgo-flavone glycosides) is the one that's of greater benefit.

Ginseng. As you may be aware, there are generally three different ginseng: American ginseng, Siberian ginseng and Korean/Chinese ginseng. The main difference among these different "nationalities" is their ginesnosides (the active chemical in ginseng) content. Since there are many different ginesnoside compounds, certain ones are more predominant in one kind than in the other and the value of the ginseng will depend on the concentration of one or a few of those compounds. Bear in mind that ginesing contains besides ginesnosides, many other substances, including vitamins and minerals that can be of benefit to you.

The most frequent concentration of ginsenosides found in ginseng varies from 1% to 3%. A ginseng extract that contains higher than these percentages means that extract is of the highest quality.

In terms of its benefits to the human body, ginseng is what is referred to as a "tonic" herb. Tonic herbs are those plants that enhance the overall performance and health of the human body. Be that as it may, in the Orient, ginseng has been used for many specific physiological or bodily functions. The following few examples illustrate some of those attributes of ginseng.

One, ginseng can help improve both mental and physical performance. This fact has been established with both human and animal studies. With this herb you're more likely to experience alertness, have enhanced memory and cope better under physically demanding situations such as exercise and athletic competition.

Ginseng may give you these benefits because of its ability to improve energy metabolism and spare glycogen (your body's stored fuel), particularly during prolonged exercise. This wonder herb may also help you deal better with fatigue and everyday stress . This is so because the herb enhances the health of the adrenal gland, which is responsible for the production of anti-stress hormones. These effects of the herb are observed after its continuous and daily usage.

In the elderly, ginseng increases cellular enzyme activity and hence helps important organs, such as the heart and the brain, function better. Many people around the world also believe ginseng to be the world's greatest aphrodisiac. Some scientists in Japan have linked this to the herb's stimulatory action on the sex hormones.

Two, when the body is properly nourished, ginseng can stimulate protein synthesis and cell proliferation.

Three, ginseng may help enhance the function of the immune system. This and all the other aspects of the herb may naturally help you build a strong and properly working body and mind.

This great herb can also be good for the digestive and circulatory systems and, as mentioned, enhance the function of the male reproductive system. In addition, ginseng may function as an antioxidant, thus helping slow down the aging process. Ginseng has many other properties and benefits, the discussion of which are beyond the scope of this book.

Perhaps the best way to summarize ginseng's overall function in the body is to describe the herb in terms of its adaptogen properties. An adaptogen is a substance that maintains and normalizes the body function regardless of external or internal stresses. Adaptogens thus are substances that make the body adaptable in extreme situations by increasing its coping mechanisms.

Goldenseal. For a long time, some healthcare professionals in this country used goldenseal in an eye drop preparation, but now its use has been predominantly to help enhance the function of the immune system because of its antibiotic and antibacterial properties. This herb is particularly effective when used in combination with echinacea, the other immune system enhancing herb discussed earlier. Like echinacea, goldenseal has tonic properties and can be effective in treating wounds and infections. When used in combination with licorice, goldenseal can help lower blood sugar, which can be beneficial for those who suffer from diabetes.

Furthermore, goldenseal may help stimulate appetite and improve digestion because it tends to sensitize or stimulate the function of the secretory cells along the digestive tract. Goldenseal also can be used to enhance the function of the nasal and throat mucous membranes.

The major active compounds in goldenseal are berberine, hydrazine and canadine. It's these compounds that have many beneficial properties. The extraction or preparation is usually made from the root or bark of the plant.

Marigold. Also called calendula by the ancient Romans, who observed that the plant bloomed on the first day or "calends" of the month, marigold is used externally to treat skin conditions. This ranges from cuts, burns and bruises to wounds and skin irritations. Internally, marigold can be used to treat conditions of the stomach, colon and liver as well as the gum. Because it has soothing properties, it can be a good mouthwash.

Milk Thistle. Milk thistle is one of those incredible herbs whose list of benefits never seems to end. Nevertheless, the primary function of the herb appears to center around the health of the liver.

For starters, milk thistle is important in removing toxins and in helping relieve liver-related chronic disorders such as hepatitis and cirrhosis. This herb also helps rejuvenate and revitalize liver function, particularly after a long and damaging period of alcohol consumption. Because it is rich in bioflavonoids, milk thistle is also an excellent antioxidant, protecting the liver and other organs of the body from free radical attacks.

The active ingredient in milk thistle is called silymarin. It's this compound that increases proteins synthesis in the liver and encourages the rejuvenation of this organ. Silymarin also has a blocking action against the absorption of toxins by the liver. Reportedly, toxic substances such as some wild mushrooms, cadmium and carbon tetrachloride (a dry-cleaning agent) can be safely processed and eliminated

Milk thistle also stimulates the production of super oxide dismutase (the body–born antioxidant enzyme) while preventing the depletion of glutathione (which is an antioxidant) from the liver. Because of its antioxidant property, milk thistle helps boost the immune system by increasing the production of T-cells and interferons (soluble proteins involved in protection of the body against foreign invaders.) The kidneys, the heart, the brain and the rest of the nervous system also benefits from milk thistle.

Passion Flower. A hairy and climbing vine, passion flower is grown mainly in southern United States. Both the fruit and the leaves are used for their medicinal properties. Because they function as a calming, soothing or sedative agent, the leaves of a passion flower are used to treat nervous disorders such as hysteria, insomnia, nervousness and restlessness. Professionally prepared dosages, given for an extended duration, reportedly can markedly improve epilepsy, Parkinson's disease, neuralgia, anxiety and hypertension.

Also, women whose hormones cause them to be irritable, the elderly who have muscular or motor control problems and hyperactive children can benefit from this plant.

Rich in bioflavonoids and many other compounds, passion flower can be used as a painkiller, an anti-inflammatory and a germicide (particularly with bacteria that cause eye irritations).

St. John's Wort. According to one legend, this plant was so named because red spots that are metaphorical for St. John's blood, appeared on the leaves of the hypericum plant on the anniversary of the saint's beheading. According to another legend, the saint had used the hypericum plant during the time of the crusades as balm to clean and heal battle wounds, and so the plant's name.

True to its legend, St. John's Wort still can be used to heal wounds, ulcers, burns, bruises and other skin problems. The other important functions of the herb are its use as a sedative or relaxing agent for those who suffer from anxiety or nervous

St. John's Wort has many benefits, including its use to treat insomnia, head-aches, anemia and bronchitis or congestion of the chest. This herb is good for viral infection, tumors, boils, bladder problems and circulation difficulties.

Caution. When taken internally, hypericin ends up accumulating in the skin. This problem makes the skin of some animals, including humans, to be extremely sensitive to sunlight and can cause it to burn. Hence, when taking the herb, stay out of strong sun.

Schisandra. A native of China, schisandra is a thorny climbing vine that has been used for a variety of applications, including as a tonic and as an adaptogen to revitalize and enhance the overall function of the body. Many of this great herb's specific benefits are as follows.

Schisandra helps you cope with stress, improve your body's ability to forestall fatigue and increase its ability to function properly. Specific organs, such as the heart, liver and kidneys, the glands and nerves and the whole body can benefit from schisandra. The herb strengthens the cells in various organs and hence helps the body cope at wider ranges of physiological state, including fortifying it against stress.

Because it normalizes and calms the body, schisandra is very useful in situations where you may have stress, anxiety or a general below-par feeling. Schisandra enhances circulation and digestion, and because it has antioxidant properties, it may boost the immune system, help with the health of the eyes and promote the well-being of other tissues in the body. In addition, schisandra helps the body use calories more efficiently. Athletes and weight watchers may find this product a useful addition to their nutritional regimen. Women have used this herb in its native country to improve their sexual interest as well as promote youthfulness.

Schisandra has pink flowers and red berries.

Spirulina. Also known as blue-green algae, spirulina has many important benefits to the human body.

One, this one-celled plant contains the highest concentration of beta-carotene and Vitamin B12 (reportedly 250% more than liver, which is one of the best sources of the vitamin) and some of the best protein (with 80%-85% bioavailability) and holds 4 times the protein found in an equivalent amount of beef. This interesting algae also houses 26 times more calcium than milk, as well as a large quantity of phosphorous and niacin. Spirulina also possesses a number of other key vitamins and minerals including linoleic acid (or omega-3 fatty acids).

Two, blue-green algae, except for its lack of carbohydrates, is considered a complete food. To have a carbohydrate energy source, the body can still convert some of the amino acids from the protein it contains into glucose and use it as fuel. This plant of the sea is beneficial for the entire body, but the brain and the nervous system seem to thrive on it. Reportedly the consumption of spirulina gives greater mental clarity and alertness. For some people though, the alertness could be too much, as it makes them feel wired.

Spirulina helps boost the immune system, normalize the cholesterol level in the body and suppress hunger or the desire to over indulge as well as help the body eliminate toxins. Whenever you get a chance, include this herb as part of your meal. It's an incredible herb indeed!

Valerian. This herb, which has been used for thousands of years has some great benefits. It can be used to calm or sedate nervous disorders such as anxiety or over excitement, headaches, hysteria and insomnia and also works as a stimulant in cases of extreme fatigue or exhaustion. In addition, valerian enhances circulation and the secretion of digestive juices and stimulates the muscular or peristaltic action of the digestive tract.

Witch Hazel. Witch hazel, whose name was derived from an Old English word that means "pliant or flexible" because the branches or twigs are highly flexible, is primarily used for external applications. Extracts of the bark, leaves or twigs can be used to alleviate pain or bruises and act as an astringent and a cleansing agent. It can also help heal wounds, bed sores, inflamed eyes, hemorrhoids and swellings. Extracts of the witch hazel plant seem to be particularly beneficial to the veins as they tend to strengthen and tone them, thus enhancing blood flow.

When prepared into a tea and taken internally, witch hazel can help stop or reduce internal bleeding, including hemorrhages and excessive menstrual flow. For women, witch hazel also helps in treating problems of the uterus, the cervix and the vagina.

A compress made of witch hazel can be used to treat irritated skin or eyes, burns, insect bites and infections. Because of its astringent properties to the skin, many cosmetic companies use witch hazel in their cleansers, hand and body lotions, massage oils and aftershaves.

CHAPTER 12
Herb Tea Samplers

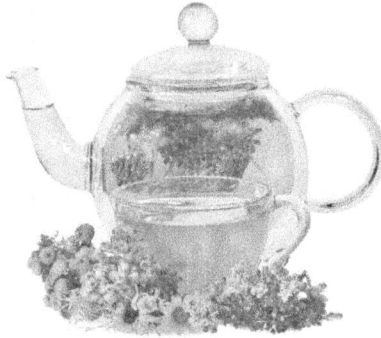

If you have browsed through the coffee and tea aisle of your supermarket or health food store, you are probably amazed at the variety of herbal teas now available to you. Not too long ago, when one thought of consuming tea, one may have considered the traditional commercial teas such as Lipton, Twining or Earl Grey. For most people, herb teas held no value or significance. Now our popular teas, such as Lipton have moved over on health food and grocery store shelves to make room for the dizzying array of herbal blends that pack these places like sardines.

Realizing the growing popularity and the many beneficial properties of herbal teas, enterprising individuals and corporations package and market an incredible assortment of such teas. These range from one or two herbs such as chamomile and peppermint to the ones whose ingredients list reads like those of multivitamin supplements.

Some of these herbs are formulated for specific conditions, and their names are as exotic as their blends: Throat Coat, Smooth Move, Gypsy Cold Care, Fast Lane and Emerald Gardens. Let's look at a sample of the different herbs you find in an herbal blend and the benefits they have to the body.

Cardamom. Cardamom is a seed herb that is also used to spice up certain dishes, particularly in Ethiopia, India and the Orient. Often combined with other herbs, cardamom's primary function in a tea blend is to warm and stimulate the body. This herb is also good for indigestion, gas, colic and headaches.

Carob. In some tea formulations, you see roasted carob. Carob pods are found in a dome-shaped evergreen tree that is native to some parts of Europe and Asia.

The tree is also grown in the Mediterranean region. Carob reportedly is very effective in treating kidney ailments and curing or preventing diarrhea. Naturally sweet, when present in a tea blend, it can help improve the taste of the tea while imparting its other benefits.

Catnip. This is another herb you are likely to see often in an herb tea. Before Lipton and other Asiatic herbs took over, catnip was the only herb tea drunk in Europe when people wanted a warm drink or a drink to treat bronchitis and diarrhea. American Indians used catnip as a sedative or calming agent. They also used it to treat colic, colds or flu in infants and children, as the herb tends to increase perspiration, which can lull a child to sleep. This herb improves circulation, which is important for the proper function of the body. It may even be a benefit to those who have a swelling under the eyes. Its primary function in an herbal tea blend is probably to help calm, relax or ease the body.

Chamomile Flower. Chamomile has many external applications that make it such a useful plant. These range from enhancing the appearance of skin and hair (particularly blond hair) to treating dryness or flakiness of the skin to diminishing lines and wrinkles. This benefit of the herb does not involve much preparation at all. Simply steep the herb for 30 to 40 minutes and wash or treat the skin with the end product. Chamomile as a compress can also be used to alleviate stiffness and muscular inflammation.

Chamomile's popularity, however, is among tea drinkers, who view the herb as a calming or soothing one. It can also be very useful with hyperactive children. For either of these benefits, simply bring one pint of water to a boil, add two teaspoonfuls of the herb and steep for 30 to 40 minutes. If you are using herb tea bags, follow the instruction on the box. The vapor bath of the tea can be a good treatment for children and adults who have asthma or a cold.

The main constituents of Chamomile are essentials oils, flavonoids and tannic acid.

Chicory. A native of Europe and now widely grown here in the U.S., chicory has been used as a purgative of mucus from the stomach and other parts of the GI tract. It's important for the health and proper function of the spleen. It can also be used as an appetizer and to stimulate and enhance digestion.

Citrus Peels. The peel of an orange or a tangerine is believed to have a health-enhancing function in the digestive tract, including aid in minimizing the formation of mucus. It is known to improve digestion as well as overall energy production in the body. Thus, as part of an herbal tea blend, it may help burn more calories and enhancing weight loss.

Hibiscus. This name is really a generic name for a whole class of plants that consist of 200 species and grow in many parts of the world. A lot of these plants have important medicinal properties. Musk-mallow reportedly is one of the most commonly used hibiscus plants that has been used to relieve stomach problems, soothe or calm the nerves and freshen the breath. Those who have a high fever can be treated with this herb because of its cooling and detoxifying properties. As part of an herbal tea blend, it can help with these and other conditions.

Hops. The beer industry has long used hops as a preservative and flavoring agent. This important plant has also had a history of use as an easing or calming substance for those who are restless or wakeful at night. This relaxing and sedative action of the herb is good for those with muscle spasms, pain or fever. This plant is also good for the health of the gallbladder and liver. It increases the production and secretion of bile. Because of its easing and calming effect, hops reportedly can be effective as an enema.

Lemon Grass. Lemon grass, also known as oil grass or fever grass, can be excellent for colds, headaches and abdominal problems. A tea of lemon grass leaves can ease dizziness, cold-related fever or stress. The presence of this herb in a tea blend can help the body ease with any of the maladies mentioned.

Licorice. The major active phytochemical in licorice is glycyrrhizin or glycyrrhizic acid, which gives most of the herb's sweet-tasting characteristics. There are, of course, also a whole variety of other compounds, including flavonoids, starch, sugars and amino acids. A native of Asia and Europe, licorice has many benefits, some of which include its ability to stimulate the adrenal glands so that they can release the necessary hormones to help metabolize calories. This herb, among other things, has a calming effect on the nervous system. When taken along with other herbs, it is reported to have a balancing or harmonizing effect on the body.

Peppermint. Peppermint has been used since ancient times particularly in Chinese, Egyptian and Native American societies. This herb now grows widely in the United States, Europe and other parts of the world. Peppermint is a very commonly used herb because it has a soothing and calming effect on the body.

The herb has other functions that range from its ability to stimulate the functioning of the digestive tract to its ability to increase the supply of oxygen to the blood, which in turn facilitates the calorie-burning, or thermic, effect of the herb. Its overall function, however, is more for its tonic properties, because the herb enhances the proper functioning of the digestive tract as well as the rest of the body.

Spearmint. Spearmint is related to peppermint in terms of its function and benefits except that this herb tends to be milder, gentler and less stimulating than peppermint. Spearmint can be used for ailments involving digestion and circulation, for colds and fever and for cramps and muscle spasms. It also helps remove gas from the gastrointestinal tract and promotes sweating, which helps to reduce fever.

Similarly, if you have a problem with nausea or vomiting, spearmint may help alleviate it. Because of its mild nature, it's often thought a better choice than peppermint for children. Women who suffer from morning sickness (as happens during pregnancy) may also find relief from this herb. Overall, spearmint is a soothing and calming herb that can be benefit you. Because its oils are volatile, it's recommended that you not boil it but steep it in a closed container.

Rose Hips. Rose hips refer to the fruit-like, fleshy hip that is left after the rose petals have fallen off. This hip is very rich in vitamin C, reportedly 60 times richer than any citrus fruit. Rose hips are also rich in bioflavonoids, a group of vitamin-like compounds that are often found along with Vitamin C and that have many important roles including their benefit as an antioxidant. This group of substances is also important for the building and repair of tissues, particularly those of the circulatory system. Besides their independent roles, bioflavonoids are helpers of vitamin C. This vitamin provides tremendous benefits to the body. Perhaps the maximum benefit of Vitamin C is attained when consumed along with its sister compounds (the bioflavonoids) and other compounds as in rose hips. The presence of these ingredients in an herbal tea preparation increases the nutritional value of the tea.

CHAPTER 13
Spice Samplers

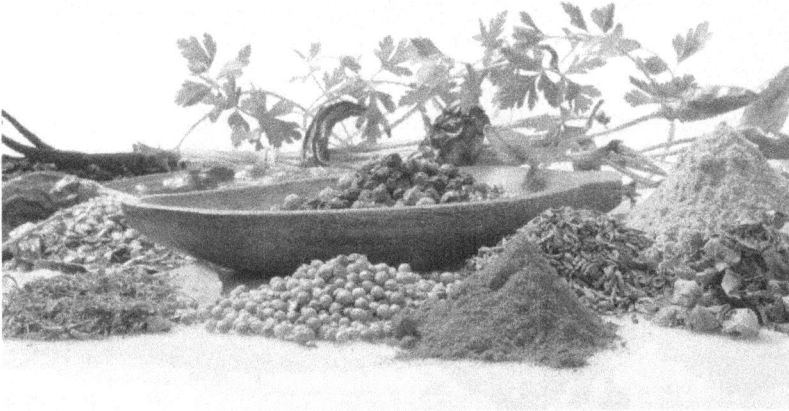

Figure 13.1 The spices in our kitchen cabinets, a storehouse of good health

For most people, spices' importance ends with their use as food flavoring agents. But as you will see below, besides their culinary function, these mostly aromatic herbs have many benefits to the body. Although the number of spices used by various cultures is extensive, the following samples may help you appreciate the role spices play in your health.

Anise. This groove-stemmed, soft-stocked herb has had many uses since ancient times. In the digestive tract, anise when consumed as tea can help prevent the formation of as well as eliminate gas, alleviate nausea, cramps and colic (or severe abdominal pain), and for nursing mothers increase the production and flow of milk. Anise can also be a nice remedy for insomnia when taken with a glass of warm milk, and when taken as an infusion, help promote menstruation. A tea made from equal combination of fennel, caraway and anise reportedly is an excellent cleanser or purifier for the digestive tract. Because of its sweetness and pleasant flavor, you often find it in cough medicines.

Basil. Although grown worldwide and used to flavor foods, it's in India where basil is highly esteemed, almost considered sacred. Basil's healthful properties are many. When steeped into tea and drank, basil can help alleviate fevers, colds, indigestion, cramps, constipation, nausea and vomiting. This sweetly aromatic herb can also relieve gas and serve as a diuretic and a stimulant, particularly when you are tired or exhausted.

If you have a fever, simmer one ounce of the herb in a pint of water for 15-20 minutes and drink. Adding black peppercorns can enhance the herbs effectiveness.

Since basil increases milk production, a nursing mother can benefit by it. Because basil increases blood circulation, a pregnant woman taking it before and after a childbirth can also benefit from it. This herb can even benefit those with yeast infection of the mouth and throat as well as those who have headaches.

Bay. Bay leaves are excellent flavor enhancers when used with certain dishes. As you will see below, bay's function in the body is more impressive than its culinary uses. Also called laurel or sweet bay, this herb can be a great remedy for liver, pancreas, spleen, kidneys and lung problems. A tea of bayberries can be effective in treating sore throat and congestion of the nose, chest and lungs and help alleviate tonsillitis. The tea is also a very good remedy for colds, influenza and fever.

On the gastrointestinal and urinary tracts, the laurel herb can be an effective agent in eliminating gas and enhancing urine flow, respectively. Women who have menstrual and womb trouble can benefit from this herb by consuming it as tea.

When externally applied, the tea as well as the oil of bayberries can be handy in treating poisonous insect and snake bites, sunburns, itches, bruises and eczema. You may even use bay oil to improve the appearance of brown and black spots on your skin. In terms of usage, the bark, berries and leaves can be used for all kinds of treatments.

Black Pepper. Besides its culinary benefits, black pepper can be excellent as an expectorant for cold-related mucous of the throat. It is more effective when made into a tea and mixed with honey.

Black pepper can also be an effective insecticide, annihilating such household pests as roaches, ants, potato bugs and moths. Simply grind and sprinkle the spice where the insects are, and you should see them disappear.

Caraway. This common spice has many benefits beyond its use in the kitchen. It can help with digestion, in the prevention of fermentation in the stomach and elimination of gas from the bowel. For this purpose, crush an ounce of the seeds and add to boiling water and let it cool and steep for 20-30 minutes. Take two tablespoon of the infusion until relief is noted. This use of the herb can be very effective in treating digestive tract disorders of infants and children as well. For women, caraway helps promote menstrual flow, alleviate cramps in the uterus and increase the production and flow of milk.

Cayenne Pepper. Cayenne or red pepper is grown widely in warm climates throughout the world, particularly in Africa, Latin America, Asia and some parts of the U.S. This deceptively hot but harmless herb has been used to spice up foods in many cultures. In terms of its health merits, cayenne is one of the few herbs that stimulate the nervous and circulatory systems and serve as an overall tonic for the body.

Some of the organs and tissues that benefit from cayenne are the spleen, kidneys, pancreas and digestive tract. Because of its stimulatory action, the glands along the digestive tract may produce more digestive juices in the presence of cayenne. So you can see the benefit of consuming red pepper along with your meals.

Capsicum is the active ingredient in whole red pepper, but the other substances include pectin, albumin, iron and phosphate compounds, magnesium and some oil.

When taken whole, all these other substances can have healthful properties as well. Because of its high Vitamin A content, capsicum is good for the eyes and can serve as an antioxidant for the rest of the body. This herb is good for the heart, as it enhances circulation and improves the health of the veins, arteries and capillaries.

In addition, it helps reduce the bad cholesterol while raising the good cholesterol. In the liver, cayenne increases fat-metabolizing enzymes and hence may help reduce fat production and deposition in the body, an important benefit for those who are struggling with their weight. Cayenne pepper has many other benefits, many of which are beyond the scope of this book.

Celery. This ancient plant has many benefits, some of which include its use as an antioxidant and calming and easing agent for the body. Because it tends to cause perspiration, some herbalists think celery may even help with weight loss. This herb has also been reported to help in balancing the acidity of the body.

A combination of celery juice and carrot juice reportedly helps ease arthritic spurs. This interesting plant is also supposed to enhance sexual drive and serve as a stimulant to the kidneys to increase urine flow. Because it contains a fair amount of sodium, it helps enhance the function of the stomach lining and is good for the joints.

Cinnamon. The use of this herb goes back to the ancient Chinese, Roman and Egyptian cultures. Cinnamon's special attribute is that it helps with indigestion, heartburn and cramps. It's also an excellent antifungal and antibacterial agent. Hence, those who have yeast infection or athlete's foot can benefit from this herb.

Add 10 or so cinnamon sticks in four cups of boiling water, simmer for 5-7 minutes, remove from heat and let cool for 40-45 minutes. Apply the solution for either of the problems mentioned.

Cloves. When steeped into tea, cloves can be good in curing nausea and relieving gas in the digestive tract. This spice is also good for circulation, digestion and treating vomiting. Clove oils can help alleviate toothaches. You may also chew cloves for this purpose. Because cloves have antibiotic properties, they can also be used as germicides.

Coriander. A small annual plant, coriander has been cultivated since ancient times. The seed is used both for its culinary and medicinal benefits.

In the digestive tract, coriander can help eliminate gas, allay cramps or griping and other disorders and enhance the muscular tone of the stomach and the rest of the GI tract. Because of its pleasant taste, coriander is often used to enhance the flavor of foods and other medicinal preparations. It also has a diuretic and alterative (capable of favorably altering disease conditions) properties.

Cumin. Primarily used to make curries, it enhances the flavor of fried foods such as beans, rice and chicken. In terms of its health merits, cumin, can be good for the heart, the uterus and the mammary glands, as it increases the production and secretion of milk.

You may use the tea or capsule of cumin powder for many of its internal benefits. Of course you can also use it with the appropriate dishes to derive the benefit of the herb. When externally applied in liniments (a thin substance rubbed onto the skin), it can stimulate circulation to the area.

Dill. Dill is an annual plant widely grown for its use as a spice; it is also found in the wild. It's a multipurpose spice that can be sprinkled on a variety of dishes.

But beyond its role in enhancing the flavor of foods, dill has a number of healthful benefits. When used as tea, it can help alleviate upset stomach and prevent the formation of gas in the intestines and has calming or quieting effect on the nerves.

It can reduce swelling and pain, stimulate appetite and fight off insomnia. When used in combination with other herbs such as anise, coriander, fennel and caraway, dill will help promote the flow of milk in nursing mothers.

Chewing the seed of this herb is also supposed to-relieve bad breath. If you have problems with hiccoughs, this herb may be the answer to the problem.

Fenugreek. The use of this spice/herb goes back to the ancient cultures of Ethiopia, Egypt, Greek and Asia. Since ancient times, fenugreek has been hailed both for its medicinal and culinary uses.

Medicinally, the seed of fenugreek can be used to remove congestion of the throat and chest, as an astringent, as a demulcent to relieve inflammation of mucous membranes and as an emollient to soothe and treat skin problems.

The tea of fenugreek can be excellent in purging excessive mucus from the throat and gut that collects when one consumes large amount of milk and cheese.

This herb can be used to treat diabetes and gout, increase milk production in wet mothers and because of its spermicide properties, even prevent pregnancy. This funny sounding herb can also be used to treat boils and carbuncles and help with anemia and rickets.

Garlic. Garlic is the reigning king of all spices in that it has been used through-out history for a number of remedies—from warding off evil spirits to protecting against the plague and helping with wound healing to fighting cancer and a number of other diseases and maladies. This amazing spice is a true wonder of nature indeed and has been used to treat many internal and external infections and other diseases.

Externally, garlic can be used to treat infections of the eye, throat, vagina and nose as well as burns and insect bites. It's also a great insect repellent. Internally, it can be used to treat parasites of the colon (when used as an enema), control fever, combat viruses and bacteria and alleviate hemorrhoids. This herb is also beneficial to the heart, stomach, lungs and spleen.

Garlic has many other benefits. These include improving blood circulation, lowering triglycerides and the bad serum cholesterol (while raising the good cholesterol), decreasing blood sugar (important for those with diabetes), reducing blood pressure and stimulating the immune system. Because it relaxes the nervous system, garlic may also help you keep insomnia at bay.

Ginger. We often use ginger as condiment to spice up or enhance the flavor of certain dishes. Ginger has, besides its culinary function, many healthful benefits. Some of these involve the elimination of gases from the intestinal tract, improved function of the liver, including its ability to increase the secretion of bile, and the processing of cholesterol. Because bile is involved in the digestion and absorption of fats and fat-soluble vitamins, it can be said that ginger may help enhance the processing of food in the body as well.

This herb, like most plant extracts, contains several different substances. These include starch, protein, lecithin, fatty acids, triglycerides, protein-digesting enzymes, volatile oils (substance that give ginger its characteristic smell), vitamins and a variety of other compounds. All these compounds together help enhance the function of the body.

Some of the specific functions of ginger are the ability to serve as an anti-oxidant, help with the digestion of protein and enhance circulation. Fresh ginger steeped in hot water (as tea) can be good for nasal and throat congestion.

Horseradish. This penetratingly pungent herb has many benefits. Some of these include serving as dilator of the nasal and bronchial channels (thus enabling the sinuses to open up and cleanse) and as an antibiotic or inhibitor of microbial and parasite growth in the body. Horseradish can also aid digestion by stimulating the cells of the gastrointestinal lining.

In addition, this root herb can be beneficial for the proper function of the kidneys and the intestines. When made into a poultice and applied externally, horseradish can stimulate blood flow to the area and help alleviate pain, such as in the case of rheumatoid arthritis.

Marjoram. In ancient Greece, marjoram was held as a symbol of love, so much so that people wore it as wreaths and garlands at weddings and called it "joy of the mountains." An ointment of the herb is supposed to enable the wearer to dream about his or her future mate. Marjoram, although native to Mediterranean countries and some parts of Asia, is now grown in the U.S. and other parts of the world.

In terms of its health merits, marjoram is used to calm the nerves, enhance digestion, treat rheumatism and sprains, relieve gas and stomach disorders and serve as tonic for the rest of the body.

Marjoram can also be used to alleviate coughs other respiratory disorders and as a mouth wash and gargle for sore throats. For women, marjoram can help relieve cramps and nausea associated with menstruation. In addition, a tea of the herb can be an excellent calming and sleep-inducing agent.

To make a tea of the herb, boil one pint of water, add one teaspoon each of marjoram and oregano (an option) and let it steep for 30 minutes. After it cools, strain and refrigerate and use any amount from this lot. You may want to reheat it before consuming it.

Also, you can add this herb to your bathwater to help you unwind and relax if you have had a long and exhausting day. Lastly, the oil of marjoram can be used as a lotion for gout, rheumatism and varicose veins and to relieve stiff joints.

Mustard Seed. Mustard seeds, which can be either black or white, have many medicinal properties. It's the white variety that is combined with vinegar and turmeric (which gives mustard its yellow color) to make the paste-like spread that we use on sandwiches, hamburgers and hotdogs.

As medicine, mustard can be used both for internal and external applications. Internally, mustard is good to ease congestion of the chest as well as an emetic to remove poison or relieve discomfort in the stomach. It can also enhance appetite and stimulate the flow of digestive juices.

Externally, a paste of the herb (prepared by mixing black mustard and cold water) can help ease pain, sprain, spasm or rheumatism by encouraging blood flow to the particular area of the body. For this purpose, the poultice is spread over a thin cloth that overlays the wound or pain and is covered with a heavier cotton cloth and left until the skin begins to irritate or burn. Upon removal, the applied area is washed thoroughly to remove any remaining mustard.

To complete the process and speed up recovery, apply grain flour such as rice or wheat on the area and wrap with dry cotton cloth. If you have sensitive or tender skin, this treatment may not work for you

Nutmeg. Nutmeg is a seed herb from the great nutmeg tree, which is native to Indonesia but now is also widely grown throughout the world. However, it's only in Indonesia and Granada of the West Indies where the tree is cultivated commercially. The nutmeg tree has spreading branches and densely packed leaves.

Besides its use as spice for a variety of dishes, nutmeg and its sister herb, mace (from the dried shell of the fruit), have been used to treat gas, digestive disorders and stomach, heart, nervous system and kidney maladies.

On the nervous system, nutmeg has a calming and soothing effect, producing a peaceful and almost euphoric state while dramatically increasing one's awareness and control. In addition, his herb reportedly heightens one's sensuality and sexual drive.

There can be some side effects with some people when taken in large quantities. These range from aching in bones and muscles to hurting eyes, sinus problems and diarrhea. For those who suffer from some mental disorder and need treatment, these inconveniences may be minor compared to the herb's benefit.

Oregano. This wonderfully aromatic herb can be added to enhance the flavor of most dishes. As for its health benefits, oregano can improve the health and function of the stomach, increase appetite and help allay congestion of the chest and throat.

As a carminative agent, it can help relieve gas from the stomach and bowel. Reportedly, oregano can alleviate deafness or pain and ringing in the ear and may even be used to get rid of a toothache. You can prepare tea, poultice or compress for many of the remedial applications. The whole plant is employed for oregano's many uses.

Parsley. This herb is the black sheep of the spice family. Although we are now finding that it contains a wide variety of excellent nutrients, in the past, parsley has been largely relegated to its use in garnishing and enhancing the appearance of foods.

In terms of its nutritional and medicinal content, parsley is a rich source of iron, beta-carotene, calcium, potassium and phosphorus. This perennial plant can be an excellent treatment for diseases of the urinary tract, such as those inflicted by venereal diseases, for problems with the liver and spleen and for gallstones.

It can also be an excellent diuretic and promoter of the health of the kidneys and of the circulatory system and can improve menstruation.

This herb can be used to treat swollen glands and breasts as well as curtail the flow of milk (particularly important to mothers who are trying to wean a child.) The roots, leaves and seeds are used for a variety of the herb's benefits. To take advantage of parsley's benefits, use it liberally in your soup, salad and sandwiches.

Caution: Those who have a kidney infection should avoid using parsley.

Rosemary. Rosemary is a Mediterranean native that is now grown throughout the world. Besides its use in spicing up various dishes, rosemary has many healthful benefits. These range from enhancing digestion to promoting liver function, including the secretion of bile. In many cultures, this herb has been used to treat maladies such as stomach and headaches and to soothe and calm the nerves.

Rosemary also promotes circulation in the capillaries (the tiniest of blood vessels), which thus helps bring more nutrients to all tissues of the body. In addition, this herb reportedly enhances memory and relieves tension and depression.

You may even see rosemary in shampoos and rinses. It's used in these products because of the herb's ability to darken and maintain a healthy scalp and youthful hair. To derive this benefit, you may make your own product by making an infusion of the herb and applying it after you shampoo your hair.

Rosemary tea can be prepared by adding a half teaspoon of the herb to a pint of boiling water and letting it steep for ten to fifteen minutes. Rosemary, which has antioxidant properties itself, can be an excellent source of vitamin E, an important neutralizer of free radicals, particularly as a protector of cell membranes, fatty tissues and fat molecules in the circulating blood.

Caution: Excessive consumption of rosemary can be fatal.

Sage. Another use of this word in the English language means a wise man or a philosopher. As the name of an herb here it means "savior of mankind." It reportedly can function as a strengthener of memory and as a promoter of wisdom and longevity.

Among its many other benefits, sage helps reduce the secretion of bodily fluids such as sweat (beneficial to menopausal women who may be experiencing hot flashes and night sweats or those with tuberculosis), breast milk (useful to women who are trying to wean a child) and saliva and mucus (beneficial to those who have a cold or chest congestion).

A tea preparation of the herb can be used for depression, nervous disorder and vertigo and trembling. You can also gargle with sage infusion to help heal sore throat, laryngitis and tonsillitis.

For these and other benefits of the herb first boil 1-1/4 cups of water. Remove from heat and add 2 tablespoons of the sage and steep for 30 to 35 minutes. Strain and add honey or sugar if necessary and drink half a cup of the infusion twice a day. For women who want to stop milk production, two cups a day of sage tea consumed over a week reportedly helps bring their milk secretion to a halt. For this purpose and to make a larger supply at a time, boil one quart of water, remove from heat add 8 tablespoons of the herb and steep for 45 minutes. Sweeten appropriately and drink two cups daily.

Sage has also been used to heal skin sores, to promote the health and regeneration of the liver and as a natural coloring agent for graying hair. In addition, sage can enhance circulation and serve as an antioxidant for the heart and the rest of the body.

Caution: Heavy and extended use of the herb may lead to poisoning.

Thyme. In ancient Greece, the name thyme conjured up power, strength and bravery. But the herb's beneficial properties lie in its ability to help ease congestion of the chest, throat and nasal cavity and alleviate gastrointestinal disorders such as stomach cramps, gastritis and gas buildup.

It also serves to soothe the nerves and can be used as a disinfectant and germicide. When applied externally, thyme can help control athlete's foot, scabies, lice and crabs. The extract of the herb can also be used to heal wounds and bruises and alleviate rheumatism. Because of its antioxidant properties, thyme may keep cells from becoming cancerous.

It is reported that alcoholics can benefit from this herb because it causes vomiting, diarrhea, sweating and hunger along with abhorrence for alcohol. For this to work, the herb has to be used repeatedly for a long period of time.

For this purpose, steep 1 to 2 teaspoons of the herb in one cup of hot water and drink this amount daily.

PART IV
The Four Pillars Recipes

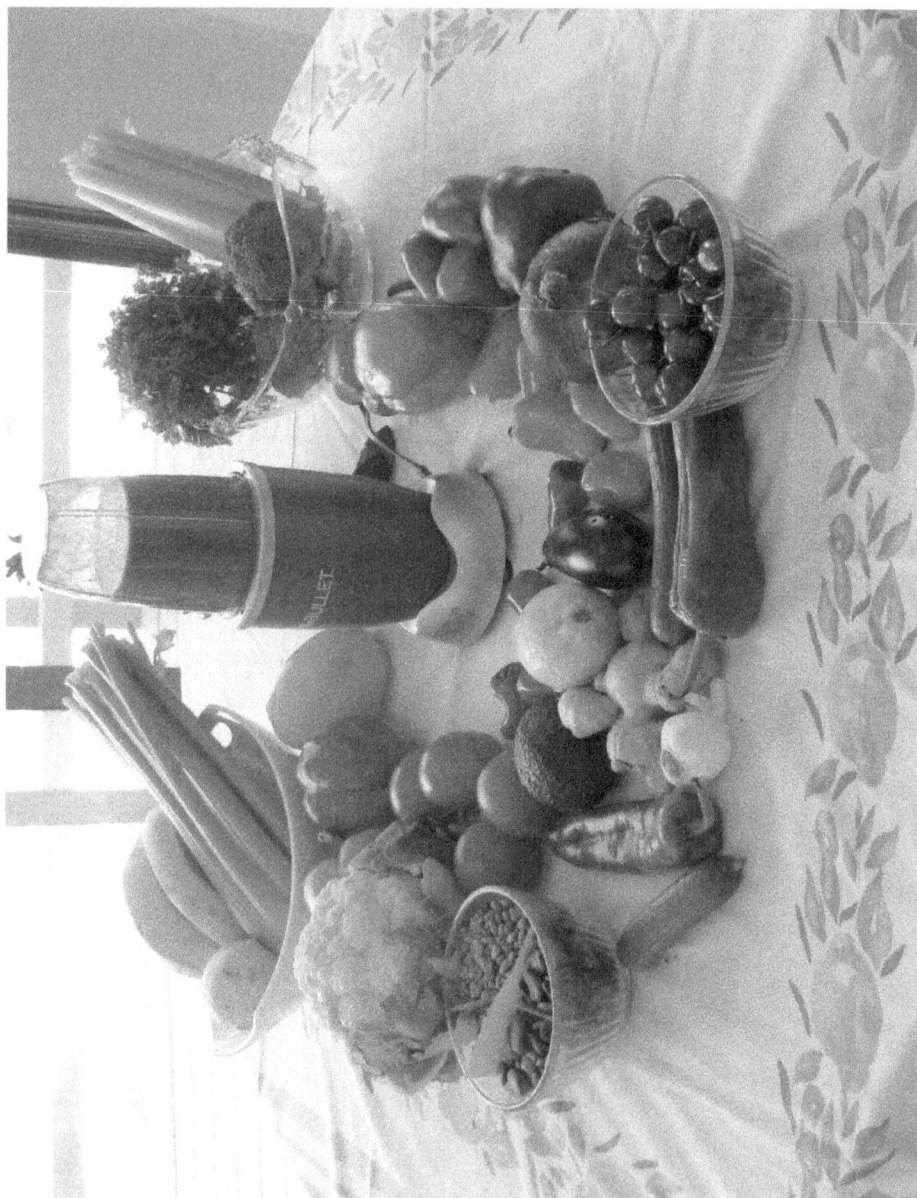

Foods rich in the Four Pillars of health

Introduction

Researchers and government agencies lament about how Americans are nutritionally impoverished when it comes to their consumption of fruits and vegetables. The United States Department of Agriculture (USDA) has long recommended that people eat 7 to 13 servings a day of these fruits and vegetables, but as the Center for Disease Control (CDC) points out, less than 15% of the population come close to consuming the recommended amounts. Knowing what we know about the importance of these nutrients in our health, this is not good news. The dearth of these important foods at the American family table in part explains the high level of degenerative diseases—cancer, diabetes, cardiovascular disease—that account for nearly 55% of all the deaths in the United States. There are a few more astounding reports about the lack of sufficient fruits and vegetables in the American households. What is missing in the USDA's recommendation is a simpler and more practical way of getting these daily servings.

The Four Pillars blends are designed to give anyone who is willing to commit two or three hours out of their week an option to meet their daily nutritional needs for fruits and vegetables. The highly concentrated and nutritionally dense drinks allow one to meet and exceed the USDA's daily recommendations.

As you will see from the assortment of fruits and vegetables, herbs and spices used to create these blends, there is no way you can consume all these things daily if you were to consume them individually. However, by combining and mixing them together you can. Depending on the quantities of the items you use, you only need to make them once a week.

Suggestions and Reminders

Some who look at the list of the produce and read the instructions below may at first believe the task for making the drinks too involved or time-consuming or even expensive.

First, when it comes to your health, nothing is more important than the time and money you spend to purchase and make the necessary foods to nourish and care for your body. I believe it's a life or death situation.

Second, once you buy the produce, it will take two to two and a half hours for one person and about one-and-a-half for two, once every seven to ten days. I think we all spend more than this amount of time in frivolous pursuits every day, let alone a week. So time should not be an issue.

Third, money-wise, if you purchase them at place like Costco and other wholesale places, the produce you need for the Super Blend will cost you roughly $70 dollars. You can make 5 gallons of the drink if you use all of the produce. This amount will last a couple of weeks and cost you only $5 dollars a day. Use even higher dollar amounts and you can see that when converted into daily expenditure, it's less than a cost of a meal at fast food places, and nutritionally you get so much more. Consider the cost if you were hospitalized because of a degenerative disease such as cancer, heart disease and diabetes. We know that these are often food-related.

Fourth, many of us balk at new things and concepts because we lack the knowledge about them. The first thing you need to do is read as much as you can about the value of good nutrition for your health and longevity. Once you make that connection, it will be so much easier for you to accept the concept of The Four Pillars drinks and foods.

After you have been on The Four Pillars drinks, you will see improvements, not only in your overall health but also in the appearance of your skin, nails and hair. This claim is not a theory. It's what happened to my wife and me. Be good to yourself and incorporate these foods into your daily menu.

Color Scheme	Phytonutrients	Benefits	Sources
Dark-Green	lutein/zeaxanthin, isoflavones, EGCG*, indoles, isothiocyanates, sulphoraphane, etc.	Good for the health of the arteries, lungs and the liver.	The greens such as kale, parsley, spinach, collard greens, Brussels sprouts, broccoli, green tea, oregano
Red-Pink	lycopene, ellagic acid, quercetin, hesperidin,	Good for the health of the prostate, the DNA and urinary tract	raspberry, strawberry, cherry, cranberry, red cabbage, red bell pepper, radishes, pomegranate, tomato, watermelon, guava, pink grapefruit, cayenne pepper
Orange-yellows	alpha-carotene, beta-carotene, beta cryptoxanthin, lutein/zeaxanthin, hesperidin	The eyes, the immune system, the skin and the overall health of the body can benefit by these compounds.	apricots, yellow grapefruit, cantaloupe, papaya, peaches, mango, bell peppers (orange and yellow), carrots, sweet potato, yams, squash, corn, turmeric, etc.
Blue-Purple	resveratrol, anthocyanidins, phenolics, flavonoids	Good for the heart, brain and bones. Also function as antioxidants.	Black berry, acai berry, blueberry, elderberry, purple grapes, plums, black beans, eggplant
Brown-White	EGCG, allicin, quercetin, indoles, glucosinolates	Good for circulations, bones, and the health of the arteries	garlic, cauliflower, mushrooms, turnips, white kidney beans, pears, apples, cocoa horseradish, ginger,

The five color groups, representing phytonutrients, their benefits and food sources
*EGCG stand for Epigallocatechin gallate
Source: http://www.vitamedica.com

Making the Four Pillars drinks

Instruction

Equipment needed:

Two large bowls

A large cutting knife

Wide/long cutting board

Several 16 ounce containers (to store the blended drink in)

A good blender NOT a juicer (we use the Nutri Bullet)

Peelers for the carrots

Spoon is good to remove the ginger skin

The preparation and blending of your Four Pillars drinks

For each one of the blends you wish to make, write down all the items before you go to the store to purchase them.

1. Wash all the fruits and vegetables thoroughly once you bring them home.
2. Use a swivel-drier or damp-dry all the leafy vegetables.
3. Place one item at a time, chop/mince finely, measure and transfer to one of the two large bowls. Do this for all the greens, carrots and ginger. The bananas you add during the blending.
4. Measure the rest of the items (berries, onions, garlic, ginger, etc.) and add them to the same bowl.
5. Squeeze the lemon into a cup, measure and sprinkle it onto the bowl's contents to minimize oxidation.
6. Wash the blender and all the containers (if they are not clean already)
7. Attach the power cord to an outlet from your kitchen counter and start to blend. Measure your filtered or distilled water and transfer to the blender. Take enough from the mixed veggies and fruits in the bowl to fill the blender half way up. Close the top and turn on the power. Blend in stages: chop, puree, and liquefy. Stop and let it cool if the motor seems to get very hot.
8. Once thoroughly blended and nearly liquified, transfer to the second bowl. Continue blending the rest of the mixed fruits, veggies, herbs and spices until they're all done.
9. Mix the liquefied blend thoroughly with the wooden spoon. If you have a hand-held blender, it would be perfect for thorough mixing. Otherwise, the spoon will be enough.

10. Fill your storage containers, cover and put them in the refrigerator. If you have made more than what you will consume in 2-3 days—most likely you will—store the rest in your freezer. You'll use them as you run out of your supply from the refrigerator.

How to constitute your drinks

The Four Pillars—cold

The batch you made is going to be concentrated and you may need to dilute each serving with 50% water. If you want to enhance the flavor even more, use carbonated water like Club Soda, Pellegrino or Perrier to dilute your Four Pillars drink. Adjust the dilution according to your taste and the concentration of the original drink. Add a dash of black pepper and ice, if you like it cold.

The Four Pillars—hot

This is an absolutely enjoyable drink but for optimum flavor, you need to add something more to it. You need to have black cumin, cardamom seeds, cinnamon powder and black pepper whole (to be ground fresh).

First, decide how many cups of the drink you're going to reconstitute. Depending on the concentration of the original, use 50% of The Four Pillars drink and 50% filtered or distilled water. Let's assume you're going to make two hot cups of the Four Pillars drink.

Heat 1 cup of water in a pot

1. Measure out 1/2 teaspoon of black cumin and 1/3rd teaspoon of cardamom seeds, if you want a richer flavor. Cardamom seeds are expensive, so half a teaspoon of the precious seeds can be enough.

2. In a mortar and pestle, grind these spices and put in the heating water.

3. Bring the water and its contents to a boil, turn the heat low, cover and let it simmer for a few minutes.

4. Add the two cups of the Four Pillars drink and bring to a near boil and immediately remove from stove.

5. Measure one tablespoon of honey (to taste) and put in each one of the cups.

6. Pour the hot drink into the cups and a dash of freshly ground (preferably) black pepper.

7. Stir completely and serve. As you drink this, your nerves prickle with joy.

To truly appreciate these and the many other spices we often use, read about them in the Ethiopian chapters. Once you realize the great benefits these condiments have for your body, you will appreciate and enjoy your foods and drinks even more.

This drink is great to have after your morning and evening meals.

Enjoy!

Four Pillars—Green

Vegetables (fresh and finely chopped)
1-1/2 cups green bell pepper
1 cup collard green
2 sticks of celery
1 cup broccoli
2 cups spinach
3 Brussels sprout
1 big green apple
1 cup cucumber
1/2 chili pepper (serrano)
3 kiwis

Herbs (fresh and finely chopped)
1/2 cup mint
1/4 cup parsley
1/4 cup cilantro

Flavoring agents
1 tsp. orange zest
1 tsp. lemon zest

Fruits
2 oranges
2 cups pineapple
4 bananas
2 large mangos
1 avocado fruit
2 tbsp. lemon juice

Spices
1 tbsp. ginger
1/2 tsp. cinnamon (powder)
2 garlic cloves
1/4 tbsp. red onion
1/2 tsp. ground cardamom seeds (optional)
1/2 tsp. ground black cumin (optional)

Absorption facilitator
2 tbsp. extra virgin olive oil

6 cups water

Four Pillars—Deep Earth

Berries
2 cups black berries
1 cup blue berries
2 cups cherries
1-1/2 cups grapes (blue)

Fruits
1 plum
4 bananas

Vegetables (fresh and finely chopped)
1 cup bell pepper (red)
2 cups Swiss chard (red)
1 cup Romano lettuce
1 cup kale
1 cup cauliflower
1/2 cup red cabbage
1 cup beets (cooked)
1/2 cup egg plant
1 tomato (medium)

Herbs (fresh and finely chopped)
1/2 cup mint
2 tbsp. basil

Spices
1 tbsp. ginger
2 cloves garlic
2 tbsp. red onion
1/2 tsp. serrano pepper
1/4 tsp. cinnamon

Enhancers
1-1/2 tbsp. lemon juice
1-1/2 tbsp. balsamic vinegar
1/2 tbsp. orange zest

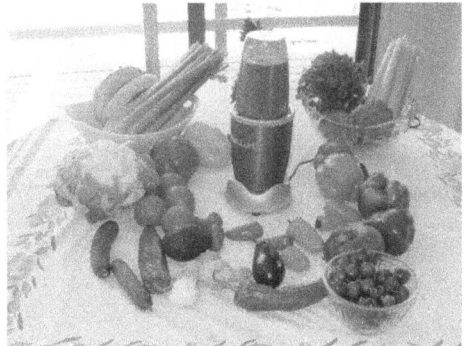

Absorption facilitator
2 tbsp. extra virgin oil
5 cups water

Four Pillars—Red

Berries
2-1/2 cups strawberries
1 cup raspberries
1/2 cup cranberries
1-1/2 cups cherries
1/2 cup pomegranates (optional)

Vegetables (fresh and finely chopped)
1/2 cup carrots
1/2 cup celery
1/3 cup beets
1/3 cup Swiss chard
1 cup red bell pepper
1/2 cup tomatoes
1/3 cup cabbage
2 tbsp. red onions

Fruits
3 bananas
1 cup pine apple
1 tbs. lemon juice
1 red apple

Herbs (fresh and finely chopped)
1/2 cup mint
1 tbsp. parsley

Spices
1 tsp. ginger
2 cloves of garlic
1 tbsp. black pepper

1 tbsp. extra virgin olive oil
4 cups of water

Four Pillars—Yellow

Vegetables (fresh and finely minced)

1 yellow bell pepper

1 orange bell pepper

2 sticks of carrots

1/2 cucumber

1 yellow zucchini

2 kiwis

1 celery stick

2 Brussels' sprouts

1 tbsp. red onion

Fruits

1 orange

5 bananas

1 cup pine apple

2-1/2 cups mangos

1 big pear

1 yellow apple

5 figs (optional)

3 tbsp. lemon juice

Herbs (fresh and finely minced)

1/4 cup mint

1 cup bean sprout

1 1/2 alpha alpha sprout

Spices

1/4 tsp. cinnamon

1/2 tsp. turmeric

1 tbsp. ginger

2 cloves of garlic

6 cups water (filtered or distilled)

3 tbsp. extra virgin olive oil

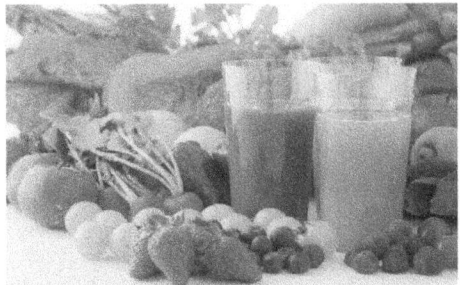

Four Pillars—Super blend

Vegetables (fresh and finely chopped)
1 cup broccoli
1/2 cup egg plant
2 celery sticks
1 cup Swiss chard
1 cup collard green
1 cup cucumber
1 cup kale
1 cup lettuce
1 cup yellow zucchini
1 cup carrots
3 Brussels sprouts
2 cups spinach
3/4 cup anise root
1 medium tomato
1 pepper—orange
1 pepper—red

Berries
2 cups strawberries
2 cups blue berry
1 cup cranberries
2 cups pink or blue grapes
1 cup black berries
2 cups cherries (if unavailable replace with raspberries)

Fruits
3 cups pine apple
1 medium apple
1 avocado
2 kiwis
4 bananas
1 large mango
2 tbsp. lemon juice

Herbs (fresh and finely chopped)
1 cup parsley
3/4 cup cilantro
1 cup mint

Spices
1/4 cup red onion
2 tbsp. garlic
1 tbsp. ginger
1 tbsp. turmeric
1 tbsp. anise seeds
2 tbsp. cinnamon
1 tbsp. black pepper

Absorption facilitator
3 tbsp. extra virgin olive oil
8 cups of filtered water

Makes 2.5 gallons
(2- 64 oz–yogurt containers
4- 48 oz–cottage containers)

The following Four Pillars recipe is to function as a base blend for a drink, loaf, kita, pizza crust and soup.

The Four Pillars Base Blend
Measurements and Ingredients:

Vegetables(fresh and finely minced)

1/2 cup spinach
1/2 cup cauliflower
3 Brussels sprout
1/2 cup celery
1/2 cup cabbage
1 cup carrot
1/2 collard green
1 cup red bell pepper
1/2 orange bell pepper
1 cup pine apple
1 banana
3 cups of water
2 tbsp. of olive oil

Herbs (fresh and finely minced)

1 tbsp. sweet basil
1/4 cup mint
1 tbsp. cilantro
1/4 cup parsley

Spices (all fresh except for turmeric and black pepper)

1 tbsp. ginger
1 tbsp. onion
1 tbsp. garlic
1 tbsp. turmeric
1 tbsp. black pepper

Makes about 1 gallon of The Four Pillars base blend.

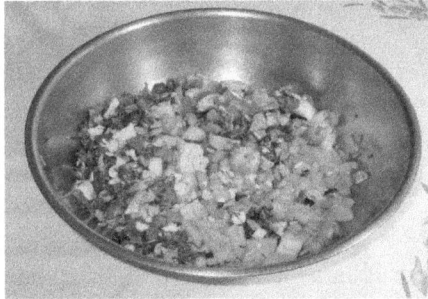

Ready for your blender

Directions:
1. Process all the ingredients in batches and collect in a big bowl.
2. Mix the contents of the bowl thoroughly.
3. Remove 2 cups of this blend and set aside; the first cup will be used as one of the dough ingredients for the loaf, kita and pizza crust, the second for the soup.

The Four Pillars vegetable, herbal and spice base blend (to be used as base the recipe for a drink, loaf, kita, pizza crust and soup.)

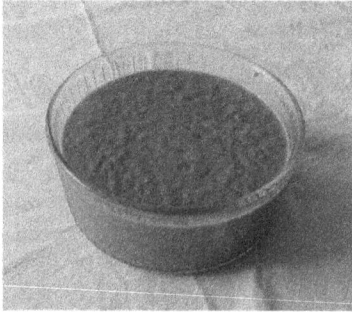

To complete the recipe for a Four Pillar drink, blend the following:

3 bananas

1 cup of strawberries

1 cup of blueberries

1 cup of mangos

2 tbsp. of lemon juice

Add to the original blend (see above), mix thoroughly and put in your refrigerator to use as your healthy drink.

Before we list the recipes for the loaf, kita and pizza crust, we need to create a master dough.

The Master Dough

Measurements and Ingredients:

3 cups of brown teff flour

2 cups of whole-wheat flour

1 cups of all-purpose flour (1/4 cup for kneading)

1 cup of the base Four Pillars blend

3 tbsp. of brown sugar or honey

2 packets or 2 tbsp. of yeast

2 tbsp. of olive oil

1 tsp. of salt (or to taste)

3 cups of distilled or filtered water (1 cup for diluting and activating the yeast)

Optional: you can add 1 tsp. of either anise seeds, or cardamom seeds or black cumin seeds to enhance the flavor of the bread.

Directions:

1. Warm 1 cup of water to 105°F to 110°F. Temperature over 120°F will kill the yeast.

2. Remove from heat and dilute the 2 packets or 2 tbsp. of yeast.

3. Add 1 tsp. of brown sugar to help start the yeast.

4. Set aside for 8-10 minutes so the yeast fully activates.

5. In a big bowl, mix all the three flours with spatula.

6. Make a well in the middle and add the olive oil and the activated yeast solution and mix thoroughly.

7. Add the 2 cups of water and the cup Four Pillars blend and knead thoroughly for 3 to 4 minutes.

8. Sprinkle cornmeal flour (if you have any, helps enhance the crust's flavor) or one of the flours on a stone or wooden board and knead the dough for 10 minutes. (See picture below.)

9. Use 1 tsp. Extra Virgin Olive oil to grease the bottom and sides of bowl.

10. Drop the rolled dough into the bowl, cover with a plastic wrap and let it rise for 1 to 2 hours.

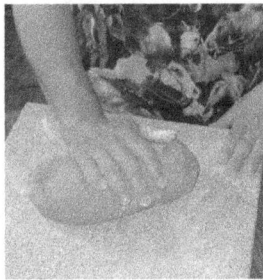

11. Deflate and work the dough for a few minutes more. If the dough is too soft, use additional flour on the kneading board to help thicken it.

12. Put it back in the bowl and let it rise for 1 to 2 hours. It depends on the ambient temperature. Once it has risen, this batter becomes the Master Dough, ready to be used for making loaf, kita or the pizza crust.

The Four Pillars Vegetarian Loaf

1. Take a chunk from the Mater Dough and fill half of a bread pan and spread it evenly.

2. Brush the top of the dough with milk to make the cooked bread shinny.

3. Preheat the oven to 350 degrees and place the pan with the dough inside the oven.

4. Close the door and let it bake for 50-60 minutes. Stick a toothpick into the baking bread to see whether or not it is cooked. If cooked, the toothpick will feel dry. If not, it will feel gooey.

5. When ready, take it out of the oven and let it cool.

6. Cut into slices and serve as part of a lunch or dinner meal. This bread is probably one of the healthiest loaves you could ever have at your table.

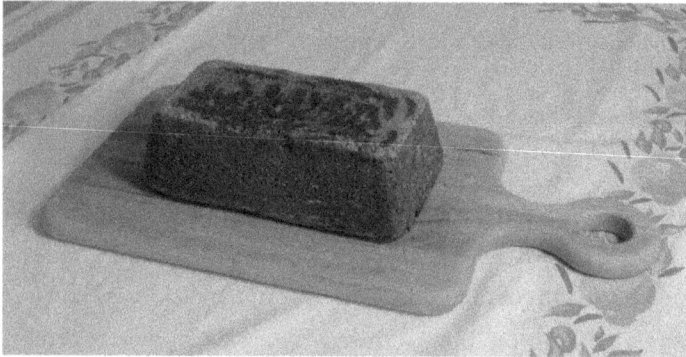

The Four Pillars loaf . . . the world's healthiest bread

Enjoy!

Kita

(Made with the portion of the dough saved from the previous recipe.)

Measurements and ingredients:

1. Preheat a large pan on a cook top and oil its bottom.

2. Take a fistful from the remaining Master Dough and drop it into the pan.

3. Spread it evenly with a spatula or your hand.

4. Bring your four fingers together and curl them to resemble a grub hoe.

5. Pierce the surface of the dough with your fingertips, walking them from one end to the other, until you have completely covered the surface with holes. (See picture next page.)

6. Let it bake for 4 to 5 minutes.

7. Once done remove the kita with a spatula and place on a tray.

8. Brush the top lightly with honey and serve with tea or coffee. Or be creative with it. We sometimes blend fresh garlic, sweet basil, pine nuts, 1 tbsp. of olive oil, making a pesto, and daub the kita surface with it. If you still want be more creative, coat the kita with a thin layer of cottage cheese and top it with the pesto. This is very good!

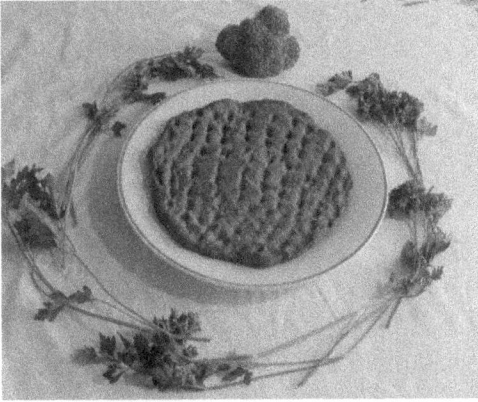

The Four Pillars kita . . . the world's healthiest kita

Enjoy!

The Four Pillars Pizza

Measurements and Ingredients:

1 cup of cottage cheese

1/2 slice of red onion, finely chopped

5 cloves of garlic, minced

7 Brussels sprouts, finely chopped

1/2 green bell pepper, finely chopped

1/2 red bell pepper, chopped

1 stick of celery

1 cup of broccoli, chopped

1 medium tomato, minced

1 tbsp. black pepper

Salt to taste

Directions:

1. Preheat oven to 425°F.

2. Take a fistful from the Master Dough (see page), knead flour on a board for a few minutes and then make a round, flat batter.

3. Oil and dust (with flour) the bottom of a baking pan and place the flattened batter on it.

4. Brush the top of the pizza dough with the olive oil. This helps minimizes from the crust becoming soggy after you layer it with the topings.

5. Add all the ingredients, one at a time, and place the pizza dough with its toppings in the oven and bake for 8 minutes.

6. Take out the pizza, add the cottage cheese in small lumps and put the pizza back in the oven and let it bake for 2 to 3 minutes more.

7. When ready take out, cut in slices and serve hot.

Alternatively:

8. Bake the crust by itself for 5-6 minutes

9. While the crust is baking, sauté the onions, garlic, ginger and Brussels sprouts together for 5 minutes. Take off the heat and transfer to a plate.

10. Next sauté the broccoli, celery, spinach, bell peppers and basil together, remove from heat and set aside.

11. When the crust is done, take it out of the oven and apply a thin layer of the cottage cheese. Top the cheese with all the sautéed ingredients, add the pepper and add salt (to taste), and serve as slice. Very healthy!

12. If you have *niter kibbeh*—spiced, clarified butter (see the Ethiopian recipes section)—sprinkle the pizza top with a little bit of it before serving can make the pizza taste sumptuous.

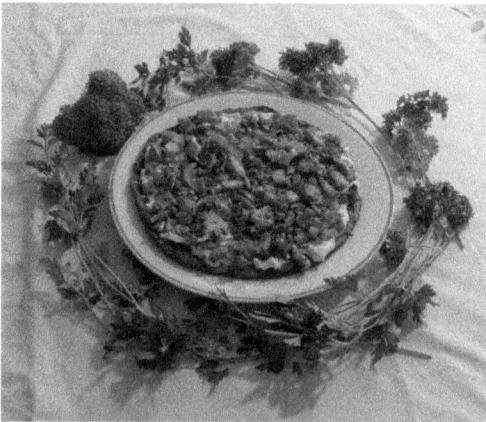

The Four Pillars Pizza . . . the world's healthiest pizza

Enjoy!

The Four Pillars Vegetarian Soup

(Made with the base Four Pillars blend, see above)

The recipe:

1 cup of the Four Pillars base blend

1 cup of cooked lentils

2 sticks of carrot

6-8 mushrooms, sliced and chopped

1 cup of spinach, finely chopped

1 cup of cauliflower, chopped

1/2 cup broccoli, chopped

1/2 cup of onions, 4 cloves of garlic, 1 tsp. of ginger

  sautéed together, then added to the soup

1 medium tomato, sliced and minced

3 dry shiitake mushrooms ground in a blender

  and then added to the soup. It enhances the soup's flavor (optional).

3-1/2 cups of chicken broth and 1 cup of water

Directions:

1. Add the chicken broth and water to a large pot.
2. Throw in the carrots and celery and let cook for 3 minutes.
3. Add the rest of the ingredients and let cook for 5 minutes at medium heat.
4. Remove from heat and serve with the Four Pillars loaf or kita for lunch or dinner.

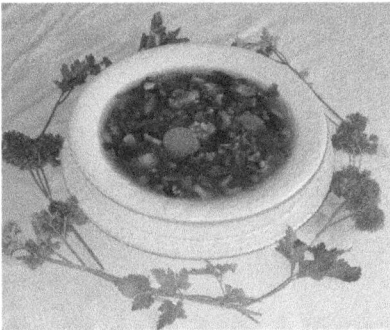

The Four Pillars soup . . . the world's healthiest soup

Enjoy!

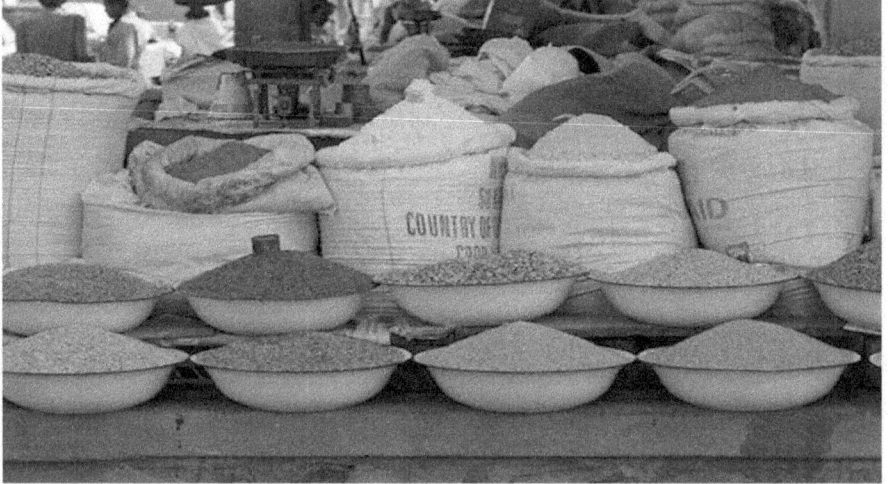

Ingredients that make Ethiopian food tasty and healthy

PART V
The Four Pillars in Ethiopian Foods

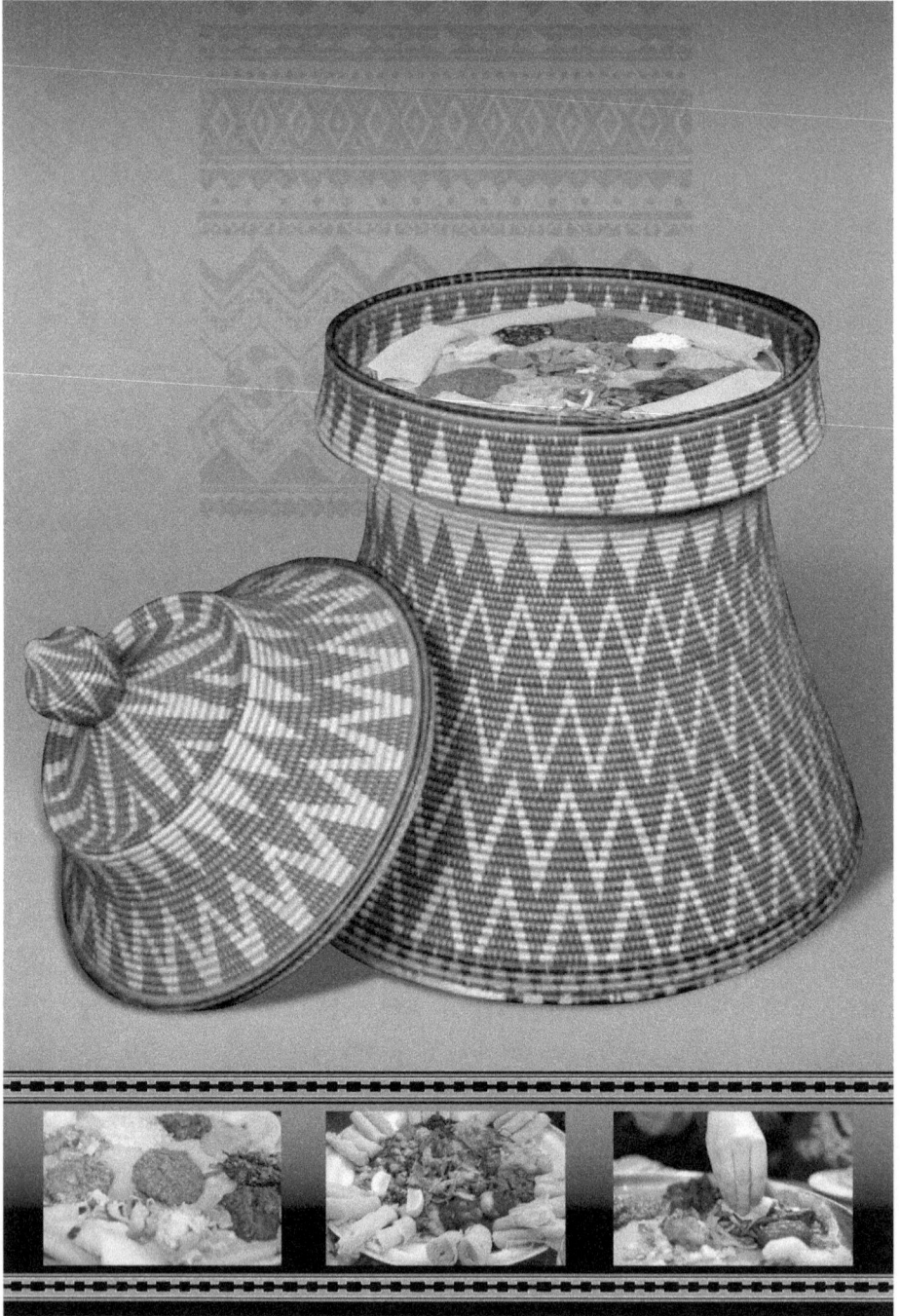

Mesob and assorted Ethiopian dishes

Ethiopian cuisine

An introduction

"Ethiopians slept for a thousand years, forgetful of the world by whom they have been forgotten." So said Edward Gibbon, the noted 18th century British historian, referring to Ethiopia's isolated existence for so many centuries.

Bounded by a scorching desert in the southeast, a deep and wide sea in the north and north-east, rugged terrain in the west, and largely inimical Muslim countries and enclaves all around, Ethiopia had led a slumberous existence, indeed, as far as its engagement with the outside world was concerned. Yes, outsiders had visited Ethiopia at different times, but rarely the other way around. A few Ethiopian emissaries had visited European cities in the late 1800s.

Some who read this quote out of context are bound to believe that Gibbons must have been referring to the country's lack of progress in the thousand years it had slept. That certainly is not the case.

Ethiopia has had progress in all its cultural elements: cuisine, religion, language, music, social customs, and the arts. Let me cite a few examples. The 6th century scholar, Yared, is a cultural icon who developed the educational system, contributed to Ethiopia's literary heritage, and composed much of the church music in use to this day.

Over the hundreds of years, the country has produced a great many artistic and literary works. Unfortunately, much of what was written or produced remained in the hands of the Orthodox Church, impacting the creativity or artistic expression of the average Ethiopian very little. Also, most of the literature was written in *Ge'ez*—an ancient language which only the learned men of the ecclesiastical institutions understood. Secular education was nonexistent until about a hundred years ago. Even after that, though, pursuing education outside of the church schools was considered sacrilegious. In this regard, Gibbon was probably right in his perception of Ethiopia's state of affairs.

Amharic (Ethiopia's national language) is perhaps one of the most sophisticated languages in the world. It has a rich vocabulary. Words can have or be made to have, depending on one's mental acuity, different shades of meaning. Through a system of poetry called *sem-ena worq*—wax and gold, the literal and figurative (or the obvious and hidden) expressions—what appears a compliment can turn out to be actually an insult or criticism. Someone's simple commentary turns out to be an observation on universal truths or wisdom. And like most poetry, it's the gold that often moves the spirit, delights or saddens the heart. This form of expression has evolved over time.

The culinary arts, on the other hand, were a different matter. The Ethiopian woman (yes, food preparation and cooking was the exclusive domain of the female gender) had no constraints. She was limited only by the extent of her talent and imagination. Because of this freedom that the women enjoyed, we have a great variety of some of the most sophisticated dishes in the world.

"Ethiopian women can make as many as seven hundred-fifty or more dishes," one woman once told me.

How?

Spices!

The Ethiopian woman combines many different spices to create dishes as distinctly different from each other as beef stroganoff is from Peking pork chops.

She also uses food preparation techniques such as aging, smoking, and drying to bring out distinct aromas and flavors in foods, and the dishes that are prepared from these ingredients are often succulent, zesty, and healthy.

As researchers around the world are finding out, spices have many beneficial properties. Their antioxidants help protect the body against cancer, heart diseases, diabetes, and other degenerative conditions. The vibrant shades of red, yellow, orange, brown and other colors that are often seen in Ethiopian spices represent their component phytonutrients. These compounds, as discussed under Pillar Four have many wonderful benefits. You can see on the back cover of this book a sample of the spice colors found in Ethiopian foods.

Traditionally, there is no standard recipe book. Nothing is written down. Each family has its own way of making its own dishes, usually inherited from the older generation. Yes, there are a few common ingredients found across the board: onions, garlic, coriander, cloves, cinnamon, etc. What a woman can add beyond these constituents, and their proportions, becomes her propriety.

The most common Ethiopian foods are *injera* and *wot*—sauce. The injera is the *crêpe*-like bread made usually from fermented *teff* flour. Particular to Ethiopia, teff is a small grain which usually comes as either white or brown or a mixture of the two, called *sergegna*. The wot can be made from the flour of legumes—pea, chickpeas, or fava beans—called *shiro*, and meats—chicken, lamb, or beef. It can be mild, middle of the road, or spicy hot. The spiciness depends on whether it was made with *berbere*, which is the foundation of many Ethiopian dishes. See the ingredient list for berbere in the Selected Ethiopian Food Recipe section.

These dishes are what may be referred to as traditional for most country folks; the dishes and how often they are prepared and consumed depends on the economic status of the household. Shiro wot and injera are the most common. Injera by itself or with a*waze*—a paste made from berbere and water—can be all that a poor person has to eat sometimes; at other times, just the injera by itself if they are in a dire situation. For vegetables, *gomen*—collard green and potatoes—are most common.

Nowadays, in cities and towns, a green salad with tomatoes, and mixed vegetables—consisting of cooked potatoes, cabbage, and carrots with homemade cheese on the side—often accompany the main dishes.

Why Ethiopian food is healthy

For those who are careful about what they eat, Ethiopian foods have many attributes that make them appealing.

The spices and herbs used to prepare Ethiopian foods are rich in antioxidants, phytonutrients, vitamins, and minerals. As you have read about these food components earlier in the book, these nutrients are very beneficial to the body.

Ethiopians fast over 200 days out of the year and break their fast only with vegetarian foods. Because of this practice, many Ethiopian cuisines appeal to vegans and also to those whose constitution is sensitive to fats and animal products. Only vegetable oils are used for cooking for the fast foods.

Ethiopians rarely eat sweet foods. Desserts are not common, although now restaurants have begun offering a few selections for those customers who have to have a dessert after their meals. You don't have to worry about loading up on too many sugar calories when you dine at an Ethiopian home or restaurant.

Regarding the absence of sweets in the Ethiopian diet, I'll share a couple of anecdotes. When I went home to visit my family several years ago, I brought with me a few Hershey's chocolate bars, thinking they would be a special treat from America for the neighborhood kids.

A couple of days after I arrived I gathered up the children and gave a chocolate bar to each. They first inspected the wrapped objects and then one by one started to tear the paper off after I urged them to do so. All the children held the bare bars and stared at them, unsure of what they should do, even after I told them what they were, emphasizing how delicious they were. To allay their concerns, I peeled off the wrapping from my own bar and started to munch on it.

One brave soul placed the end of his bar into his mouth and took a bite. Seconds later, his face went sour. His lips twisted. "Ughhh." He immediately turned his head away and spat it out. Others took a bite of their bars, sank their teeth into them, but just as quickly their expressions also went sour, and they, too, spat their bites out. After I calmed down from hearty laughter, I asked each what it was they didn't like. They all said the candy was too sweet.

The other testament about the excessively sweet American diet concerns my own experience with dental caries. I had never had cavities before I came to the United States at 19 years of age, but within six month of my arrival, I got two of them.

The only time white sugar is used in Ethiopia is with tea or coffee. Even this practice is a recent phenomenon. Where I grew up, we either drank our coffee without any sweeteners or with fragments of a salt bar. Sugar was just not available to folks who lived in remote places.

The low calorie, low fat diet, together with the use of spices and herbs in food preparation are major factors why Ethiopians, on the whole, are healthy people. Obesity, heart disease, cancer, and diabetes are almost unheard of. With the introduction of Western-type diets, however, the health picture of the population is bound to change for the worse in due time. In the cities this is happening already. And Ethiopians who live in Western societies have been getting these food-related diseases in greater numbers. For example, one study of the Ethiopian community in Israel found "within just a decade a relatively high prevalence of diabetes (10 to 17%), which was literally unknown to it prior to (their) immigration."

Ethiopians don't use processed or frozen foods. These things are a product of modern technology. To taste good and wholesome, the foods have to be prepared fresh from whole grains and vegetables. However, because pure teff flour is sometimes finicky to turn into good injera in the Unites States, some restaurants may constitute the teff dough with white wheat flour. Temperature, humidity, baking temperature and even altitude can affect the fermenting dough from which injera is made.

Ethiopian foods have a good amount of fiber—teff, as you will see later, contains a great amount of roughage, providing you one of the four pillars of health.

This book is to serve the reader primarily as an educational tool. Although I have included recipes for foods, it's not meant to be used as a major reference source for a wide range of dishes. There are other books for that and I've included the titles of a couple as well as links to web sites at the end. This book is about the benefits of the most common ingredients found in Ethiopian dishes.

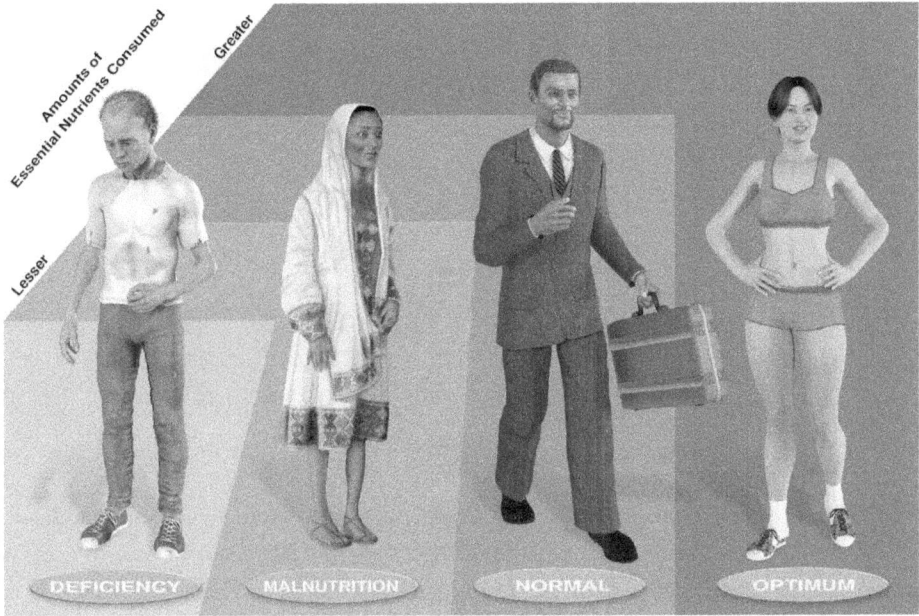

White sugar, white flour, soft drinks   Teff, Mitten Shiro, Berbere, 4 Pillars Foods & Drinks

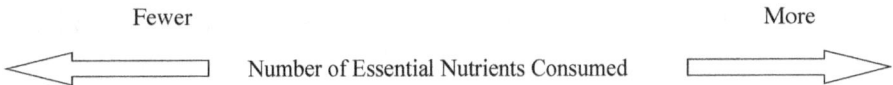

Fewer   More

Number of Essential Nutrients Consumed

Nutrition Continuum

This nutrition continuum illustrates the four possible levels of nutrition and serves as a model that accommodates individual differences and nutritional need variabilities among humans.

CHAPTER 14
Teff

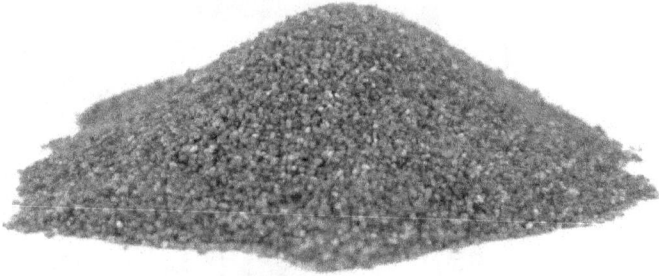

Teff is a highly nutritious grain that has been cultivated in the highlands of Ethiopia starting sometime between 1000 B.C and 4000 B.C. Now it's also grown in the United States and Australia, and probably in other countries as well. It's a tiny grain—150 granules of teff is equivalent to one kernel of wheat—yet, nutritionally, as you will see below, teff offers so much. Teff comes in many different varieties, but the most common are brown and carmine red. The white variety is more expensive than the others but in the homes of well-to-do families in Ethiopia, it's the most desired. Nutritionally, though, the brown and red varieties offer much more than the white teff.

Teff is a very good source of protein, including some of the essential amino acids that one usually finds in animal products like whey or eggs. Reportedly, a 2-ounce serving of teff can contain as many as 7 grams of protein, which is equivalent to that found in an extra-large egg. It's said that daily consumption of one injera crêpe supplies enough of the amino acids to sustain life without another protein source. This explains why many Ethiopians who don't consume milk or eggs or meat during fasting or even non-fasting times, show no sign of nutritional deficiency.

Furthermore, a cup of teff can provide 14.7 mg or 82% of the daily value (DV) of iron and 347 mg or 35% DV of calcium. Reportedly the iron from teff is better absorbed than that found in other grains. Teff therefore can be good for menstruating women or anybody who doesn't get sufficient iron from their normal diet.

That same cup of teff can contain up to 356 mg or 89% DV of magnesium and 828 mg or 83% DV of potassium. And it has a whopping 17.8 mg or 892% DV of manganese. This quantity of teff also contains high amounts of copper and zinc—78% and 47% of DV, respectively, and smaller amounts of selenium and sodium. A cup of teff provides 16 grams of fiber.

Vitamin-wise, this same cup of teff was found to contain between 30% and 50% DV for thiamin, riboflavin, niacin, and Vitamin B6. Interestingly, we also expect to find 261 mg of omega-3 fatty acids and 1807 mg of omega-6 fatty acids. These fatty acids, as you saw earlier, are very important for good health and vitality.

Teff has a low glycemic index, only 84. Twenty to forty percent of the carbohydrate contained in teff is resistant starch, meaning that much of the carbohydrate is not available to the body. Both these attributes should be appealing to diabetics and those who wish to lose or manage weight. Teff is gluten free, which make it a desirable food for people who are sensitive to gluten (a form of protein found in wheat, barley, and rye), a condition referred to as celiac disease. When people with celiac disease consume foods that have gluten, their body mounts an immune response that attacks the small intestine. These attacks disrupt the normal absorption of nutrients into the body.

One writer described the white teff as having a chestnut-like flavor and the brown, a slight taste of hazelnut. I'd describe the white as somewhat nutty and the brown as slightly tart and sweet.

You should now see why teff is indeed such a remarkable grain. In the years I have been reading and writing about nutrition, I often wonder about the good health of my family from Ethiopian highlands, where there are no fruits or vegetables, which are normally the good sources of vitamins, minerals, phytonutrients, and fiber. Yet these people seem healthy and fit. All this has to do with the four pillars of health they find in teff, and in the peppers and spices. Nearly all of them are lean because they work hard and walk a lot.

How you prepare and consume teff

Traditionally, the teff dough is fermented to make injera. Because certain vitamins are produced during the fermentation process, the nutritional value of the food is enhanced during this process.

Ethiopians generally use teff flour. You can use the whole teff with soups, cereals, and other such dishes. Even then, you will be better served if you use teff flour. You shouldn't try to make flour by grinding whole teff in your blender or coffee grinder. The grains are way too small for these machines. It's better if you purchase teff flour at a health food store or an Ethiopian market and use it to make bread by itself or to replace a quarter to a third of the wheat flour you use to make loaves, cakes, and other bread products. You can also make porridge out of teff flour: sprinkle it with berbere or salt and red pepper powder (to taste), and serve.

In a recipe, if you're substituting teff for nuts, other grains, or seeds, use only half as much teff as the full measure of the item you're replacing, because the teff granule is so small.

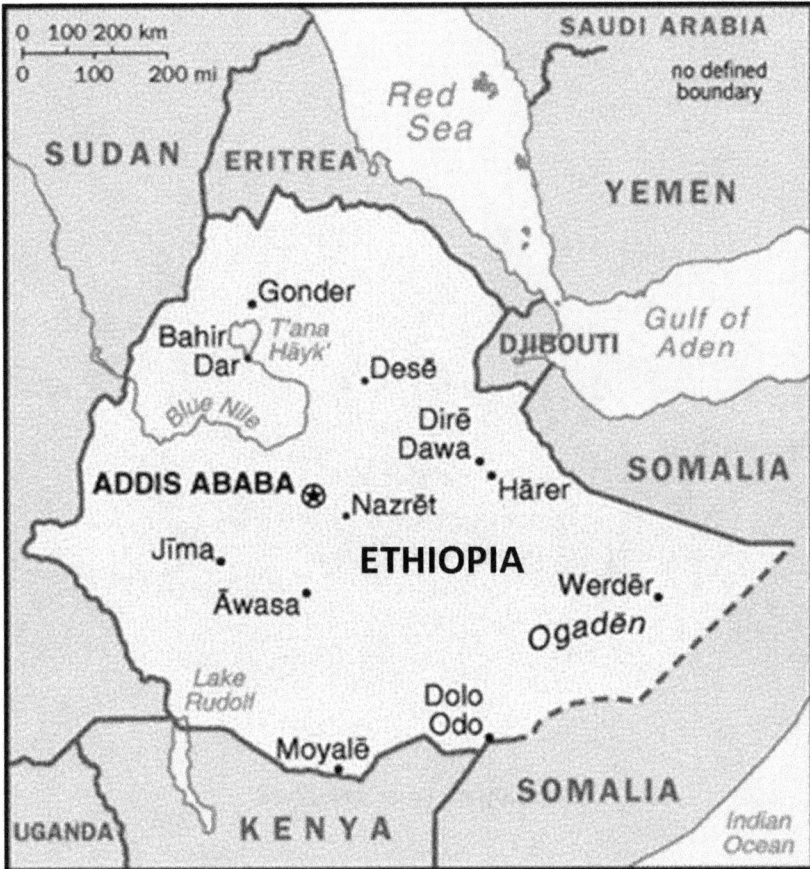

An ancient country, rich with history and traditions,
the birthplace of coffee, teff and many flavorful and healthy foods.

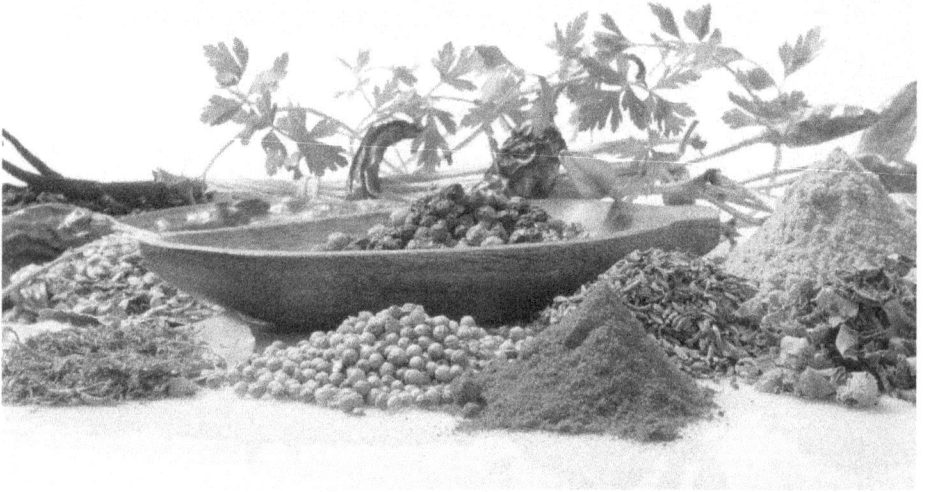

Ethiopian spice samplers

Ethiopian spices

Chapter 15
Abesh (Fenugreek)

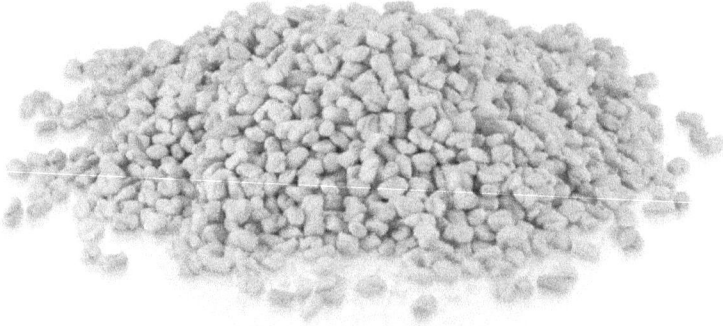

Abesh is one of the main ingredients in many Ethiopian spice formulations. By itself it's used to flavor injera, and as part of other spices, wot and other dishes. As you will see below it's also often made into a drink.

Like all the spices we use in our foods, most people may think that abesh's role in dishes is merely as a food-flavoring agent and a beverage. As you will soon see, abesh actually has many benefits for your health, good looks, and longevity. The great flavor you're trying to impart to your dish by including abesh and other ingredients in it is only part of the full story.

First, let me just say that abesh seeds have intrigued me since I was a boy. A groove runs nearly diagonal across its rectangular slab-like shape. A hook drops down onto one edge of the seed, which used to remind me of a bird's beak. The seeds appear neither true gold nor yellow but somewhere in between, with a texture of marble.

These seeds are rock-hard to chew on and taste bitter if you manage to crack one of them. As if to make up for the deficiency in taste, though, they smell somewhat sweet. I often wondered what the deal was with abesh, that my mother always included them in her spice concoctions. Now, from the studies I have done, I know that abesh's hardened exterior and unpleasant taste are only a facade. These golden-yellow seeds, which Westerners call Fenugreek, have many health benefits.

Abesh grows worldwide in semi-arid regions such as the Mediterranean, western Asia, northern Africa, the Middle East, and in the United States. The plant grows 1-2 feet tall and its pale green leaves come in three parts, like clover. Near the base of the leaves' long pods shoot out, each containing 10-20 seeds.

Abesh is an intriguing plant that has a multi-faceted, if paradoxical, aspect. Here is a more or less complete list.

1. In the literature, the seeds are described as smelling like maple syrup, celery, or burnt sugar. Yet their taste is bitter and unappealing. Roasting can usually soften the edge of the unpleasant flavor.

2. Abesh can be used as an herb (leaves) or a spice (seeds).

3. The fresh leaves are mild and pleasant, the dried ones are bitter.

4. Abesh has all the characteristic of a legume—it's rich in fiber and protein—but it's treated like a spice.

5. Abesh is probably one of the few spices that contains all four pillars of health—vitamins, minerals, phytonutrients, and fiber.

6. Like many spices and herbs, abesh has a long history of use as both a culinary and medicinal plant since ancient times. It was one of the spices that ancient Egyptians used to embalm mummies and one of the items found in King Tut's tomb. Ancient Greeks and Romans had a less lofty yet practical use for the plant: they fed it to their cattle.

The benefits of abesh

Let's see what abesh hides behind its hard seeds and bitter taste. As I mentioned above, abesh contains a variety of nutrients, phytochemicals, and fiber. It's these constituents that make it beneficial to the body.

Internal benefits

In one human study, abesh was found to lower the bad cholesterol (LDL) and sugar levels in the blood. This study was done with persons who had type-2, non-insulin dependent diabetes. In another controlled, double-blind trial, researchers found that Fenugreek lowered elevated cholesterol and triglyceride levels in patients who had type-1, insulin-dependent diabetes.

Here is list of internal benefits attributed to abesh:

Managing cholesterol Abesh seeds contain alkaloids and steroidal saponins (soap-like substances), which are believed to inhibit cholesterol synthesis and absorption from the digestive tract. The fibers in abesh can help purge excess cholesterol, fat, and sugar as the spice's bulk goes through the GI (gastro-intestinal) tract. It's also been discovered that an amino acid compound called 4-hydroxy isoleucine found in abesh seeds increases the production of insulin in the body. For this reason, abesh is often included in the diet of diabetics. Abesh does not affect the good (HDL) cholesterol.

An associated benefit is that this spice can also help reduce high blood pressure and the risk of heart disease.

Heart burn/acid reflux If you suffer from this condition, soak abesh in warm water overnight then take a teaspoon of it with your meal. The mucilage (water soluble fiber) coats the lining of the stomach, thereby soothing and minimizing the problem.

Manage or lose weight Galactomannan is the name of the soluble fiber found in abesh. This substance, when soaked, absorbs water and swells up. The same thing happens in the GI tract when abesh is consumed, making the person feel full and causing him or her to eat less. This effect should allow a person to lose weight over time.

Good remedy for sore throat Drink a warm solution of abesh, honey, and lemon and this should help sooth your sore throat.

Eliminate excess fat, sugar, and toxins The high mucilage content of abesh should help purge any excessive and harmful substances from the GI tract. For example, 100 grams of abesh seed provides 24.6 grams or 65% of the recommended daily fiber intake.

The non-starch polysaccharides found in abesh include saponins, mucilage, tannin, pectin, and hemicellulose. It's these compounds that remove cholesterol and excess sugar and toxins from the body, thereby protecting the colon from cancer.

For your skin and hair Abesh, when used as a pack and applied on the face and elsewhere on the body, is thought to help lessen blackheads and pimples and reduce lines and wrinkles. You can wash the skin and hair with water that contains abesh soaked overnight. Alternatively, you can use an abesh paste both on the hair and face. Leave it on for 10-15 minutes and then wash off. Abesh boiled in coconut oil, cooled, and applied to the scalp is supposed to help with thinning hair.

For women issues Abesh is known to reduce menstrual discomfort, help induce labor, and increase milk production in lactating women. This spice is also known to increase breast size, help with hot flashes, increase libido, and reduce the vaginal dryness associated with menopause.

For men issues Abesh is a known natural aphrodisiac. It is supposed to increase sexual desire, virility, and performance. The sexual benefits are derived from the phytochemicals found in the abesh seeds, which convert into sex hormones in our bodies. And there are a great number of these chemicals in abesh.

Abesh is a rich source of copper, magnesium, calcium, iron, selenium, zinc, and manganese.

It's also a good source of potassium, which is an antagonistic partner with sodium in the body fluids and helps regulate heart rate and blood pressure. Abesh contains a good number of vitamins, including Vitamin B6, thiamin, folic acid, niacin, riboflavin, Vitamin A, and Vitamin C. These nutrients, along with phytochemicals and fiber, work as synergistic Four Pillars partners to keep your body at optimum health.

You can drink ground abesh mixed with water and honey added to taste, or soak the whole seed in water overnight and drink the resulting gelatinous mixture. You can apply a warm poultice (bandage) of the spice over eczema or irritated skin to find relief and sooth the area.

For tea preparation: add 7 tablespoons of abesh seeds to 4 cups of boiling water and let steep for about 20 minutes. Filter, add honey or sugar and drink.

In Ethiopia it's the flour that's commonly used to make a drink. For this purpose, abesh flour is poured slowly onto water and allowed to steep overnight. This practice is to remove the spice's bitterness. In the morning, the liquid is drained carefully and the residue beaten for several minutes by adding water and sugar or honey alternatively. The resulting beverage is considered very healthy and nourishing and is often drunk during the long fasting days.

I hope the next time you make your abesh drink or use it as a flavoring agent in foods, you keep its many benefits in mind.

Caveat: Abesh can cause the release of a distinct body odor in sweat or urine.

CHAPTER 16
Allspice

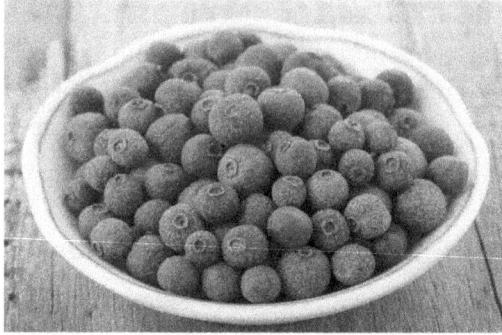

Allspice, also called Jamaica pepper, pimento, English pepper, to mention a few of the names it's known by, is from the *Pimenta dioica* tree native to southern Mexico, and Central America. Now it also grows in many countries where the climate is warm. It was named allspice by the English in the early sixteen hundreds because they thought it contained the combined flavor of cloves, cinnamon and nutmeg.

The allspice fruit is picked while it's still green and traditionally dried in the sun. This causes the outer skin to shrivel like prunes. In fact, they resemble the larger version of black pepper when they dry, which also goes through the same process. The leaves are used sometimes as an infusion into sauces, but they are removed before serving. Both the wood and leaves are often used to smoke and impart flavor to meats.

Allspice is a regular ingredient in Caribbean dishes, and in *moles* (pronounced molaye)—a common Mexican cuisine made with red chilies, almond, peanuts, cinnamon and chicken. In India and elsewhere, allspice is also found in curries, in pickled foods, and in the Middle East, in stews and meat dishes. In the United States and many European countries, allspice is mostly found in desserts and commercial sausages.

In Ethiopian cooking, allspice is found in berbere and meklesha (see recipe pages). When ground, allspice does live out its namesake. It gives off the combined aroma of cloves, cinnamon and nutmeg.

Allspice's essential oils—eugenol and a class of compounds called, phenyl-propanoids—have had many medicinal uses. These compounds and others are responsible for the medley of aromas found in allspice. When used as tea, allspice is known to help with excessive gas in the GI tract, and with indigestion problems as well as serving as tonic to the overall health of the body. It's also known to aid with circulation.

This exotic herb of the Americas reportedly brings relief to muscle aches and pains, fights infection and helps normalize blood sugar (important for diabetics). It's also known to have antifungal, anti-microbial and anti-inflammatory properties. As antioxidants, the compounds of allspice may help with heart health, fight cancer and slow the aging of our bodies. Furthermore, in Ayurvedic medicine, allspice is used to treat colds, diarrhea, hysterical paroxysms and fatigue as well as in muscle and joint pains. For tooth aches allspice can have a numbing effect.

Finally, all spice also contains a number of minerals and vitamins, which add to its nutritional value.

CHAPTER 17
Beso Bela (Sacred Basil)

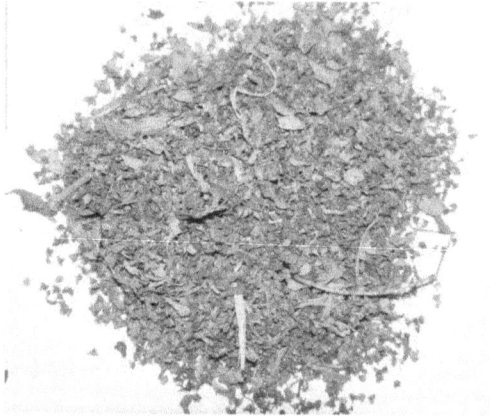

Beso bela was one of the perennial herbs in my mother's garden. It has a beautiful aroma, close to sweet basil, but beso bela is more refined and delicate. Just about every Ethiopian dish worth its salt has to have beso bela—the leaves, flowers, and seeds are used. It's in berbere, mitmita, and is a crucial component of the herbs used to impart aroma and taste to *niter kibbeh*—clarified butter.

Beso bela's stems are often straight and hardy and snap like kindling when you break them. Small, parchment-like pink blossoms grow at discrete points along the top portion of closely grown stems, making them appear like a collection of minarets. The leaves are hairy and grow out of the stems at discreet points, too, like shelves.

In Ethiopia, beso bela is revered for its aroma and flavor but in India, it's venerated for its holiness. Just about every Hindu home has a shrine built outside for the plant and they worship it every morning. They call the plant *Tulsi*—meaning The Incomparable One. This plant symbolizes the goddess Lakshmi, wife of Vishnu, one of India's important deities. Beyond beso bela's association with Hindu's divinity, it has also been esteemed for its power, as one writer puts it, to heal "the body, mind and spirit."

Beso bela's healing properties

In Ayurvedic medicine—a traditional Hindu system of medicinal treatment—beso bela has been used as a remedy for a number of ailments, including the common cold, fevers, respiratory disorders, sore throats, and kidney stones. As part of cough syrup, it helps remove mucus and relieve congestion. Drinking a decoction of the herb with honey and ginger is an effective preparation for bronchitis, asthma, and influenza. Furthermore, this holy herb has been used to heal ulcers and infections of the mouth, skin disorders such as ringworms, dermatitis, and loss of pigment, headaches, stress, sore eyes, and digestive disorders.

While many of these claims come out the traditional practices, modern science has also begun exploring beso bela's health benefits. A number of researchers believe that the herb indeed has great promise. For example, in one study, diabetic rats fed powdered beso bela leaves showed a significant drop in serum sugar as well as triglycerides and the LDL (bad) cholesterol levels, while at the same time substantially increasing the HDL (good) cholesterol level. Whether this result is transferable to human subjects is not known, however.

In another experiment, beso bela was tested for whether it helped to manage stress. In 1991 an animal study was published in the *Indian Journal of Pharmacology* where scientists showed that beso bela does indeed work in managing stress. In fact, it was more effective in treating stress than Asian ginseng and Siberian ginseng—both known remedies for the bodily condition.

A 2011 randomized, double-blind, placebo-controlled study on humans showed that beso bela was found 1.6 times or 39% more effective in the management of stress symptoms compared to the placebo group. And beso bela supplements, according to the study, were tolerated by all patients for the duration of the experiment.

We all experience stress in our lives. In fact, biologically, it's an important and necessary component of life. It causes us to react—to stop and fight or flee in time of danger, or when we're called upon to perform at our best—like studying for an exam or working on a project. There is also the type of stress where what's demanded of us is beyond our ability to cope. It can be an everyday traffic jam, a bad relationship with a boss or significant other, or any other challenge or hardship we might be going through.

When we are stressed, our body produces a number of hormones (cortisol, adrenaline, corticosterone, catecholamines, and others). If you need to flee from danger or your body is called upon to function at its best, these hormones are fine, but when they are released chronically, day after day, they can become toxic to our body. In these kinds of situations, our immune system can be weakened, our blood sugar can be out of whack, our body age faster, and we can become depressed. To cope with the problem, some people may resort to overeating or drinking or using drugs.

Those who practice herbal medicine have identified certain plants that can help the body cope or adapt to stressful situations. One of these plants is beso bela. It is used as a tonic—to enhance the overall health and function of the body, and as an adaptogen—enabling the body to adapt and thrive under physical and emotional stress. The phytochemicals eugenol and caryophyllene found in beso bela help normalize the stress hormone levels in the body and assist the person to cope and thrive in demanding situations. These aromatic essential oils reportedly "elevate both mood and spirit . . . and help combat stress," as one writer put it.

Beso bela contains many phenolic bioflavonoids, carotenoids, vitamin A, and other compounds that fight the oxygen and hydroxyl free radicals (see Appendix A), which are some of the deadliest chemical elements, contributing to the aging of our bodies and making us susceptible to cancer and heart disease.

In addition, beso bela comprises other essential oil compounds that were found to be anti-inflammatory, anti-fungal, anti-viral, and anti-bacterial.

This wonderful plant has vitamins A and C and K, and minerals such as zinc, iron, calcium, iron, and manganese.

The point of all this discussion is for you to realize that spices like beso bela and others you use in food preparations are not just for aroma and flavor. They can have many health benefits as well.

CHAPTER 18
Dimbilal (Coriandor)

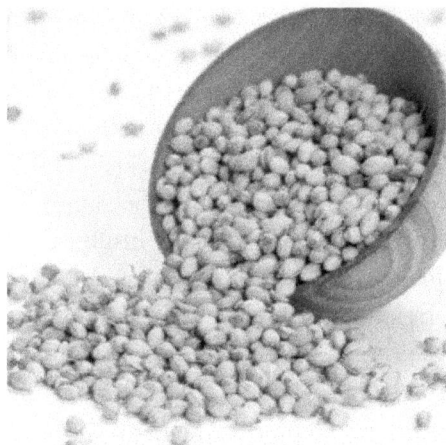

Dimbilal, or coriander as it's called in English, is one of the staple spices in Ethiopian cooking. It's one of the spices that make up berbere, shiro, niter kibbeh. Wonderfully aromatic, if you're accustomed to it, ground dimbilal can be added to stews and soups and even used in the making of breads. Although ground dimbilal is now readily available, when I was growing up, my mother always bought the pods and cracked them open to get to the two seeds. She often powdered them and combined them with other ingredients to make berbere.

Nobody knows when dimbilal came to Ethiopia but it's one of the oldest spices, which traces back to 5000 B.C. Its history is rooted in the countries of southern Europe, northern Africa, and southwestern Asia. Dimbilal is mentioned in the Bible and was found in the burial chambers of some of the pharaohs of Egypt. In ancient Greece, it was valued for its medicinal properties as much as for its culinary functions.

For those of us who live in North America, dimbilal has two different names. I'll clarify here for Ethiopians who may not be familiar. The European Spanish term for coriander is cilantro. In North America, however, particularly in Mexico, cilantro generally refers to the leaves. The Mexicans refer to the seed as *semilla* (pronounced, sey-me-ya) *de cilantro*—the seed of cilantro. In the English-speaking world, coriander refers strictly to the seeds.

In ancient cultures (even in some parts of the world at present) dimbilal was valued for its medicinal properties as much as for its benefit in food seasoning. Now modern science has identified the real benefits of dimbilal's volatile oils and aromatic substances.

In January 2011, the *Indian Journal of Experimental Biology* reported that diabetic laboratory animals fed dimbilal powder showed a significant drop in the blood sugar level while there was an increase in the insulin level. The researchers also noted a higher level of antioxidant activity in the tissues of these animals. In research done by Islamic Azad University of Iran and published in the March 2009 issue of *Phytotherapy Research*, lab animals fed dimbilal seed extract showed a drop in blood sugar and increased levels of insulin production. Although we cannot say that these findings apply to humans as well, the fact that these research-ers found a definite correlation between the consumption of dimbilal seeds and a drop in blood sugar is a good indication that humans can potentially benefit from including dimbilal in their diet.

Dimbilal also reduced the bad cholesterol and triglyceride levels in the blood, which means regular consumption of this spice, can potentially help with the health of the heart and the blood vessels. Additionally, Dimbilal was found to sooth inflammations, and to improve the health of the nervous system and the digestive tract. Dimbilal's antioxidant compounds are also believed to help with the health of the eyes, particularly with conjunctivitis (pink eye) and macular degeneration.

Traditionally, dimbilal has likewise been used to treat nausea, seasonal fever, stomach problems, vomiting, bed cold, rheumatism, and joint pain. Dimbilal seed oil has been used as an analgesic (substance that relieves pain) and for its fungicidal and anti-bacterial properties, as a deodorant, and even as an aphro-disiac. Speaking of dimbilal's antibacterial property, it is supposed to be one of the better natural treatments for Salmonella poisoning, and for diarrhea caused by fungal infection.

All these benefits come from dimbilal's many essential volatile oils and antioxi-dant compounds. Its leaves can be good natural cleansing agents as well.

Dimbilal's leaves and seeds are good sources of vitamins and minerals, fiber (especially the leaves), and phytonutrients. A bunch of home-grown dimbilal leaves can reportedly offer 225% and 258% of the daily allowances of Vitamin A and Vitamin K , respectively. Regarding minerals, dimbilal contains good amounts of potassium, calcium, manganese, iron, and magnesium.

For some of the benefits mentioned above, you can blend dimbilal leaves and/ or seeds in water and drink or boil them in water and drink as tea. We blend ours along with the Four Pillar fruits and vegetables. The rich flavor, aroma, and nutrients found in dimbilal can help you to lead a healthy and happy life. How about this: if you can go along with the Chinese belief, dimbilal may even endow you with immortality.

Bon appetit!

CHAPTER 19
Inslal (Anise)

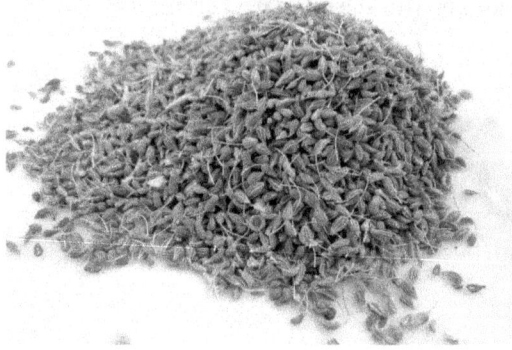

Inslal was the other herb in my mother's garden. She used the delicate green branches and fuzzy, cattail-like leaves mostly to enhance the flavor/aroma of *areqee*—homemade whiskey. She also boiled the leaves in water to drink as tea to lessen the effect of a cold. I think she also added a small amount inslal seeds in some of her bread recipes as well as in her stews.

Outside of Ethiopia, anise traditionally has been used as a remedy for asthma, bronchitis, cold-related congestion of the chest and throat, and disorders of the digestive tract, such as bloating, flatulence, nausea, and dyspepsia.

Anise has moreover been used to stimulate appetite and promote digestion. The herb does this by stimulating the production of enzymes and digestive juices. To take advantage this herb's benefits, people customarily chew anise seeds, drink hot anise tea, and eat appetizers or desserts made with anise seeds.

Anise's essential oils have both sedative (in high doses) and stimulatory (in low doses) effects. This dose-dependent property of the herb's oils has found uses in the treatment of epileptic and hysteric attacks, and by those who suffer from spells of anxiety, anger, and insomnia. Anise can have a tranquilizing effect on these persons. Those who are in low spirits for whatever reason can be helped if they take a concentrated anise tea or drink water containing two or three drops of the herb's essential oils. Anise can similarly improve circulation and increase blood flow in the remote tissues. This means that people who are diabetic, rheumatic, and arthritic can find relief by increased blood circulation.

Anise has also been used as diuretic, allowing the body to remove toxins and fluid build-up from the tissues.

Additionally, this sweet and fragrant herb has had varied uses by women: to increase milk production and flow while nursing, to kick-start menstruation, to alleviate the pain and discomfort associated with menstruation, and as an aphrodisiac.

The essential oils in anise have antibacterial, antispasmodic, and purgative properties. This means if you have wounds, scabies, or even lice, drops of the herb's oils can protect the affected areas and speed up their healing. If you have excessive contraction of the respiratory tract, blood vessels, nerves, muscles, or even internal organs that turn into cramps and convulsions and similar symptoms, anise oil can be a good palliative and anti-spasmodic agent for these conditions.

Anise oil's purgative or carminative benefits come from the herb's ability to minimize bloating and remove gas from the GI tract. For those who suffer from pain and cramps associated with excessive gas build-up, an herbal remedy like anise seeds can be a welcome source of relief.

Anise seeds contain a number of phytochemicals, predominant among which is anethole, a volatile essential oil that gives anise its aroma and flavor. The seeds are also rich in B-complex vitamins and a great many minerals. From reading the earlier chapters you know how important these nutrients are to the body's proper day-to-day functioning as well as long-term health. Herbs and spices are important sources of these key components of wellness.

Anise has traditionally been used, in many different cultures, to flavor various dishes and alcoholic beverages. Anise is found in Anisette (most Mediterranean countries), Arak (the traditional alcoholic beverage of many Middle Eastern countries), Raki (Turkey), Ouzo (Greece), Mastika (Balkans), Patis (France), Absinthe (originally from Switzerland, but now available throughout Europe), Sambuca (Italy), Xtabentún (Mexico), and others.

Nowadays, anise is also used in dairy products, candies, meats, and gelatins. It's likewise used in creams, soaps, perfumes, and sachets.

Do you want to have fresh and pleasant breath? Chew a few anise seeds before you go out.

To get anise's many benefits, boil 2-3 tablespoons of the seeds in 3 cups of water for 3 minutes. Let it cool and then blend. Filter the liquid with a fine mesh sieve or cheesecloth, and serve with ice cubes. Alternatively, you can also consume it as a hot drink. You can be creative with anise seeds. People often add it to breads, soups, sauces, cookies, and other foods. We do, too.

Anise's other benefits: A cloth soaked in a tincture of anise can be used as a compress to sooth the eyes, to treat scabies, psoriasis and lice.

Caveat: very high doses of anise oil can slow down circulation and respiration, and can cause vomiting, pulmonary edema, and seizures. Anise can be poisonous to small animals and even to children in high amounts. Pregnant women should not consume excessive levels of the herb. Anise can cause an allergic reaction to skin and some internal organs such as the respiratory and GI tracts.

CHAPTER 20
Ird (Turmeric)

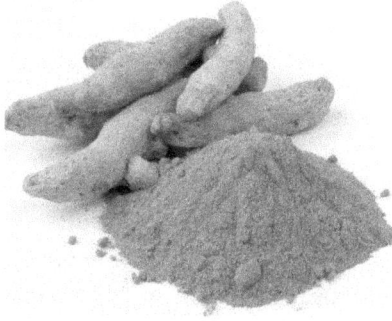

This pile of golden flour (for those who are reading this book with color digital devices) doesn't come from dried and powdered Maskel daisies, the fruit of mangos or papaws, or from bell peppers of the same hue. The sun has no direct hand in its creation, unlike all the other colorful phytonutrients synthesized in leaves and petals or within the flesh of fruits and vegetables. It comes from the turmeric plant's finger-like underground stems (shown above), which are similar in growth to ginger, kratchai, and glangal.

Turmeric (also known as *curcuma longa*) is a spice native to India, where it's been used for 4000 years, as a condiment and medicine, and for certain ceremonial events. Now turmeric is widely grown in nearly all Southeast Asian countries and other tropical places. Its uses—both as spice and medicine—have been exported to other countries over the past several centuries.

Turmeric was introduced to China around 700 A.D., to Ethiopia and the rest of eastern Africa around 800 A.D., and from the 1200s A.D onward to eastern Africa and Europe.

Traditionally, in India, China, and most other Asian countries, turmeric is used as a food flavoring and color agent, as a dye for fabrics, and as medicine to treat the body for a number of ailments and diseases.

Curry, the most famous of the Indian spices, is partly turmeric—it imparts the deep orange color and heady smell to the condiment. The other components are ground coriander, cumin, abesh (fenugreek), ginger, mustard, cinnamon, and black pepper. In many of these countries, turmeric also has much religious and cultural significance.

In Hinduism, turmeric powder is a symbol of purity of mind and spirit as well as one's inner pride and security. For many, the herb also signifies fertility, prosperity, chastity, and sensuality. For all these reasons, worshipers often anoint their sacred images with turmeric paste.

Similarly, in Buddhism, yellow is tied to generosity, prosperity, and purity—this is the reason Buddhist monks wear robes dyed deep orange. Because of turmeric's association with fertility and good luck, Hindus and Buddhists use it in religious and wedding ceremonies.

Equally significant is turmeric's long-time use to treat and heal the body. Traditionally, turmeric has been used to relieve arthritis, dissolve gallstones, treat bloating, and as tonic to improve the overall health of the body. Furthermore, turmeric has been used to alleviate or heal asthma, allergies, rheumatism, diabetic wounds, runny nose, cough, and sinusitis.

In many Asian countries, turmeric is used as a disinfectant for burns, cuts, and bruises. When applied as a paste, turmeric can be effective in treating these conditions and in enhancing the appearance of the skin. Many cosmetics companies now use turmeric in the manufacture of their products.

The science behind the traditional uses of turmeric

Out of its traditional uses came the discovery that turmeric indeed has many healthful properties. Hundreds of research studies have been done on the benefit of turmeric to human health. In test tube studies and lab animal models as well as on humans, turmeric has been found to treat chronic inflammation of the colon or large intestine (a condition known as ulcerative colitis), chronic disease of the air passages, asthma, and rheumatoid arthritis, to name but just a few.

In other studies, turmeric was found to help fight cancer of the colon, skin, pancreas, blood (childhood leukemia), and liver. Similarly, there have been studies documenting the benefit of the spice on psoriasis, Alzheimer's disease, arthritis, and even depression. These findings have not been without controversy, however. Because some of the experiments were in test tube and animal models, there are those who suggest that what worked in a lab and in animals may not work when applied to human subjects.

What contributes to turmeric's beneficial properties?

So far, more than 100 compounds have been isolated from turmeric, including the main coloring agents, volatile oils known as turmerone and curcuminoids. Of all these, curcumin is the most studied. Turmeric's anti-cancer property comes largely from this chemical and its relatives' antioxidants. As you may have read earlier in the book (more in Appendix A), antioxidants help neutralize free radicals, which are believed to be one of the main causes of cancers. The other antioxidants found in Turmeric are vitamins C and E and several carotenoids.

Curcumin moreover has the capacity to neutralize cancer-causing substances and in stopping mutated cells from turning cancerous. This compound is good for the heart. As an antiviral, curcumin can help speed up the healing of wounds.

How to use turmeric

In Ethiopia turmeric is used to color foods and as a part of spice blends. You can increase your intake of turmeric by adding it to meat stews and even shiro wot.

I'll leave it up to your ingenuity to determine how much of the spice you want to add to the different dishes. The key is to make sure that the additional turmeric doesn't lessen or exaggerate the flavor of the other ingredients. You can add turmeric to rice, lentils, *nifro* (a cooked mixture of wheat berries and legumes), egg salad, and other dishes that don't already have spices in them. One writer recommends adding turmeric to sautéed apples, steamed cauliflower, and green beans and onions. She also suggests mixing brown rice with raisins and cashews and seasoning them with turmeric, cumin, and coriander.

Turmeric has no known toxicity.

Enjoy!

CHAPTER 21
Kewrerima (False Cardamom)

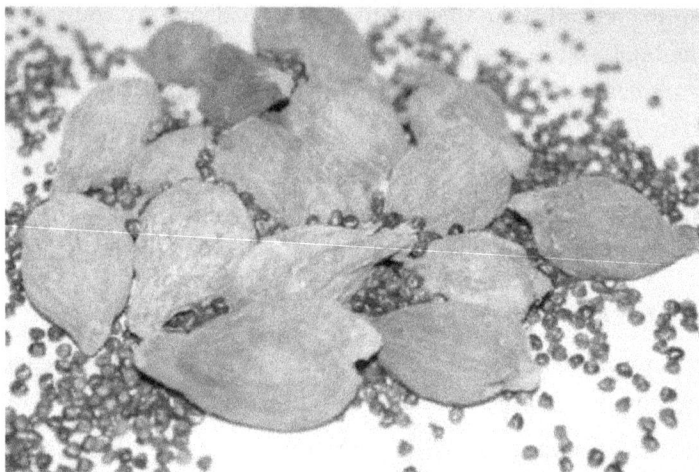

Kewrerima is one of our prized spices. Its aroma is rich and beguiling, and for those who are used to Ethiopian foods, mouth-watering. Kewrerima is found in just about every base spice blend, including berbere, mitmita, niter kibbeh, and other mixes constituted to create elaborate or rare dishes. Kewrerima is sometimes used to flavor and give an extra kick to the aroma of freshly made coffee and tea.

What's in a name?

Ethiopians who know this wonderful spice as kewrerima may be confused when they notice the English name. They might even be a little taken aback. Why would someone call one of their favorite spices *false* cardamom—an imposter? Incidentally, it's also called Ethiopian cardamom, which would be more fitting, but it's not widely known by this moniker. The distinction in name actually started during ancient Roman and Greek times, when spices began to come from India. I'll explain this in just a bit.

The various cardamoms that exist in the world today belong to the ginger family, *Zingiberaceae*. There are two genera in this family, to use a biology term. One is *Elettaria*, consisting of the smaller straw green pods, called green cardamom or *true* cardamom.

A native of southwest India, green cardamom also grows in Guatemala, Sri Lanka, Malaysia, Thailand, Tanzania, and in a few other tropical countries. India, Guatemala, and Sri Lanka are, respectively the number 1, 2, and 3 producers and exporters of green cardamom.

The Middle East, the Scandinavian countries, and India itself are the greatest consumers of green cardamom. This spice is the third most expensive in the world of spices, after saffron and vanilla, because cardamom's crop yield is so low— only 40 to 120 pounds per acre. Comparatively, 2,000 pounds of caraway seeds can be harvested in a similar acreage.

With its long luxuriant leaves and reedy stems, green, or true, cardamom grows in clumps like bamboo to a height of 10 to 15 feet. The production is labor intensive, as it needs constant care and the pods have to be picked individually by hand. (See next page for more info.)

The second type of cardamom is called *amomum*. It has a larger pod and comes in shades of black, dark brown, red, and white, and has many different regional names. Amomum grows mainly in Asia, Africa, and Australia.

The "true" and "false" names assigned to the cardamoms were supposedly coined by a 4th century B.C. Greek botanist named Theophrastus, who had been given conflicting information as to the sources of the two varieties. One of his sources said they came from the land of Mendes, in northern Persia. A second said they came from India. Hence, he named the green kind *true* cardamom, and the others *false* cardamom.

To further complicate matters, the amomum genus has hundreds of species, one of which is *aframomum*, which is kewrerima or Ethiopian cardamom. Kewrerima grows in western Ethiopia (around Lake Tana), in southern Sudan, and in Uganda. As most of you know and I mentioned above, kewrerima is one of the major ingredients in berbere, mekelesha, mitten shiro and mitmita. Unfortunately, there has not been much compositional analysis done on kewrerima (that I could find) to determine the level of vitamins and minerals and the diverse phytonutrients and volatile oils it comprises.

The western African species is known as *Aframomum melegueta* but its every-day name is alligator pepper or grains of paradise. Its seeds are hotter than the Ethiopian variety. A Japanese study found that grains of paradise can lower body fat and decrease waist to hip ratio. Besides its culinary uses, this spice has also been esteemed as an aphrodisiac.

CHAPTER 22
Cardamom

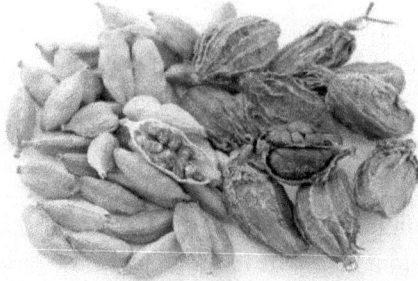

Green and brown cardamom

Green cardamom is one of the four key ingredients in the freshly made Ethiopian tea. The others are cinnamon, cloves and black tea but it is the third member that the ancient Silk Road traders once called the Queen of Spices that gives the tea its distinct and luscious flavor. Drinking this tea can be as pleasurable an experience as drinking coffee produced in certain regions of Ethiopia; it is that rich, smooth and savory hot beverage we all enjoy so much. I've covered cloves and cinnamon in the spices section of this book. Let's talk about the green cardamom in detail and some basic information about one of the Asian amomum cardamoms.

Green Cardamom's nutritional profile and benefits

All cardamoms have been valued for both their culinary and medicinal benefits. In western countries the green cardamom has been esteemed more than others because of its distinct bouquet and flavor—intensely aromatic, but not pungent or spicy tangy, yet warm and tasty. And somehow, like fine prose or poetry, green cardamom appears to contain layers of flavor and aroma, each fine and delicate. Because of these qualities, green cardamom has versatile application in savory dishes.

In India and the Arab countries green cardamom is used in various sweets, teas and coffees as well as spice mixes like curry and Garam Masala—a blend used in rice dishes and snacks. In the United States, green cardamom is often used in flans, soups, stews, purees, and rice dishes, as well as ice creams and fresh fruit salad. Scandinavian countries use ground cardamom in baked foods such as breads, buns, biscuits, and cakes, as well as in meatballs.

The brown or black cardamoms are bigger in size and have a different aroma and flavor than their smaller green cousins. They give off a smoky fragrance with a slightly mint and pepper overtone. Some have described their aroma as camphor-like. The seeds are somewhat sweetish and not as strongly pungent as the green ones. In India, they are used in several spice mixes and flavorsome dishes—ranging from curries to stews, lentil dishes and pilafs. They can also be found in rice pudding, tea and even coffee beverages. Historically black and brown cardamoms have also been employed to treat various stomach ailments, common infections and dental problems.

True Cardamom can help with digestive disorders (bloating, acidity, heartburn, nausea, and constipation). It has diuretic properties and, therefore, can aid in removing toxins and other bodily waste efficiently. In time-honored Ayurvedic medicine, cardamom is used to fight depression and bad breath. It's similarly known to help with infection of the mouth and throat.

Spicy drinks are great to drive away the common cold and flu. Cardamom with kundo berbere (black pepper) and turmeric can do the trick. I often also add, pinches of rosemary, anise and a tablespoon full of honey and lemon for this purpose.

The phytochemicals in cardamom work as an antioxidants and anti-inflammatory. In some studies, these compounds have been found to inhibit the growth of cancer cells, bacteria and fungus. Cardamom is also good at keeping the platelets in the blood fully dispersed. It's anti-spasmodic, meaning it can help with muscle and gastro-intestinal cramps as well as hiccups.

Additionally, green cardamom houses a range of minerals consisting of calcium, magnesium, manganese, copper, iron, phosphorous and zinc. The manganese content is astounding. In a hundred grams of the green cardamom, there are 28 mg or 1,217% of the daily value of the mineral. Manganese is involved in many enzyme reactions, including those that fight free radicals in the body and help minimize the incidence of cancer and heart diseases. Lastly, cardamom contains a fair amount of vitamins, including, pyridoxine, riboflavin, niacin and Vitamin C.

Now you can see why those ancient Silk Road merchants crowned it "the queen of spices," just as they had bestowed black pepper as the King of Spices. The next time you sit down to eat your Ethiopian food or drink tea or your Four Pillar hot beverage constituted with cardamom seeds and other spices, you should think of all the good things they bring to your health and wellness.

Enjoy!

CHAPTER 23
Koseret *(Lippia Javanica)*

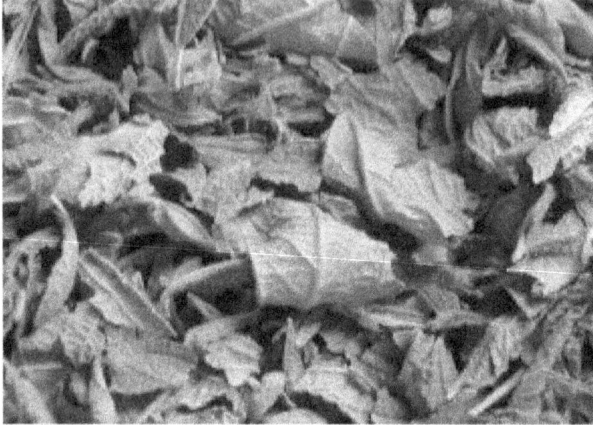

Koseret is one of the spices that impart aroma and good taste to Ethiopian clarified butter. It's also used in many spice blends, including berbere, mitmita and mitten shiro. In the countryside, farmers often feed their cattle koseret leaves because the herb reportedly makes their meat tender and flavorful.

Botanically, koseret or lippia javanica belongs to *verbenaceae* family. Koseret is one of 200 species distributed throughout tropical and southern Africa, eastern India, and South and Central America. It grows 3 to 6 feet high, with large aromatic leaves and white flowers. Koseret mostly grows in the wild. It is sometimes cultivated and grown in private home gardens—both for aesthetics and its aroma as well as for its culinary and medicinal values.

Wherever it grows in the world, the locals have their own name for the plant, just as Ethiopians do. In English, koseret is known as lemon bush or fever tea. Its botanical name, *lippia javanica*, however, has a bit of history. The first part of the name, lippia, was given by the French physician and natural historian, Augustin Lippi (1678-1705) who was sent by Louis XIV as part of a delegation to start trade relations with Ethiopia. The second part, javanica, was given by a German botanist called Nicolaas Laurens Burman (1734-1793), who believed that the plant came from Java.

Medical uses of koseret

It is reported that some tribal groups in southern Africa use a tea of koseret leaves and stems to treat coughs, colds, and fevers. A poultice of the plant extract is employed to treat skin conditions such as scabies and scalp infection. The smoke of the dry plant is supposed to alleviate asthma and chronic cough and chest congestion. Koseret is used to kill insects, lice and mites and provides protection against mosquitos.

To ascertain traditional claims, modern researchers have done experiments with lab animals and human subjects and have demonstrated that koseret has undeniable anti-inflammatory, anti-microbial and decongestant properties. Koseret is an effective repellant against mosquitoes and insects.

Outside of Ethiopia, koseret's culinary use is very limited. Some cultures use the lemon bush oil extract as flavoring agent, or add the dried leaves to fresh fruit and cooked dishes.

CHAPTER 24
Kundo Berbere (Black Pepper)

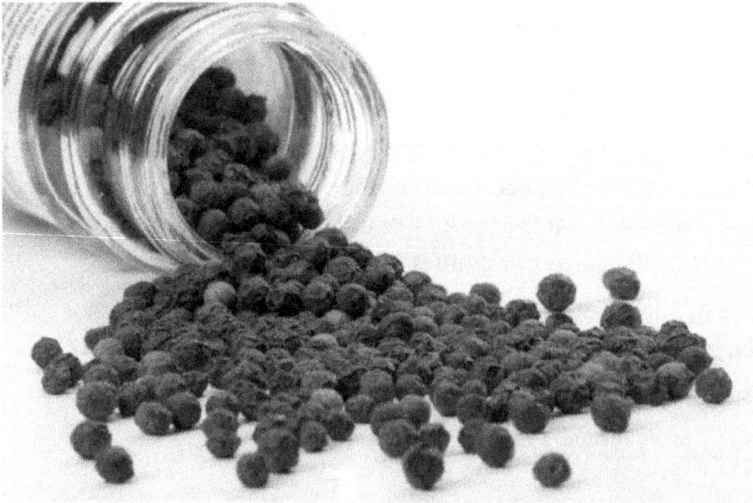

Kundo berbere or black pepper is one of the oldest and widely used spices in the world— so much so that it's often referred to as the King of All Spices. During the Middle Ages kundo berbere was used as currency. People paid rent, dowries, and taxes with black pepper seeds. It's no wonder it used to be called "black gold."

Kundo berbere originated in southern India and Sri Lanka, and it is now grown in countries such as Indonesia, Malaysia, Vietnam, Brazil, China and Thailand. Kundo berbere comes from a climbing vine called piper nigrum, one of a thousand varieties of a larger plant family called *piperaceae*. The plant can grow up to 30 feet high. It produces round berries that turn red upon full ripening.

The kundo berbere we consume is generally picked when the berries are still green. Then it is dried under the sun, which causes them to shrink and shrivel like prunes. The white kundo berbere comes from the same plant but a mechanical or chemical process is used to remove the outer skin of the berries. White pepper tastes milder and is used in light colored dishes and condiments such as soufflés, white sauces and mayonnaise.

No definitive record exists to show when kundo berbere came to Ethiopia. Historians, such as the famed Richard Pankhurst says it might have come during the height of the Axumite era, around the first century A.D., when Ethiopia was a powerful trading partner with India. But if the spice had such an ancient introduction into the country, why was it not widely used? According to reports, as recently as Emperor Lebna Dingle's rule (1508-1540 A.D.) kundo berbere was available only to the royal household.

No matter, this gentle and zesty spice has had a much longer foothold in Ethiopian soil than the red or cayenne pepper, introduced into the country in the 18th century. Cayenne pepper and its relatives claim South and Central America as their historical home. In Ethiopian cooking, kundo berbere is used mostly by itself or as part of the mekelesha in stews and soups that need extra gentle heat and flavor.

Just as important, if not more so, is kundo berbere's benefit to the human body. Kundo berbere contains a number of phytonutrients that define its characteristics—odor, color, heat, and aroma—and its health benefits.

Kundo berbere contains essential oils, flavonoids, lignans, alkaloids, aromatic compounds and amids. Compounds called chavicine and piperine are responsible for kundo berbere's spice and flavor.

In the vitamin area, kundo berbere contains choline, folic acid, niacin, pyridoxine, riboflavin, thiamin, vitamin A, Vitamin C and Vitamin K.

Mineral-wise, calcium, copper, iron, magnesium, manganese, phosphorus, and zinc are the main ones found in The King of All Spices.

Kundo berbere's health benefits

Based on research findings as well as traditional uses, the literature accounts quite extensive health benefits to this spice, which occupies our kitchen cabinets unsung and unadmired. We use the spice on a whim or when compelled to use kundo berbere and others spices in a special dish.

Kundo berbere can enhance appetite, clean out chest congestion, speed up recovery from a cold, heal sore throats, help with fever, improve digestion and calmly normalize a malfunctioning GI tract. Piperine, one of the phytonutrients found in kundo berbere, is the compound responsible for all of these benefits. Black pepper can also help with conditions associated with stomach pain, chills, blood poisoning, intestinal gas (bloating), nausea, strep throat, headache, hypothermia-induced vomiting, malaria, dysentery, cholera and even arthritis.

Black pepper improves circulation, kills a wide spectrum of microbes, alleviates pain, and calms and sooths inflamed tissues and organs. As you will see be-low, kundo berbere has a wide range of anti-cancer properties. The compounds in kundo berbere have been found to be superior antioxidants in neutralizing free radicals and protecting the body from carcinogenic substances.

Applied externally, a mixture of black pepper powder and cream and oil, can help ease problems associated with nasal congestion, skin eruptions, sinusitis and epilepsy. Because kundo berbere has antibacterial properties, it can be used as a food preservative.

Bioavailability

The compounds found in kundo berbere have other unique properties; they can increase the absorption, assimilation and function of foods in our bodies. Piperine not only increases the bioavailability of other phytonutrients to the body but also boosts their activity once they are in the tissues. Piperine does this by enhancing the phytonutrient's absorption across the intestinal wall. Once they are absorbed into the blood stream, piperine can protect them against oxidative damage until finally they get into the cells where they are needed to do their own protective work. The function of this ancient spice is truly remarkable!

By including black pepper with your meals often, you can increase the effica-cy of the phytonutrients in the food you consume as well as benefit from kundo berbere's own antioxidants. This is the reason you see black pepper in all the Four Pillars recipes. The piperine enables active compounds from other foods to stay in the body's cells longer. Researchers who found this correlation applied piperine and curcumin (the compound found in turmeric) to both animal and human models. They concluded that piperine increased curcumin's absorption, its serum concentration and bioavailability.

We often add extra kundo berbere to our glass of Four Pillars drink. It gives character, zest and heat to the beverage.

Cancer prevention

By increasing the availability of other cancer-fighting phytonutrients and using its own antioxidant compounds, black pepper can help minimize the incidence of cancer and the aging of our bodies. Piperine also thwarts communication between existing cancer cells, thereby limiting their growth and proliferation.

Additionally, by stimulating the production of the body's specialized enzymes, black pepper can help neutralize and eliminate cancer-causing chemicals from the body. Rancidity, caused by the oxidation of fats and cholesterol, is a common problem with fats—both within and outside the body. It is generally a result of a free radical attack on fat and cholesterol molecules. The black pepper compounds can serve as effective natural antioxidants and as a food preservative. So perhaps the next time you plan to store your meat you may want to treat it with black pepper powder first.

Black pepper's other benefits

Black pepper can serve as an anti-inflammatory for those who suffer from rheumatoid arthritis, inflammation of the bronchioles of the lungs, inflammation of the stomach lining, and a great many similar problems.

Black pepper may help improve brain health, particularly in those who are suffering from reduced memory, cognitive malfunction, Alzheimer's disease, dementia or other age-related brain conditions.

Black pepper can help lower cholesterol by increasing the breakdown and utilization of fats in the body. This King of All Spices can also help boost the immune system and treat problems with intermittent fever such as those induced by malaria, colds, and neuritis. Black pepper can assist with the efficient digestion and processing of foods by stimulating the taste buds and increasing the secretion of digestive juices in the stomach. As you can see, kundo berbere indeed is a remarkable spice, fitting of its royal status.

Medicinal uses of black pepper

Include this great spice with your daily meals as a general protection of your health. You may want to take a concentrated amount. Grind the berries, boil them in water and drink the decoction. I generally add a teaspoon of turmeric, the juice from a slice of lemon and honey to taste. You'll feel great afterwards.

Caveat and disclaimer: Avoid excessive topical application of black pepper, as it can stimulate the kidneys. Pregnant women should not take concentrated amounts of black pepper—the pungent compounds can cause burns to the fetus.

Finally, by all means, don't treat kundo berbere/black pepper as medicine, although it does have medicinal properties. Consult with your physician if you have health problems or are on medication before including the spice as part of your daily nutrition.

Enjoy!

CHAPTER 25
Mitmita (Bird's Eye Chili)

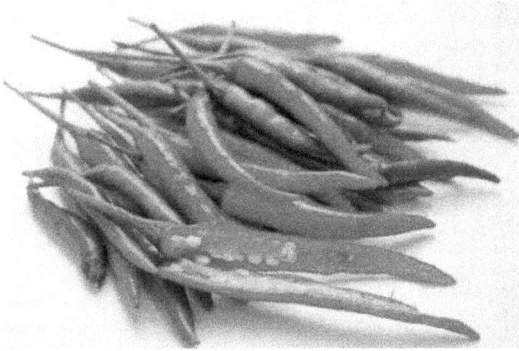

It's hard to believe that the peppers grown and used as part of our berbere or mitmita are not native to Ethiopia. According to reports, all the peppers used around the world today originated in the Americas—Mexico, Central America, and South America. Although some say Columbus, who discovered America, might have brought chili peppers to Europe even earlier, it was the Spanish and Portuguese traders who introduced the peppers to the rest of the world in the 16th and 17th centuries. Tomatoes, corn (or maize), pineapple and potatoes came from the Americas, too.

How did Ethiopians survive up to that time without their precious peppers? For that matter, how did the rest of the world survive, depending on peppers for so many different cuisines?

I have no answers, except to say that people made use of whatever herbs they had, like watercress in the case of Ethiopia. Long before computers were introduced, we depended on the typewriter. Long before cars and airplanes came into existence, we depended on horses, carriages and our feet to get to and from places. Now, it seems hard to believe that humans once existed without all these conveniences.

I guess the same goes for our wonderful herbs and spices that have been spread around the world from their places of origin. We need to share what we've got with the rest of the world. East Indians are the purveyors of many of spices we use today. In a limited way, I guess the rest of the world might say the same about coffee and probably in years to come about teff, too. Coffee and teff are Ethiopia's gift to the world.

Mitmita, or bird's eye chili to use its English name, is one of the hottest peppers from Ethiopia. Outside their native land, there are several other peppers a lot hotter than mitmita, so much so that people have to wear masks and suits when they pick them.

To clarify, mitmita refers both to the bird's eye chili pepper and to a powdered seasoning mix that usually contains, in addition to the chili, cardamom, cloves and salt. Some people enrich it by adding ginger, cinnamon, cumin and other ingredients to increase mitmita's range of use.

The final mixture varies from bright to dark orange, depending on the number and kind of spices that have been included along with the base four (cardamom, cloves, salt and chili). Its aroma and flavor also change from formulation to formulation. No matter what it has in it, mitmita is still fiery hot.

Beyond aroma, flavor and spiciness, let's talk about the benefit of mitmita to your health. This discussion refers just to the chili itself.

The benefits of mitmita

First of all, remember that almost all peppers go from green to red if left on the vine. When peppers become red, it means they are rich in phytonutrients—carotenoids, bioflavonoids and vitamins. Red pepper has 8 times more Vitamin A than green pepper. Their beta -carotene content is significantly greater too, going from –137% of DV in green pepper to 841% of DV in red.

Capsaicin is the compound that gives peppers their fiery taste. It is an odor-less, colorless and oily chemical. The "heat" in capsaicin that we feel on our tongue or when it comes in contact with our skin is more apparent than real. There is no actual physical damage but the chemical tricks the brain into believing that the tissue is being burned. The brain responds by releasing endorphins to relieve the pain and also give the body an overall euphoric feeling. The side effect of this is that when endorphins are floating in your system, your desire to eat is suppressed. For those who are trying to lose or manage weight, these cascading events will cause the person to eat less.

Here are some of the other advantages of capsaicin

Capsaicin can stimulate cells along the lining of your stomach to produce more digestive juice, which means this compound can speed up the breakdown and processing of foods. It's an anti-inflammatory—important for those who have joint problems or tenderness in their nasal cavity or elsewhere in their bodies. The beta-carotene and flavonoids found in chili and all other red peppers can be good antioxidants, neutralizing tissue-damaging free radicals and shielding our genetic material.

Additionally, chili peppers have been found to reduce bad cholesterol, which means that if you're a regular consumer of chili peppers, you can keep your heart and vascular system healthy. Because of the antioxidant properties of the compounds found in chili and other peppers, studies have shown that these red phytonutrients can potentially help in treating lung and prostate cancer.

When you consume chili peppers, your body's metabolism is enhanced. This is more good news for those who are trying to lose or manage their weight. Chili has been found to help with arthritis and even as an insect repellant and sleep aid. Researchers in Australia reported that those who consumed spicy food before they went to bed slept well, longer, and felt completely rested when they woke. The study also found that these people had more energy and felt more awake. This benefit of chili is probably connected to the incidental release of endorphins, induced by capsaicin, which relaxes and calms the body.

Chilies are good in fighting congestion of the chest and blocked nose, relieving chronic joint and muscle pain and, according a Duke University study, can kill cancer-causing bacteria known as *H. pylori*. Chilies can help prevent the microbial contamination of food, an important advantage in countries where people have no refrigerators.

Those who consume the berbere and powdered mitmita blend can also benefit from the many other spices found in them. See berbere and mitmita's ingredient list under the Ethiopian recipes.

In short, I hope that when you think of chilies and other spices, you will think of their health benefits, in addition to their importance to enhance the flavor, aroma, and taste of your foods.

Bona appetit!

CHAPTER 26
Netch Azmud (Bishop's Weed aka Ajwain)

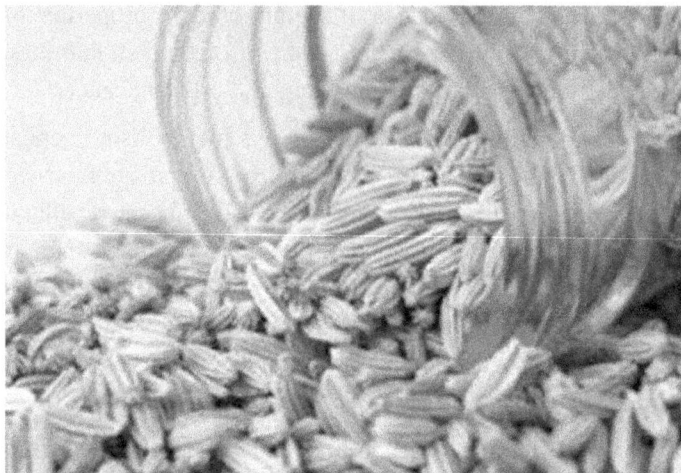

If you're like me, you probably thought *netch azmud* (also called bishop's weed or ajwain) and *tikur azmud* are related, a variation of each other. One is netch (white), the other tikur (black). As you will see below, they are not related at all, although in some of the Ethiopian dishes they can be used interchangeably.

Ethiopians who cook with these spices know how they taste and smell. For those who are not familiar with these spices, here is the difference.

Some nutrition writers describe netch azmud as having a thyme-like aroma with a cumin undertone. Tikur azmud's whole seed aroma is subtle at the first whiff but becomes pungent when you pulverize them. Aroma, like taste, is an individual thing. Some writers refer to tikur azmud as having a bitter aroma. I think this herb smells rather pleasant, particularly in baked bread but even when the seeds are chewed alone.

Tikur azmud is a native of India. Netch azmud has Ethiopia as one of its homes. It supposedly originated in Egypt and spread to northern Africa, the Middle East, India, and southeastern Asia.

The health benefits of the spice were never thought about because most Ethiopians, like people everywhere else, think of spices and herbs merely as devices to make foods flavorful and enjoyable. What happens to these spices and herbs once they enter the body—whether or not they have any benefits to their health—is never a consideration.

Netch azmud's benefits

Traditionally, the seeds of netch azmud have been used to treat ailments associated with the digestive tract, such as bloating, indigestion, gastrosis, diarrhea, and cholera. This spice has similarly been used for conditions related to the respiratory system, such as asthma, chest pain (angina), common cold, bronchitis, pneumonia and emphysema.

Netch azmud is known to be anti-inflammatory, anti-parasitic, anti-spasmodic, diuretic, and even aphrodisiac. According to one report, a combination of netch azmud, fennel seeds, dried ginger, and salt increases appetite and enhances digestion.

Additionally, a poultice of netch azmud over psoriasis and vitiligo (a chronic disease where the skin loses its pigmentation) can bring relief and healing. Methoxsalen is a prescription drug used to treat psoriasis. It was once made from netch azmud, until the synthetic version took over.

Finally, netch azmud is thought to be an excellent tonic spice, improving the body's overall health.

CHAPTER 27
Netch Shinkoort (Garlic)

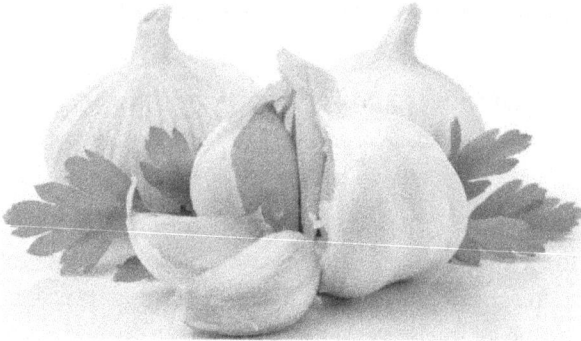

Netch shinkoort is the king in Ethiopian cooking. It's a major ingredient in berbere and mitten shiro. Ground garlic and black pepper are combined and powdered and used as finishing touches to sega (meat), doro, and lentil wots (stews). You sprinkle a teaspoonful of it for ten or so minutes before you remove the pot from the fire. Alternatively, you can use mekelesha (see the recipes section.) Again, like all the spices and herbs, garlic's role in Ethiopian dishes is mainly to enhance flavor, taste, character and depth to the foods. Like others, most people don't make a conscious association between the consumption of garlic and its benefit to health and well-being. Let's see what garlic can do for you.

One, garlic contains a group of phytochemicals called organo-sulfur compounds which give the spice both its color and smell. Although modern researchers don't exactly know how these compounds work in the human body, there have been a good number of laboratory and epidemiological studies to show that consuming garlic regularly may be beneficial to our health.

Two, garlic has been valued for its culinary as well medicinal properties since ancient times in many different cultures. Researchers from around the world have identified many of garlic's unique characteristics and benefits to the human body.

Garlic and its sulfur compounds have been found to help control cholesterol production in the body. In a laboratory study, these compounds have also been shown to have blood-thinning properties, one of garlic's traditionally known attributes. Garlic's phytochemicals have been found to promote the health and function of the blood vessels, by making them more supple and pliable. These phytochemicals also have an anti-inflammatory function, important to those who suffer from joint aches and pains. They do this by inhibiting the activities of the enzymes responsible for the condition in the circulating fluids. For those who are concerned about their heart, vascular and circulatory health, regular consumption of garlic can be a benefit.

Garlic compounds have been shown to have antioxidant activity in laboratory tests and some researchers think that it may play the same role in the body. These substances are believed to stimulate the production of glutathione, the body's natural antioxidant and help boost the immune system.

Furthermore, garlic's compounds are believed to disrupt the replication of cancer cells, while at the same time increase their apoptosis or death. In some case-controlled studies, in countries where people consume a higher amount of garlic in their diet had a significantly lower incidence of gastric cancer than those who consume little or none. In a similar study, researchers found that those who have a high intake of garlic in their diets had far less incidence of colorectal cancer than the control group.

Garlic has antibacterial and anti-fungal properties as well. Those who suffer from ring worms of the body and feet can benefit if they use a garlic solution on their skin or soak their feet in it.

A few practical details

Allicin is a key active ingredient in garlic. When you crash garlic you release the enzyme that catalyzes the production of Allicin. Allicin, in turn, rapidly changes into organo-sulfur compounds, some of which are the volatile oils that permeate the air and enter your nostrils.

Cooking reportedly makes the enzyme inactive. It is therefore recommended to let the crashed garlic sit for 10 minutes or more before you cook it. That way, the allicin-producing enzymes would have run through their courses. If your food ingredient calls for garlic, add it near the completion of the cooking. It's also said that if you added garlic toward the end of the cooking, the heat will impact the enzymes less. And never use a microwave oven with all fruits, vegetables and spices. (Microwave ovens use radio waves to agitate and vibrate water molecules in food. As these molecules continue to vibrate and shake they generate heat at atomic level. It's this heat that cooks the food. My concern is when you disturb molecules like this, there is a chance of breaking the bonds and creating free radicals.)

In Ethiopian cooking, the berbere spice blend contains the most amount of garlic. The garlic we find in berbere comes from the crushed, dried and powdered garlic. It has minimal direct heat exposure. So, technically the organo-sulfur compounds of garlic in berbere should be relatively intact.

Then from the comparative case studies done in other countries, those who eat garlic regularly had a low incidence of certain type of cancers than others. You can still benefit even from cooked garlic.

As you will see later, many of the spices found in the Ethiopian cooking have antioxidant and anti-cancer characteristics. The combined effect of the spices found in the stews and the vegetarian and meat dishes should be a benefit to you.

Caveat

Garlic naturally has a strong odor, which can be noticed on one's breath and sweat. It can be offensive if the person doesn't keep good hygiene—take a regular bath, brush and wash their mouth and freshen their breath before coming in contact with people. If too much garlic is consumed, the person could experience heartburn, nausea, flatulence, abdominal pain and diarrhea. Prolonged exposure of garlic to one's skin can cause blisters, contact dermatitis and lesions.

CHAPTER 28
Senafich (Mustard Seeds)

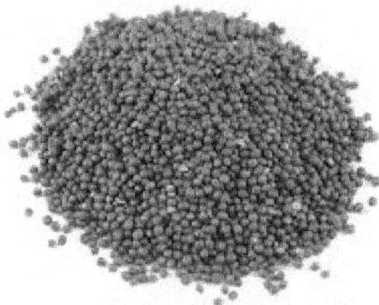

Ground mustard seeds are one of the most common spices in Ethiopian cooking. Their uses vary according to the creativity and imagination of the person using them. The most common use, however, is a dip prepared with vinegar, salt, and garlic. Ground mustard seeds are also one of the ingredients in *siljo*—a fermented puree made from *bakela duket* (fava bean flour), the milk of sunflower seeds, garlic, abesh (fenugreek), ginger, lemon juice and water.

Like most spices added to Ethiopian cooking, ground mustard seeds are used to enhance the flavor and aroma of the foods. And like most spices that are used in their cooking, the nutritional and health benefits of mustard seeds are not in the forefront of the cooks' thoughts. The spices and herbs are just part of the food blend. As you have already read, these herbs and spices also have many great health benefits.

Mustard seeds contain a good amount of vitamins, minerals, essential fatty acids and fiber, as well as phytonutrients. Of the vitamins, the predominating ones are the B-complex, those nutrients are important in energy production and nerve impulse transmission. These are: niacin, thiamine, riboflavin, folates, pyridoxine (Vitamin B6), and pantothenic acid. To a limited extent, mustard seeds also contain vitamins A, C, E, and K. Vitamin A and Vitamin E are fat-soluble antioxidants that help protect the body's cells and fat molecules against free radicals.

Of the minerals in mustard seeds, the most concentrated are calcium, copper, manganese, iron, selenium and zinc. As you may have read in the earlier chapters, these nutrients are essential for the proper functioning and protection of the body. Some of these minerals—manganese, zinc, copper, and selenium—are among the antioxidant enzymes (glutathione peroxidase, superoxide dismutase, and catalase) that help protect the body against cancer and cardiovascular diseases.

This wonderful condiment holds a good number of phytonutrients as well—sterols, curcuminoids, isothiocyanates, phenols, bioflavonoids, and carotenoids. All of these, as you may have read in this book or elsewhere, are important compounds in fighting cancer, in minimizing problems associated with heart diseases, and in slowing the aging of our bodies.

Sterols, found in all plants, are the equivalent of cholesterol. They don't harm your body but they help it. When ingested as part of the plant, sterols block cholesterol absorption in the intestine, thereby helping to lower blood cholesterol and lessen the health problems associated with this substance.

Curcuminoids are compounds that give plants their yellow color, like turmeric and some fruits and vegetables, for example. They, too, are important antioxidants. So are isothiocyanates, flavonoids, and carotenoids. Isothiocyanates are sulfur-containing molecules that occur naturally as glucosinolate compounds in all cruciferous vegetables such as broccoli, Brussels sprouts, cabbage, kale, turnips, collard greens and watercress. Research has shown that isothiocyanates can minimize the incidence of esophageal and lung cancers as well as others, including gastrointestinal cancer. A 2002 study published in the *International Journal for Vitamin and Nutrition Research* showed that isothiocyanates inhibited the replication of human cancer cells and accelerated their deaths. Similar compounds, also found in mustard seeds, were discovered to inhibit the growth of bladder cancer cells.

Mustard seeds contain a fair amount of essential amino acids as well as essential oils. The selenium level in mustard seeds is particularly high. This mineral, as was discussed earlier in the book, is good for heart health and in the prevention of cancer. Although, in western countries, mustard leaves and oils are also used in food preparation. In Ethiopia, it's mostly the seeds that are used. There are generally three types of mustard seeds: the black, white (in reality, it is a straw yellow), and brown. Brown is the most commonly used in Ethiopia.

Cited health benefits

In addition to their role in cancer prevention, mustard seeds are known to aid with the health of the cardiovascular system and as a treatment to respiratory disorders, such as chronic bronchitis, cold and sinus problems and asthma attacks. A poultice (bandage) made with mustard paste and applied to aching tissues and joints (as in rheumatism) can bring relief and comfort. A decoction made from mustard can help remove alcohol- and narcotic-related toxins from the body. Mustard seed oil has been found to increase lipid and glucose metabolism, which can be a benefit for diabetics.

People who suffer from psoriasis, acne, ringworms, contact dermatitis and other skin conditions can profit from the ingestion and application of mustard seeds. Mustard seeds are known to rejuvenate hair, enhance skin tone and invigorate the nerves.

In short, mustard seeds can contribute to your health, as well as enhance flavor and aroma in foods.

Caveat: Use mustard seeds in moderation. Anything in excess can be toxic. Consult your physician before you treat this spice like medicine.

Enjoy!

CHAPTER 29
Shinkoort (Red, Yellow, or White Onions)

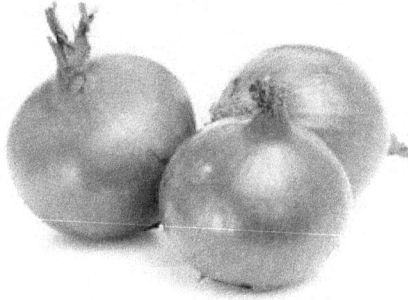

Onions are the mainstays of nearly every Ethiopian dishes. They are one of the base ingredients in meats and legume foods. Sliced raw onions are also served with green salads and other vegetarian dishes. These layered, round objects make the food sweet, rich and tasty. In all these situations, onions are used to enhance flavor and give body or character to the foods. Most of us don't associate our consumption of onions to their value in our body. As you will see below, onions offer many great benefits to our health.

Onions contain a number of phytonutrients, many of which have been studied and found to help with several disease conditions. Let's look at the different areas that onions have been useful to us.

For starters, just like garlic, onions contain a great number of sulfur compounds and flavonoids called polyphenols. These compounds provide several benefits. Quercetin, anthocyanins and kaempferol are three well-studied flavonoids. They serve as antioxidants, antihistamine, anti-asthmatic and anti-inflammatory in our bodies. Incidentally, as with garlic, it's the sulfur compounds that give onions their characteristic smells and cause you to cry every time you chop them.

According to a 2012 study by the University of Colorado, quercetin can inhibit the growth of certain cancer cells. Another study published in the *International Journal of Nanomedicine* showed that kaempferol may inhibit the formation and growth of ovarian cancer. The sulfur compounds in onion are also known to kill bacteria, enhance circulation and lower the bad cholesterol level in the body.

These so called organo-sulfur compounds are also believed to minimize the risk from certain types of cancer. A November 2006 publication in the "*American Journal of Clinical Nutrition* found a positive correlation between the consumption of sulfur-rich foods and the lowering cancer incidence to the ovary, the colon and the esophagus. When onions are combined with turmeric, the synergy of the two substances can be great. Another 2006 study in *Clinical Gastroenterology and Hepatology* showed that when patients were given onion and turmeric together, they found that the two substances helped reduce the size and the number of pre-cancerous cells in the intestine. According to one doctor, regular consumption of onion can help detoxify the body. Ethiopians and those who cater to Ethiopian foods should find this revelation reassuring. Both turmeric (*ird*) and onion *(shinkoort)* are part of our daily diet.

High consumption of onions reportedly helps the body produce insulin, consequently lowering the blood sugar level. This theory was confirmed in a study published back in 1975 in the journal Clinica *Chemic Acta: The International Journal of Clinical Chemistry*. Additionally, onions are good for the heart. They can help lower blood pressure, inhibit the hardening of the arteries and keep the blood vessels supple and elastic, according Dr. Jonathan Stegall, an integrative medicine practitioner from John Creak, Georgia. Because of their antioxidant properties, onions also can help boost the immune system and protect the overall health of the body.

Yet, in another study, a regular consumption of onions was found to increase bone mass in post-menopausal women. The fibers in the onions should help with bowel movement, while their antioxidants help reduce the risk of gastric ulcer.

Onions also contain a number of vitamins and minerals. The highest concentration of the phytonutrients is found in the first layers of skins. Make sure you keep as many of the usable top layers as you can.

In closing, I couldn't help but think of the amount of onions used in Ethiopian foods, particularly with all of those meat dishes. After reading this chapter, you should be thinking beyond flavor and aroma, when you add or eat onion-based dishes. You should savor these foods. Think how much good they do for you every time you sit down to eat a meal with onions in them.

Caveats

For those sensitive individuals, onions may cause gas and bloating. For those with heartburn, consuming raw onions can worsen the condition. Consuming a large amount of green onions may interfere with a drug-thinning medicine, if you are on one.

CHAPTER 30
Tena Adam (Rue)

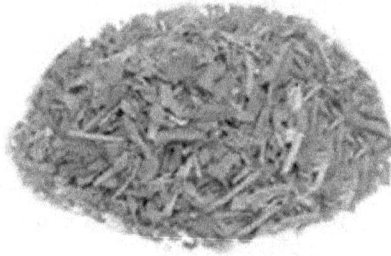

Tena Adam, or rue, is one more herb my mother grew in our garden. The strongly aromatic, pale green plant used to mystify and fascinate me. I think this was primarily because of its unusual, pungent smell, its clubbed leaves, and dainty, rounded yellow petals. Somehow, tena Adam seemed to me to have mystical and magical properties beyond its culinary uses. As you will see below, tena Adam has historically been associated with magic, mysticism, and witchcraft—my intuition was not imaginary.

Since ancient times, tena Adam has had many uses, both in food preparation and medicine, as well as in witchcraft. What I found fascinating as I read various articles in preparing to write this piece was that my childhood perception of tena Adam had historical antecedents.

During the European Middle Ages, people hung rue on their doors and windows as a protection against evil spirits. They rubbed their floors with it to kill fleas and to protect against plagues and pestilence. Christians sprinkled church entrances with the herb before performing mass and during exorcisms. Rue was considered sacred and the precious herb was planted around temples and churchyards. People carried bundles of rue twigs with them as they went about to ward off spells by witches. In courts and law offices, rue was strewn as a protection against diseases that might be carried by criminals. Even today there are people who believe that a rue plant in their garden can be protective of their home and bring harmony, prosperity and happiness.

Although rue is still used in many cultures as a flavoring agent, most people in the West are afraid to consume it. While the volatile oils extracted from rue are concentrated and can be poisonous if taken in large doses, some people believe that the rue leaves and berries are also poisonous.

Ethiopians have used rue berries in powdered berbere blend, in mitten shiro, and the leaves or berries in clarified butter for centuries. Rue berries are also often added to coffee and tea drinks. In all these situations, the dried and ground rue berries or leaves impart pungency and a pleasant aroma and flavor. The fresh leaves are sometimes added to boiling water or milk and given to children who have *kurtet* (pain) in their stomach and poor bowel movements. I have never heard or read stories about people who were poisoned by the use of tena Adam.

Like I mentioned, that concern should apply only to the concentrated volatile oil extract, which can be poisonous if taken in large doses. I suppose the same could happen if someone consumed too much of the berries or the leaves of tena Adam. For that matter, even water can be poisonous if consumed in excess.

Tena Adam's medical application

Medicinally, tena Adam is used as an antidote (corrective measure) against poisons, pestilences, and afflictions. The oil extract of tena Adam is used to counter the deadly effect of poisonous snakebites (like that of cobra and king cobra). The venom produced by these snakes' attacks is called neurotoxin because it affects the nervous system of the victim, causing them to suffocate and die. The venom released by vipers—such as copperheads, cottonmouths and most rattlesnakes—on the other hand, damages the blood vessels, causing the blood to become very thin and the victim eventually bleeds to death. This venom is called hemotoxic. Rue has no effect on hemotoxic venom.

To continue with rue's "anti-" effects, the herb is also known to be anti-arthritic, anti-rheumatic, anti-epileptic and anti-hysteric, to name but just a few. Rue's essential oils function as an anesthetic to all the affected bodily parts. These oils are also effective anti-bacterial and anti-fungal agents. Therefore these substances can help prevent infections both internally—like the colon, intestines and urinary tract, and externally—those that appear on the skin, such as ringworm, athlete's foot, and dermatitis. Furthermore, these oils have antiviral, anti-inflammatory, and antioxidant properties. In small amounts, these compounds can alleviate headaches.

The main active ingredient responsible for all these activities is called rutin, found as 7% to 8% in dried leaves. It's this compound that is the cause of the strong aroma and bitter taste when eaten in larger quantities. In small amounts, both the smell and taste are rather pleasant.

Tena Adam is also an excellent insect repellant; it discourages the presence of beetles and slugs and other vermin. Other uses include treatment in intestinal worms, mouth cancer, hepatitis, hemorrhage and fever. It's similarly used to treat arthritis, dislocations, swellings, sprains, tumors, warts, and aches associated with the ears, teeth and head.

In foods and beverages, rue and its oil are used as flavoring agents. In manufacturing, rue oil is used as fragrance in soaps and cosmetics.

Caveat: Ethiopians who read this reminder might find it surprising because, as mentioned, tena Adam is used in various dishes without having to worry about toxicity. Nonetheless, the literature warns that tena Adam (or rue), particularly the oil, can be poisonous when taken in excess. Pregnant women should never take tena Adam because it might cause uterine contractions, leading to abortion.

CHAPTER 31
Tikur Azmud (Black Cumin)

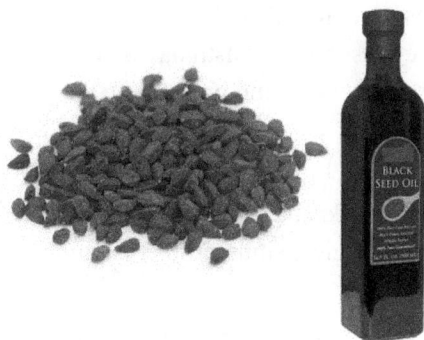

One of my favorite homemade loaves is one that is made with these black seeds in it. The English-speaking world calls it black cumin. Its technical name is *nigella sativa*. In Ethiopia, we endearingly call it tikur azmud. You will be astounded to know that these precious and wonderfully toothsome seeds have many health benefits besides their use to enhance the flavor of breads and other dishes.

Since olden times (more than 2000 years ago), black cumin seeds have been used to heal and improve the health of the body. Just to give you a perspective Hippocrates, the famed Greek medicine man, used black cumin to treat people with digestive disorders and other conditions. King Tutankhamen valued black cumin so much that it was one of the items found in his tomb. Supposedly, Cleopatra was a big fan of the herb not only for its remedial properties but also as a beauty aid. A continuous use of the black seed oil is found to improve the appearance of the skin, hair and nails. The Prophet Muhammad was more divinatory when he called black cumin "a remedy for every illness except death."

Modern researchers have discovered so many health benefits to black cumin that the founder of Islam's claim cannot be taken as mere exaggeration. In the last fifty-plus years, there have been over 200 different studies of the benefit of black cumin to the human body.

One study, conducted at the Cancer Research Laboratory of Hilton Head Island in South Carolina, showed that black cumin oil inhibited cancer growth by 50%, and stimulated immune cells and the production of interferon (protein molecules that protect the cells from the damaging effects of viruses). Additionally, black cumin oil increased the production of bone marrow cells by as much as 250%.

The bone marrow cells consist of the red cells, white cells and platelets. As you may know, white cells are one of our immune forces that fight viruses, bacteria and fungi. The red cells carry oxygen, the element that helps burn the food we eat into energy. Platelets are cells that help our blood to clot.

Black cumin oil was also found to be beneficial in treating cardiovascular diseases, diabetes, kidney disease, and asthma, as well as cancer of the pancreas, lungs, kidneys, liver, prostate, skin, and breast. The list goes on.

Black cumin oil is known to help fight colds and flu, stress, tired legs and muscles, arthritis, rheumatism, bruises, high blood pressure, diarrhea, hair loss, all types of aches (headache, backache, earache, etc.), stomach and intestinal problems, skin fungus, acne, allergies, sinus problems, and even in subduing a baby that cries uncontrollably.

Regarding the use of black cumin seeds to treat aches and pains, I recently had a tooth pulled out. I chewed a pinch of the herb on the good side of my mouth every so often and the relief I got was almost magical. What else?

In several animal models, this remarkable herb was found to be a potent agent against inflammations of the brain and spinal cord (encephalomyelitis), the swelling of soft tissues from excessive accumulation of fluid (edema), inflammation of the colon (colitis), inflammation of the silk-like membrane of the abdominal wall and that covers the organs (peritonitis), and arthritis. Black cumin seed oil can also be used to treat hemorrhoids, hepatitis, fever, cough and tapeworm, as well as nasal dryness.

Furthermore, you can use black cumin oil to enhance your physical appearance. This can be achieved by consuming the oil, a teaspoon of it with your warm tea or soup, or by adding the same amount into your personal cream and applying it on your face and hands. It's known to help with skin blemishes and conditions like eczema, psoriasis, acne, lines and wrinkles. For lasting effect, though, it's better if you consume the seeds or oil for a protracted time. Then, according to the reports, you are supposed to have lustrous hair, nails and skin.

What makes black cumin seeds and oil such versatile curative agents?

The most studied active ingredient in black cumin seed is called thymoquinone. It's this compound, which acts as an antioxidant, fighting and killing cancer cells and bacteria and fungus that cause inflammations in the body. There are many other compounds in black cumin seeds, including vitamins, minerals, and fatty acids, which together have a powerful effect on the health and wellness of the body.

Other researchers who studied tikur azmud's oil suggest that one should take a teaspoon of the oil, alone or with warm tea, an hour before a meal once or twice a day.

If you have access to tikur azmud oil capsules, which are sold in Indian or Middle Eastern as well as some Ethiopian food stores (see caveat below), use this version of the spice. However, consuming ground tikur azmud with your favorite food in similar amounts can also have positive results. Alternatively, you can soak the seeds overnight, then warm over a stove, filter, and drink as tea.

If you purchase black cumin oil, heed this warning. According to Tony Isaacs, natural health researcher and author of *Cancer's Natural Enemy*, there are many different products sold under the umbrella of black (black cumin seed oil, black onion seed, black caraway seed, and black sesame seed), but the true product is the one labeled as *nigella sativa*.

All these accounts are not just products of folklore or old wives' tales. As you will see from the list of references at the end of the book, most of what we have discussed here are results of scientific studies that have been conducted in various institutions around the world.

Black cumin seeds and oil indeed appear to be a cure for nearly everything and anything under the sun except death.

How to used tikur azmud

Most of you know the various recipes for loaves and as blends with other spices. For those who don't, when you make dough for loaf or other breads, put in a dash of the black seeds and mix thoroughly. A pinch or two will be sufficient, depending on the amount of batter you have.

For teas: Boil hot water, throw in a teaspoon of tikur azmud, steep for 15-20 minutes, filter and drink. You can also add honey, lemon and black pepper to enhance the flavor.

Add ground black cumin to stir-fry dishes, salads and casseroles to give these foods a new twist in flavor and taste. Include lemon and cilantro for maximum effect.

Caveats

1.   Pregnant woman should not take black cumin oil or the seeds in large quantities. They should consult their doctor before using it.

2.   Black cum seeds have blood pressure lowering effect and therefore not recommended to those who suffer from low blood pressure.

3.   Black cumin oil should not be taken plain and with a full stomach. It should be mixed in water, tea, juice or honey and taken and 1-2 hours before a meal.

4.   Never mix the intake of black cumin with prescription or other drugs.

If taking the seeds, they must be heated. Never take the seeds that have not been heated as they will upset the stomach.

CHAPTER 32
Timiz (Long Pepper)

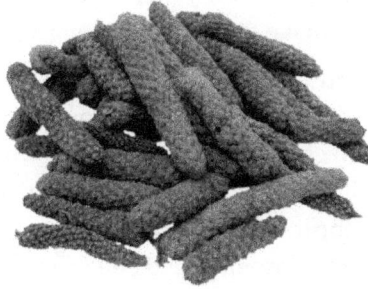

Timiz (botanically known as *Piper Carpense*) is generally found as part of the spice blends like mekelesha and berbere. It has a pungent smell with properties of both coriander and black pepper, but hotter and sweeter. Timiz is used to enrich the flavor of meat dishes and sometimes coffee and tea.

Timiz is produced by a climbing vine shrub with heart-shape, luxuriant leaves and white flowers that resemble a bottle-cleaning brush on a stick. Upon maturity, tiny poppy-seed size berries are embedded like cornrows on an ear but in a winding pattern, giving rise to its Amharic name, *timiz* or twisted. These berries or fruits are yellowish-orange but the individual spikes (the whole ear of corn structure) are red when ripe but turn black upon drying.

In Ethiopia, timiz grows in the Bonga coffee forest of the South-west section of the country. Despite its high demand, its production is reportedly low. There is also an imported timiz, which is referred to as *yeferenge*—a white person's— timiz, to distinguish it from the homegrown, *yehabehsa* (a generic name for Ethiopians) variety. Yeferenge timiz actually comes from India and in the general literature it bears its name of origin or it's known is simply as "long pepper". This variety has a stronger aroma and more spicy than the Ethiopian version. The Indian timiz (which incidentally also grows in Malaysia, Indonesia, Singapore, Sri Lanka, Nepal, and South-East Asia) is a lot more expensive, both because of the tariff levied on it and because of its supposed superior quality.

Interestingly, timiz is not popular elsewhere in the world other than the countries where it's grown. It's an old spice. During the Roman Empire, it was the preferred food flavoring-agent. When the black pepper was introduced, timiz fell out of favor.

Besides its culinary uses, timiz has many health benefits. In Ethiopia, it's used to alleviate *kurtmat*—the stinging aches in the bones and muscles, *wugat*—sharp pains in chest and abdomen or *kurtet*—the cutting sensations in the intestines and stomach. In other countries, long pepper has traditionally been used to relieve congestion in the chest and respiratory tract (such as asthma, bronchitis and coughs). It's also used to facilitate digestion and improve bowel movement.

Long pepper oils have antiseptic properties and can help heal wounds and cuts, suppress pain and reduce inflammation. Have involuntary muscle spasms like hiccups? Drink a tea of timiz or mix the powder of it with honey and swallow it. It can help stop it. Since timiz stimulates the reproductive system, it's often used as an aphrodisiac. Long pepper has similarly been used as a calming or sedative agent to those who suffer from insomnia and epilepsy.

Moreover, This interesting spice has been used to treat a host of other conditions: headaches, toothaches, intestinal worms and snakebites. In addition, long pepper has been used to treat Vitamin B1 deficiency, stroke and as a remedy to ministerial cramps, infertility and as an aid during and after childbirth.

Many of us, who live in cities and towns where modern medicine is readily available, probably won't reach for the timiz bottle in our kitchen cabinets to treat or cure many of the maladies listed above, but the point is as we have already seen, all the herbs and spices we use to enhance flavor and taste house many wonderful benefits to our health. They may help you live a healthy, long life.

Enjoy!

CHAPTER 33
Tosign (Savory)

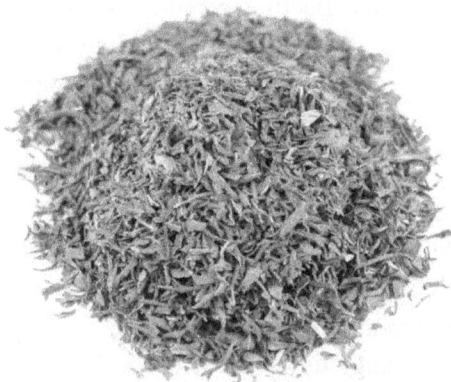

In Ethiopian cooking, tosign, can appear both in the berbere and mitten shiro blends. It's also added to boiling water and drank as tea. Besides its overall tonic effect on the body, tosign tea reportedly can also help lower an abnormally high blood pressure.

In western societies and a number of other cultures, tosign (or savory) has been used as a spice and, more commonly, as an herb. Savory is employed to stimulate appetite and improve digestion, as palliative for sore throat, and as carminative to bloating and gas. It's also used to treat headaches and lessen the problems associated with coughing.

Tea made of savory can be effective against the flu, particularly when taken together with chamomile, colt's foot and honey. A combination of savory and black currant tea is supposed to alleviate or even cure severe and spasmodic cough.

The leaves of savory are rich in vitamins, minerals, fiber and phytonutrients. Many of these phytochemicals are antioxidants that can help boost the immune system, reduce bad cholesterol levels, and protect the heart and blood vessels.

The aroma, color and flavor found in herbs and spices are often a result of the complex organic compounds contained in them. The aromas they emit come from volatile essential oils.

Savory, like most herbs, has a number of these smelly substances and they include thymol, carvacrol, aslinalool, camphene and a few others. The first two compounds are the most studied. Thymol has been shown to have antiseptic and antifungal properties. Carvacrol has been shown to control the growth of several bacteria, including E. coli and Bacillus cereus. Carvacrol reportedly imparts a pleasant, tangy taste. Because of these attributes and its anti-microbial properties, carvacrol has been used in food preparation and preservation.

Savory is a storehouse of vitamins, minerals and fibers. In 100 hundred grams of dry savory, you can expect to find 474% of the DV for iron, 265% of DV for manganese, 210% of DV for calcium, and 94% of DV for magnesium. And you can get 120% of DV for dietary fiber. Its content of potassium, zinc selenium, and vitamins A, B6 and C are reported to be high as well.

Savory can be used to treat problems affecting the urinary tract and when you have sore throat, diarrhea, indigestion or diabetes to relieve the problems associated with frequent thirst. The juice of savory can be applied directly on the skin to treat insect bites. This herb can function as a tonic to enhance the overall health of the body. In some cultures, savory is even used as an aphrodisiac.

For many of savory's benefits, you can add it to your favorite dishes, or make it into a tea and drink it periodically. You want to add honey or sugar to taste, to sweeten the infusion. The Addition of black currant to savory tea can stop a severe bout of coughing.

Gamma aminoburyic acid (GABA) is a natural chemical and neurotransmitter that calms and normalizes your brain and the nervous system. Its primary function is as an inhibitor, preventing over overstimulation. It does this by counteracting glutamate—the brain's major excitatory neurotransmitter. When GABA binds to a receptor, it prevents stimulation by glutamate. When GABA levels are inadequate, overstimulation due to high levels of glutamate can occur. A low level of GABA can lead to anxiety, insomnia, depression, moodiness and a number of other disorders. There are many ways you can correct these problems nutritionally, as well as with medication. Reportedly, savory can have a positive impact on your GABA level.

As mentioned above, you can add savory to your favorite foods or make into a tea and consume regularly when you have conditions that the herb is known to treat. You can also use this herb as part of your everyday diet to take advantage of its tonic properties.

Enjoy!

PART VI
Selected Ethiopian Food Recipes

The Super Spice Blends Found in Most Ethiopian Cooking

These spice mixes are used in hot meat dishes as well as serve as flavor enhancers in other foods.

1. Berbere (the classic blend)

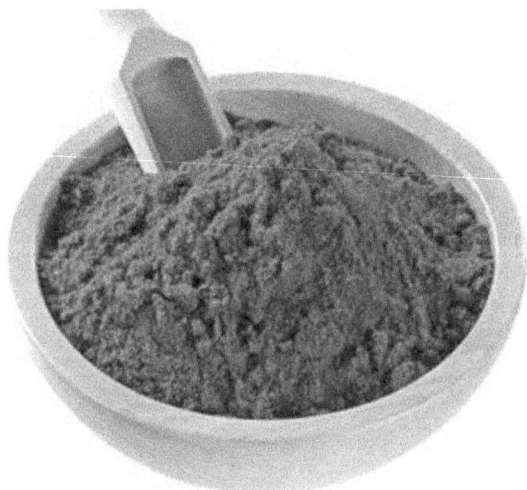

Berbere is the foundation of all the red meat and vegetable stews as well as the raw material for *awaze*—a paste—in Ethiopian cuisine. Berbere is a blend of many spices, many of which have been already described in this book. Berbere is a nutritionally dense food—rich in vitamins, minerals, phytonutrients and fiber. Traditionally, making berbere is a long and involved process—taking several days and often the help of family members or neighbors, particularly with removing the wood part of the dried jalapeno peppers. It's made in large batches to last six months to a year.

Customarily, there are no measuring cups or scales. A woman's eyes, hand, fingers or imagination serve as measuring devices. A large canvas or skin mat is necessary to dry some of the ingredients individually. A woman would often gather the jalapeno pepper and try to guess how many hand-cups or pinches of the small ingredients it would take to create the proper blend of the berbere blend.

Berbere preparation for a family of four will last one year

1. Snip the stalks of the jalapeno with one's fingers

2. Wash the final trimmed peppers and spread on canvas to dry in the sun

3. Mill the dried jalapeno and keep aside.

    a. Measure one or two handfuls of tena adam (rue) berries and place in a wooden mortar.

    b. De-shell 30-40 garlic cloves and add to the mortar.

    c. Measure a handful of beso bela and add to the mortar.

    d. Peel and mince ginger and measure in a cupped hand and add to the mortar.

    e. Pound the above items together into a paste.

4. Combine the paste with milled pepper (step 3) and mix thoroughly in a large bowl.

5. Cover tightly and leave it aside for two days, for the aroma and flavor of each ingredient to infuse into each other.

6. On the third day open the bowl, transfer the blend on to a matt and let it dry for a day or two in the sun.

7. In a heated skillet toast lightly the dried mixture to bring out the flavors and make sure that it has dried completely.

8. Cool down and mill the mixture.

9. In a separate batch, measure out coriander seeds, fenugreek seeds, black peppercorns, allspice, cardamom pods, and cloves and toast in a pan, mixing continuously with a wooden spoon for about 4 minutes. Take away from fire and let cool.

10. In a separate container mix beso bela, netch azmud, tikur azmud and tosign and grind.

11. Combine the blends from #8, #9 and #10 and mix thoroughly.

The final product should be fire red, wonderfully aromatic and flavorful, ready to be used as the base spice blend for chicken, meat and legume dishes as well as for a number of other foods. Because in the traditional way of making berbere measuring devices are not used, the flavor, aroma and color can be as individual as the person making it.

Below is the modern, standardized berbere recipe.

Measurements and Ingredients:

2 tsp. coriander seeds

1 tsp. fenugreek seeds

1⁄2 tsp. black peppercorns

1⁄4 tsp. whole allspice

6 white cardamom pods

4 whole cloves

1⁄2 cup dried onion flakes

12 garlic cloves

5 dried chilies de árbol, stemmed, seeded,

and broken into small pieces

3 tbsp. paprika powder (to deepen the color)

1⁄2 tsp. ground nutmeg

1⁄2 tsp. ground ginger

1⁄2 tsp. ground cinnamon

Directions:

1. In a small skillet, combine coriander seeds, fenugreek seeds, black pepper-corns, allspice, cardamom pods, and cloves. Toast spices over medium heat, swirling skillet constantly until fragrant for about 4 minutes.

2. Let cool slightly.

3. Transfer to a spice grinder along with onion flakes and mill until they turn into fine powder. Add chilies, and mill with the other spices until fine.

4. Transfer the mixture to a bowl and stir in the paprika powder, salt, nutmeg, ginger, and cinnamon. Store in an airtight container and use as needed.

5. Store in an airtight container and use as needed.

2. Mekelesha –The finishing spice for wots

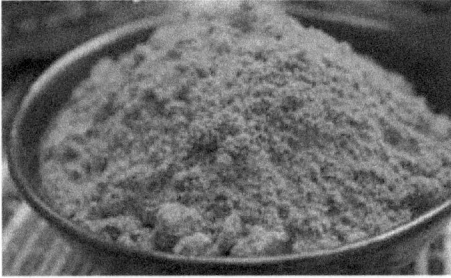

Measurements and Ingredients:

1/2 tsp. coriander seeds

5 cloves of garlic

1/2 tsp. cumin

1/4 tsp. nutmeg, freshly ground

1/2 tsp. cinnamon powder

1 tsp. black pepper

1/2 tsp. Indian long pepper

Mill these together to produce a wonderful aroma and a gray, nutmeg-like blend. Store in a tightly covered container and use as needed.

3. Mitmita

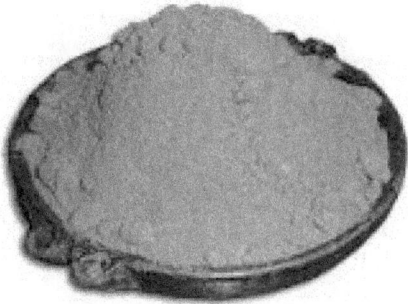

Mitmita is a classic hot spice blend used with kitfo and raw beef cubes. It's also frequently served as condiment with main course dishes. It can be eaten with plain injera or sprinkled over bean dishes before serving.

In Ethiopia, the bird's eye chili is usually collected from the garden, and sun-dried and combined with the ingredients below and milled.

Measurements and Ingredients:

2 lbs. bird's eye chilies

1/2 tsp. black mustard seeds

2 tbsp. whole cloves

1/4 cup kewrerima (Ethiopian cardamom) seeds

3/4 cup sea salt

2 tbsp. ground cinnamon (optional)

1 tbsp. cumin seeds (optional)

1 tbsp. ground ginger (optional)

Directions:

1. Combine the seed and whole chilies and dry roast, making sure some of the seeds don't pop and fly away.

2. Remove from fire and let cool

3. Combined the powered options with the chilies and seeds

4. Grind to a fine powder in a coffee grinder or mortar and pestle

5. Store in an airtight container

The resulting powder is light or dark orange, depending upon which ingredients you have included.

4. Mitten Shiro

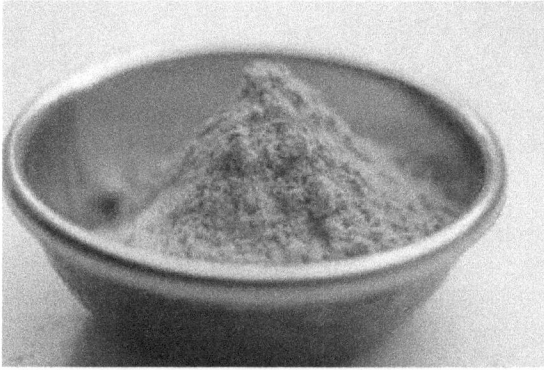

Making mitten shiro is as tedious and involved as creating the berbere blend. Like berbere, once you make it, it will last you for six months or more. As we mentioned before, there is no standardized recipe, as each household creates its own. Although most of the ingredients listed below are used across the board, there are also creative women who take away one or two ingredients and add their own. Since traditionally there have not been measuring devices for the ingredients, the quantity and therefore the taste of the mitten shiro may vary from one formulation to another. The following recipe is created in approximation to what most women use to make the mitten shiro blend.

There are generally four types of legumes consumed in Ethiopia. These are peas, lentils, wide beans, also known as fava beans, and chickpeas. When we talk about shiro wot, we usually mean the sauce made from peas flour. However, for mitten shiro all four legumes can be used, in part, because peas, as the most consumed, can be expensive.

Measurements and Ingredients:

    8 cups peas
    3 cups fava beans
    4 cups chickpeas
    4 cups lentils
    3 cups berbere
    1 cup tena adam (rue) seeds
    1 koseret (oregano, a substitute)
    3 heads of garlic, peeled and finely chopped

1 cup red onion

2 tbsp. fenugreek

1 cup ginger, finely chopped

1 cup beso bela (sacred basil)

12 kewrerima pods (just the seeds)

2 tbsp. coriander powder

1 tbsp. bishop's weed (netch azmud)

2 tbsp. cloves

2 tbsp. cinnamon

Salt as needed

2.5 cups water

Making the mitten shiro

1.   Wash peas, chickpeas, beans and lentils individually and boil each in water. You need to do them this way because these legumes cook at different rates.

2.   On a large canvas spread each item in its own lot and let dry in the sun or in the oven at low heat. Grind to powder at home or send out to be milled.

3.   De-shell the cardamom pods and grind the seeds.

4.   Combine the onion, garlic, ginger and koseret and smash in mortar and pestle into a paste. Spread on mat and let dry in the sun. Once the mixture/blend is completely dry, grind at home or send out to be milled.

5.   In a heavy skillet, roast in low heat the fenugreek, cloves, coriander, sacred basil, cinnamon bark, bishop's weed for 3 minutes. Take off heat, cool and grind these as well.

6.   In large bowl, mix the berbere, the shiro powder and the spice blends (3-5 above). This is your mitten shiro. Transfer to a container with tight lid and store in a dry place.

Mitten shiro's 20-30% of total weight reportedly is spices and salt.

There is also Netch shiro. It's used to make alicha shiro wot. With Netch shiro, the pea flour is combined with ground garlic, ginger, mekelesha and salt. Fifteen to twenty percent the weight of netch shiro is purportedly spices and salt.

You can see, just as with berbere, these seemingly simple food ingredients, are packed with many good things that are healthy for you. This is so particularly in light of all the spices and their associated benefits we discussed in the previous chapters.

No pure sugars, excessive amounts of fat and salt and there are no extraneous fillers, artificial colors or preservatives in these foods. Both the colors and preservatives are part of the natural spices and herbs.

5.   Niter Kibbeh (Clarified Butter)

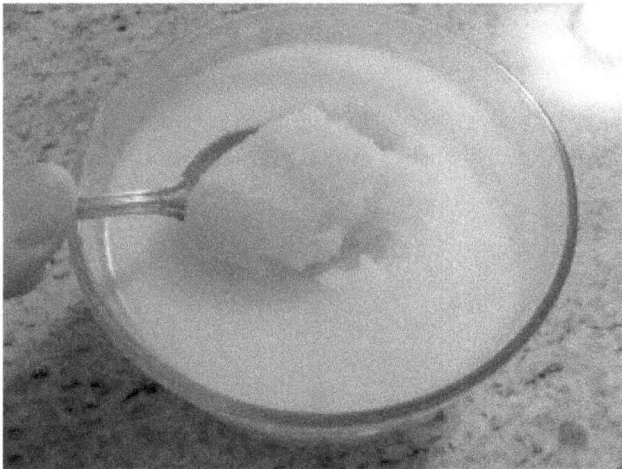

Clarified, spiced butter is one of the major components of the Ethiopian cooking. It enhances the flavor, taste and aroma of foods. Traditionally, it's used in cooked meats, vegetables, as well as legume dishes. During the fast days, women use only oils to prepare non-dairy and meat foods. As you can see from the Measurements and Ingredients, it is beautifully aromatic and tasty and you can't eat enough of it once you start. It can go with anything.

. Makes 1-1/2 cups

Measurements and Ingredients:

1 pound unsalted butter

1/2 medium red onion, chopped

1 garlic clove, minced

1 tbsp. minced ginger

1 tsp. fenugreek seeds

1 tsp. ground cumin

1 tsp. kewrerima or green cardamom seeds

1 tsp. dried beso bela (or oregano)

1/2 tsp. ground turmeric

7 sweet basil leaves

Directions:

1. Melt the butter in a saucepan over low heat, stirring frequently. As it cooks, it begins to froth, bubbles building on top. Skim and discard the foam, do so continuously until you see no more of the bubbles. Make sure to stir occasionally so it won't turn brown on you.

2. Add the onion, ginger, fenugreek, cumin, garlic, cardamom, oregano, turmeric, and basil and let it simmer for 15 minutes but still stir occasionally.

3. Remove from the heat and let it cool.

4. Strain into a container using a finely meshed sieve.

5. Cover the lid and store in the fridge.

Clarified butter's unique features:

1. It has a longer shelf-life than regular butter.

2. It has a high smoke point. This means you can cook foods with it at higher temperatures than you would with regular butter. It's ideal for stir-fried dishes. This is because clarifying the butter removes a lot of the milk solids and other salts, which cause the regular butter to burn.

Food Recipes

Injera (Ethiopian Flat, Leaven Bread)

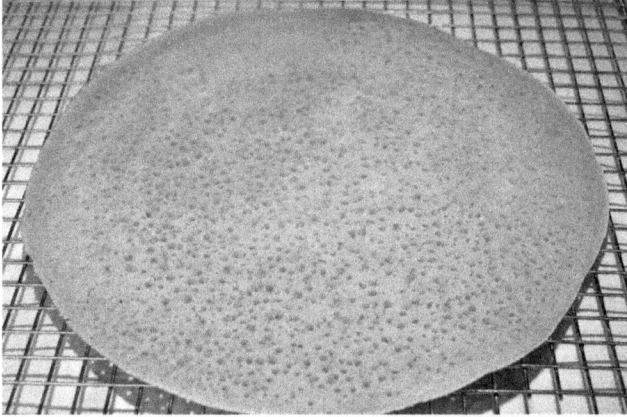

So you think you can make injera, eh?

As you have read in the previous chapters, why Ethiopian food is textured, tasty and healthy is due to the spices, the whole-grain foods and preparation techniques. Making many of the dishes given below is very easy once you have berbere, Mekelesha, the necessary spices to make niter kebbeh and other specialized dishes. Producing authentic injera from pure teff, however, will take a keen understanding of the temperature and time needed to ferment the dough or batter, your patience and willingness to try and try again if you didn't succeed the first time. Although it's relatively simple to make teff injera in Ethiopia, people in the United States find it difficult to do so. For this reason they often had to add barley, whole wheat or self-rising flour.

Anybody can make flat bread out of the teff dough, but to be called injera, it has to meet certain expected standards.

1. The top of the injera has to stare at you with its thousand eyes, steady and unblinking. And there should never be closed ones anywhere on the surface—more or less.

2. This injera has to feel spongy, stretchy, and delicate to the touch.

3. Since it's generally made from fermented batter, it characteristically must taste sour and tart.

From this list, the first two are often the hardest to achieve on the first try, particularly to those who don't know about the nuances of preparing and fermenting the teff dough and making the injera from it. This is so because there are some processes and conditions to be met in order to make a credible injera. How well have you kneaded and prepared the dough? What is the ambient temperature where you keep the fermenting dough? What is the quality of the flour? Is the *mitad* (grill) clay or metal? Is mitad sufficiently heated before you pour the dough on it? And is the dough runny enough when you pour it onto the mitad?

Once you understand these requirements, you're ready to try the recipe below.

The perfect injera

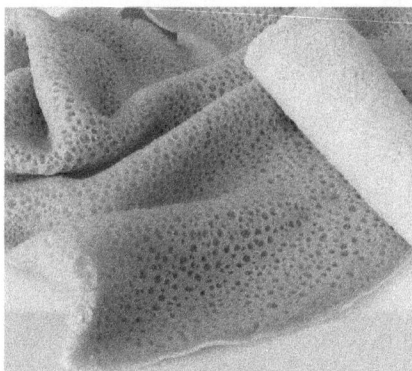

Spongy, stretchy and delicate like a fine fabric

An advice and wisdom

Regardless of how the injera comes out—flat and soulless as a tortilla or bold and wide-eyed like someone high in caffeine—what ultimately matters is the nutritional value of the injera. And as you saw earlier, teff has a lot of good things for your health. If it's for your own consumption, the aesthetic details of the injera are probably not that important. If you have dinner guests, one of whom is the Royal Highness of Ethiopia, then I'd keep it locked in my *madd-bet*—kitchen house. On a serious note, let's talk about our teff injera recipe.

Cooking items:

A large metal or plastic bowl

Flat-end wooden spoon (optional)

A measuring cup

A 10- to 12-inch skillet with a glass cover (ideally)

A large plate or tray

Yeast powder

A dish towel

A small clean cloth or paper napkin

1 tbsp. of vegetable oil

The recipe:

3.5 cups brown teff flour

1 cup whole wheat flour

1/2 cup all-purpose flour

4 cups filtered or distilled water

1 tbsp. yeast powder

Preparation:

1. Combine the three flours in the bowl

2. Add the water and mix the content with the spatula or your washed hand.

3. Keep adding the water until the mixture is thick and moist enough for kneading. Beat it with the spatula or your hand for a minute or so.

4. Heat 1 cup of water till hot. Remove from stove and add the yeast and Mix it thoroughly.

5. Set aside for 15-20 minutes to activate the yeast. Adding half a teaspoon of brown sugar can help speed up the activation.

6. Add the yeast-water mixture to the dough and blend thoroughly. Cover it with the dish towel (or a plate) and leave it overnight or until evening time if you made it in the morning. If you place the dough near a warm stove, it can rise quicker. If you use natural yeast, generated from a previous batch of dough, fermenting the new batter generally takes 3-5 days.

Baking:

1. Heat the skillet at the medium setting of your cook top plate dial.

2. Mix the dough with spoon or a washed hand.

3. Add 1/2 a cup of water (if it needs it) so the dough becomes runny.

4. Apply the vegetable oil onto the cloth or napkin and rub the skillet bottom and sides with it, so the baking injera won't stick to the bottom.

5. Pour half a cup of the dough onto the center of the skillet. After quickly putting down the cup, grab the skillet by the handle, lift and swirl it, until the dough spreads and covers the bottom evenly. Put it back down on the hot plate or grill. If the skillet is sufficiently heated, the dough hisses as it touches the pan and you swirl it around. This is a good indication, assuming you have met all the other requirements the injera is probably going to come out alright.

6. Cover immediately and wait for 2.5 to 3 minutes. If the cover is clear you can watch as the white dough turns brown progressively, until it eventually fades completely.

7. Remove the lid and check to see if the edges have begun to lift. If they have, pry one end with the spatula, insert it all the way and lift and transfer the freshly-baked injera on to the plate. Now you made your first perfect injera, the rest is history. Keep baking until all the dough is used up.

Sometimes the edges of the baking injera may not lift. In this case, pick them with a spatula until you have access to the whole bread to lift it.

There are many other recipes for making injera. In the United States, the Ethiopian restaurants that make those beautiful and delicate injeras, use higher amounts of wheat or barley flours—60% to70%—than I've included in the recipe above. Nothing is wrong with these injeras. It's just you're not getting the benefits of teff as much as you would when preparing the injera or loaf from the brown grain. Whole barley and whole wheat flours have their own beneficial nutrients as well.

Making a loaf out of teff flour

Use the same recipe but make the batter thicker like regular injera dough. You can add half a cup of brown sugar and a tea spoon of anise seeds. You can let it ferment for a few hours or can make it right away. If you bake it shortly after you make the dough, the loaf will be heavy and hardens when it cools down. If you baked yeast-risen dough it will be lighter and spongy. You can also make kita out of the freshly made dough. This bread is thin like a pizza crust. If you're sweet-toothed, you can sprinkle it with honey or a little bit of brown sugar and serve. You don't need the sweetener; the plain kita is just as tasty.

Another remarkable thing about teff is, it's filling. You can have just a loaf made from teff flour and tea or coffee and go about your task in the morning without feeling hungry. And you will have so much energy, too. If you're trying to lose or manage weight, replacing your regular breads with teff injera, kita or loaf can be the best alternative to achieving your goal or desire.

Meat Dishes

Doro Wot (Red Chicken Stew)

One of the most popular Ethiopian dishes

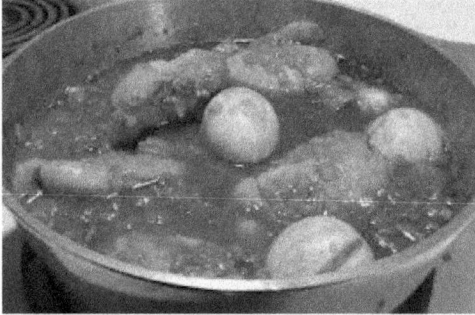

Measurements and Ingredients:

3 finely chopped red onions (preferably)

1/3 cup berbere

4 cloves of garlic

1 tsp. of finely chopped ginger root

1/4 tsp. ground cardamom

1/8 tsp. ground nutmeg

1/4 tsp. ground fenugreek

1 tsp. freshly ground black pepper[14]

1 tsp. table salt

1/4 cup niter kibbeh or ½ cup extra virgin olive oil

1-3 cups filtered or distilled water

4-6 hard-boiled eggs

6-8 pieces of chicken (legs, drumstick or thighs and wings), thoroughly washed, squeezed and dab-dried

(Serves 6-8 people)

Trivia: In Ethiopia getting the chicken ready for cooking is as elaborate and as making the stew itself. Every trace of fat or tissue that is not meat has to be removed. Then the chicken pieces are washed several times.

---

14   If you have mekelesha, use it instead.

Making the doro wot

1. In a large pot (preferably clay or enamel) sauté the onions in medium heat, till they turn brown. This can take 3- 4 minutes

2. Add 1/2 a cup of water to dissolve the onion its constituents and simmer for 3-4 minutes for 3-4 minutes.

3. Add the berbere and let it simmer for 5 minutes.

4. Add the niter kebbeh or the oil and let it cook for 3 minutes.

5. Add the garlic and the rest of the spices (except black pepper) and let it cook for 3-4 minutes.

6. Add the rest of the water and let the contents cook for 5 minutes more.

7. Add the chicken pieces and make sure they are beneath the surface of the simmering sauce. If not, add enough water to cover them.

8. Lower the heat and let it cook for 15-20 minutes.

9. De-shell the eggs and poke them with a fork or straw, creating as many holes as you can.

10. Check to see if the chicken pieces are well cooked. They must feel tender.

11. Now add the eggs, and stir the content well so the eggs get coated with the sauce.

12. Cover and simmer for 4 to 6 minutes more.

13. Finally, add the salt and black pepper or mekelesha and stir.

14. Remove from heat and let it cool.

You're now ready to reward yourself: feast over one of Ethiopia's classic meat dishes known as doro wot! Ideally, you would want to eat your doro wot with injera. If you don't have one, you can still enjoy it over rice or with regular bread, together with salad and other vegetables on the side.

Enjoy!

Sega Wot

Measurements and Ingredients:

2-3 lbs. lean, cubed beef

3 red onions, finely minced

3 cloves of garlic, finely minced

2 tsp. minced or powdered ginger

1/2 cup berbere

1/4 cup niter kibbeh or extra virgin olive oil

1 tsp. cardamom seeds or powder

1 tsp. black pepper (or mekelesha)

Making the sega wot:

1. Add the onion to a large pot with a lid and let it simmer for 15 minutes. Don't over stir.
2. Add 1 tbsp. of the niter kebbeh or oil and cook for 5 minutes or so, until the onion turns dark brown, but not burnt dark.
3. Add the berbere, 1/4 cup of hot water and the rest of the niter kebbeh or oil and let the mixture simmer at low heat for 15 minutes or so. Add the beef (a piece at a time), the garlic and 1/4 cup of hot water, put back the cover and let it cook for 12 minutes. Stir occasionally.
4. Add the garlic, reduce heat and let everything cook for 7-10 minutes, until the meat is tender.
5. Add salt (to taste), cardamom and black pepper (or mekelesha) and continue to simmer for another 5 minutes, still at low heat.

Remove from fire, cool to a comfortable temperature and sever over injera or rice. This wot can serve 6-8 people.

Doro Alicha (chicken stewed in turmeric sauce)

Measurements and Ingredients:

- 4 yellow onions, finely chopped
- 1/4 cup olive oil or
- 1/4 cup niter kibbeh
- 3 tbsp. of finely minced garlic
- 1 tbsp. finely chopped ginger root
- 1/2 cup dry white wine or honey wine
- 3 cups of water
- 4 hard-boiled eggs
- 6 drumsticks and 6 thigh bone-in chicken meat
- 1/4 tsp. turmeric (for light amber color)
- 1 freshly ground black pepper
- 1 tsp. ground cardamom

Preparing the doro alicha

1. In a heavy enamel or iron stewpot, cook the onions over moderate heat for about 5 minutes or until translucent by adding water as needed.

2. Add the garlic and ginger and continue to sauté for 5 more minutes, adding water as needed.

3. Add the niter kibbeh and stir for another 5 minutes, till everything is well blended.

4. Add the dry white wine, bring to a boil.

5. Cook briskly, uncovered, for about 5 minutes, stirring occasionally.

6. Gently drop the chicken into the simmering sauce. Stir carefully until the chicken is well coated with the sauce. Add water if needed.

7. Reduce heat, cover, and simmer for 10 minutes.

8. Remove from heat, let it cool down and serve with injera or over rice.

Courtesy: Brundo Ethiopian spices

Kitfo (Steak Tartar)

Measurements and Ingredients:

3 pounds freshly ground, very lean beef

1 tsp. mitmita

1 tsp. kowrerima

1 tsp. salt (as needed)

1/4 cup of niter kibbeh

Preparing the kitfo

Mix ground beef and the rest of the ingredients thoroughly. Heat pan and sear lightly and serve with Injera.

Vegetarian Dishes

There are many vegetarian dishes in Ethiopian cooking. The most common ones are shiro wot (prepared from pea or a combination of 3 or 4 legume flours), kik wot (made from split peas), miser wot (from split or whole lentils), mixed vegetables and Ethiopian salad (see below). You find these in nearly all Ethiopian restaurants. The most complex dishes are generally made at home for special occasions like a wedding, during the fast days or big annual festivals.

Here are a few vegetarian recipes.

Shiro Wot

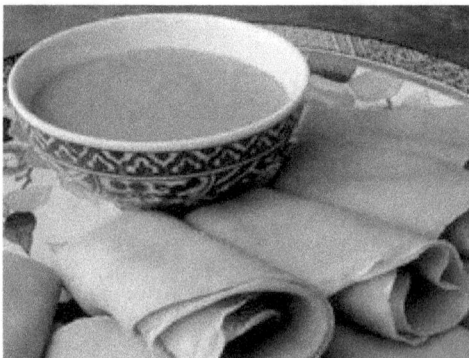

Measurements and Ingredients:

1.5 cup shiro (ground pea or chickpea flour)

(Normally purchased from an Ethiopian store. You can also make your own following the recipes given on Page 243.)

1 large onion, finely chopped

1/2 cup olive oil or niter kebbeh (if you have one)

4 cloves of garlic

1 tbsp. berbere

1 tsp. salt (to taste)

3 cups of water

Making the shiro wot:

1. Sauté the onion in the oil in a medium-size pot for 3 minutes.

2. Add the berbere, a little bit of water, cover top and let the contents simmer.

3. In a bowl, dissolve the shiro in the remaining water completely by adding the flour gradually. Transfer the resulting mixture into the cooking pot. Alternatively, you can add the shiro directly but slowly to the pot as you continue to stir the content. Just make sure it doesn't become lumpy.

4. Add the salt to taste and cook for 25-30 minutes at low heat. The shiro wot can be served runny or thick. If the latter, add more shiro powder (or a thickener like corn starch) and let it cook longer.

5. If you have niter kebbeh, add a table spoon of it to further enhance the flavor.

6. Serve on injera or with rice.

Misir Wot (Lintel Stew)

Measurements and Ingredients:

4 cups of lintel

1 large onion finely minced

2 tbsp. niter kebbeh or 1/2 cup extra virgin oil

5 cloves of garlic finely minced

2 tbsp. Berbere

2 tbsp. salt (as needed)

8-10 cups of water

Making the misir wot:

1. In a large pot simmer onion, garlic, and berbere with the butter or oil for 8-10 minutes.

2. Add the lintels and water and continue to simmer at low heat for about 25 minutes. Stir occasionally and check to see if the lintels are completely cooked. If done, turn off heat source.

3. Serve with injera or over rice.

Kik Wot (split yellow peas stew)

Measurements and Ingredients:

3 cups of split yellow peas

2 large onions fine minced

2 tbsp. niter kebbeh or ½ cup of extra virgin olive oil

4 cloves of garlic

2 tsp. turmeric

2 tsp. salt (as needed)

8-10 cups of water

Making the kik wot

1. Add onions, garlic, turmeric and the butter or oil and simmer for 8-10 minutes.

2. Add the split peas and water and continue to simmer at low heat for 20-30 minutes.

3. Stir often to make sure the contents don't stick to the bottom of pot.

4. Once the peas are completely cooked, remove pot and serve hot.

Mixed Vegetables

Measurements and Ingredients:

1 large onion, minced

1/4 of cabbage head

3 cloves garlic, minced

1 tsp ginger, minced

2 medium potatoes, chopped

2 medium carrots, chopped

2 tbsp. extra virgin olive oil

1 tsp. salt (to taste)

1 tbsp. turmeric

Making the mixed vegetables

1. Sauté onion, garlic, ginger and chilies in oil for 10 minutes.

2. Add potatoes, carrots and cabbage and cook for 25 minutes

3. Add salt and turmeric and simmer for 5 minutes

4. Once done remove from heat. Serve with injera or over rice.

Gomen (Collard Green)

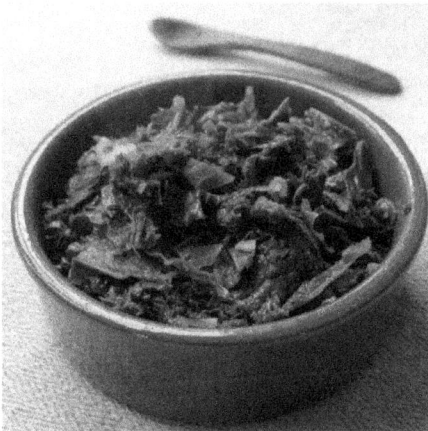

Measurements and Ingredients:

2 bunches collard greens, finely chopped

2 red, yellow or white onions, minced

1 tbsp. niter kebbeh or 1/4 extra virgin olive oil

3 medium size tomatoes minced

3 cloves of garlic minced

2 jalapenos, chopped (optional)

2 cups of filtered or distilled water

Making the gomen

1. Wash the collard green thoroughly and run through a spinner or dab-dry with towel.

2. Snip and discard the stalks.

3. Chop the leaves finely.

4. Heat a deep skillet, sauté onions and tomatoes in the niter kebbeh or oil for 4-6 minutes.

5. Add the minced garlic and cook for 4 minutes, cover pot and cook at medium heat.

6. Add the sliced jalapenos and salt as needed.

Serve hot with injera or use as a side dish to a main course.

The Ethiopian Green Salad

Measurements and Ingredients:

1/2 a head of green lettuce

1 thinly sliced tomato

2 garlic cloves, finely minced

1 tbsp. each: extra-virgin olive oil and white wine vinegar (mixed and shaken together)

1 medium onion (red, yellow or white), chopped in short thin trips

3 tbsp. parsley, chopped

3 tbsp. freshly squeezed lemon juice

1 tsp. black pepper, freshly ground

1/4 tsp. ginger, finely minced

1/2 red bell pepper

Salt to taste

Making the Ethiopian green salad

1. In large salad bowl, mix vinegar, garlic, oil, ginger and black pepper and whisk gently

2. Add lettuce, onion slices, tomatoes, bell pepper and parsley.

3. Add lemon and toss well. Serve as a regular side dish.

All five vegetarian dishes are served over injera.

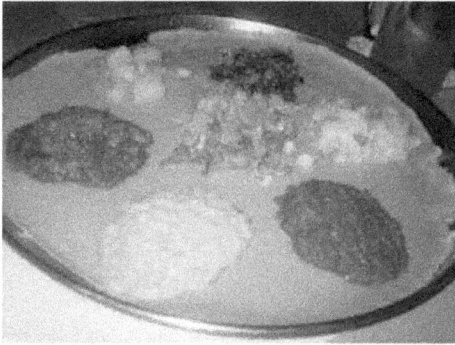

Misir wot, kik wot, gomen, mixed vegetables and the Ethiopian salad.

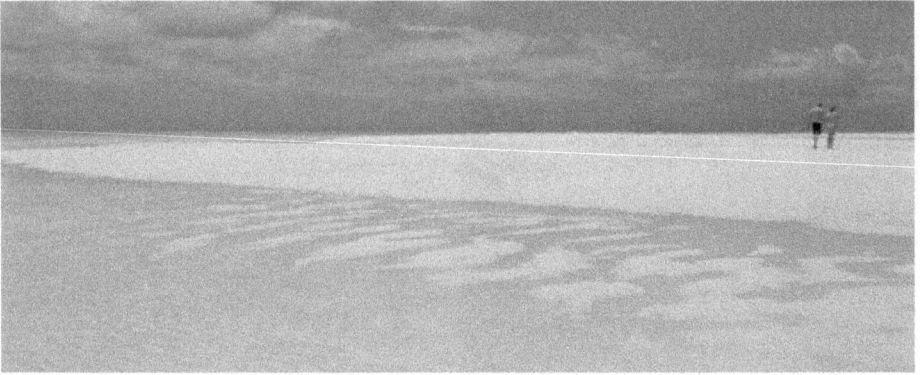

May you have a happy and healthy life to the very end!

PART VII
Appendices

APPENDIX A
Free Radicals and Antioxidants

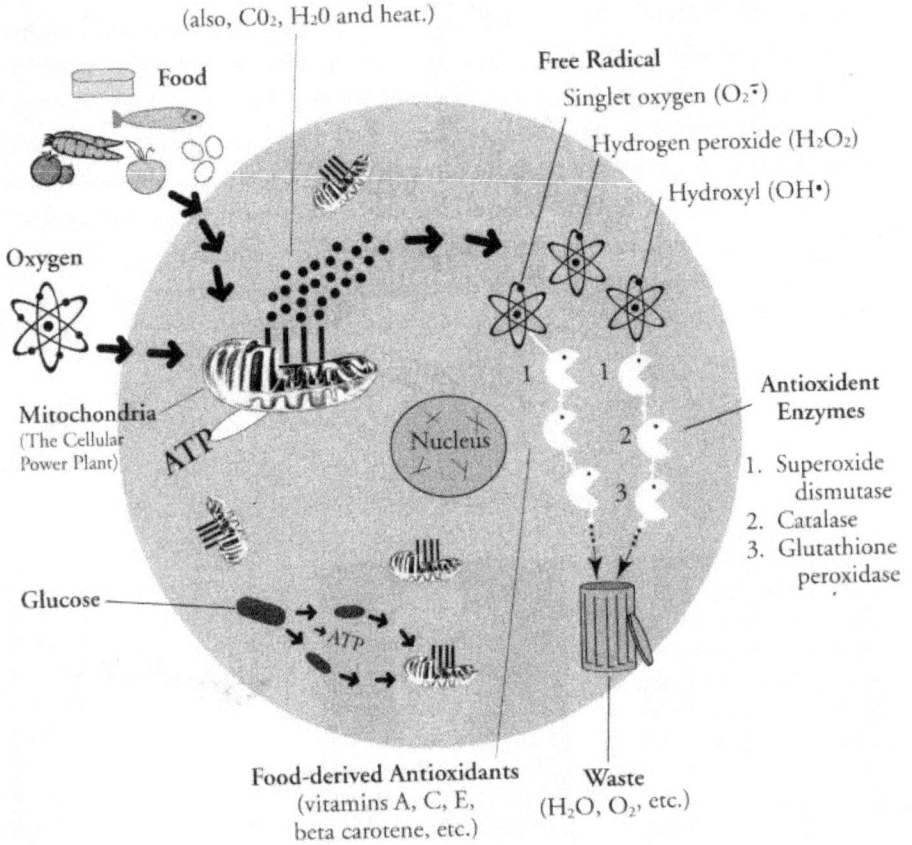

(also, CO_2, H_2O and heat.)

Food

Free Radical
Singlet oxygen (O_2^-)
Hydrogen peroxide (H_2O_2)
Hydroxyl (OH•)

Oxygen

Mitochondria
(The Cellular
Power Plant)

ATP

Nucleus

Glucose

ATP

Antioxident
Enzymes

1. Superoxide
   dismutase
2. Catalase
3. Glutathione
   peroxidase

Food-derived Antioxidants
(vitamins A, C, E,
beta carotene, etc.)

Waste
(H_2O, O_2, etc.)

Figure A.1 Free Radical Generation and Cellular Energy Production

Within this orb lies everything that you are or are able to do.

Free Radicals

Atoms are the basic building blocks of any substance. When atoms combine, they form stable molecules, like oxygen in our atmosphere (two oxygen atoms combined as one molecule) or water (two hydrogen atoms and one oxygen atom). When certain molecules combine, they form long chain substances (or polymers) like proteins, fats and carbohydrates—just to name a few.

Atoms or molecules are bonded together by electrons. In organic compounds, the most frequent number of electrons shared between atoms is two. These bonds are not permanent. Depending on the presence of other forces (temperature, radiation and chemical agents), these bonds can break and separate from each other, leading to an uneven number of electrons in each molecule or atom. As shown in Figure A1, the same situation can result when a molecule is stripped off one of its outer electrons. In either case, the resulting molecule or atom is referred to as a free radical. In the body, free radicals are generated during the normal course of metabolism, or they may be induced by environmental factors, such as radiation and pollution.

Free radicals are unstable substances that cause havoc in the area in which they roam or with the things they encounter. A free radical's ultimate goal is to find another atom or molecule with which to pair up or from which to steal an electron to become stable again. When this happens, however, new free radicals are formed that go around attacking more molecules to generate still more free radicals. Such a chain reaction could millions of free radicals. If this reaction goes unchecked, it can lead to major complications in the body.

Cell membranes are damaged. Collagen and elastin proteins cross-link, causing wrinkles or lines to form in the skin. Fats become rancid. Contacts between nerve cells are severed, and the DNA malfunctions. The cumulative effect is physical and mental aging, as well as the onset of various degenerative diseases like cancer, stroke, arthritis, arteriosclerosis, diabetes and senility.

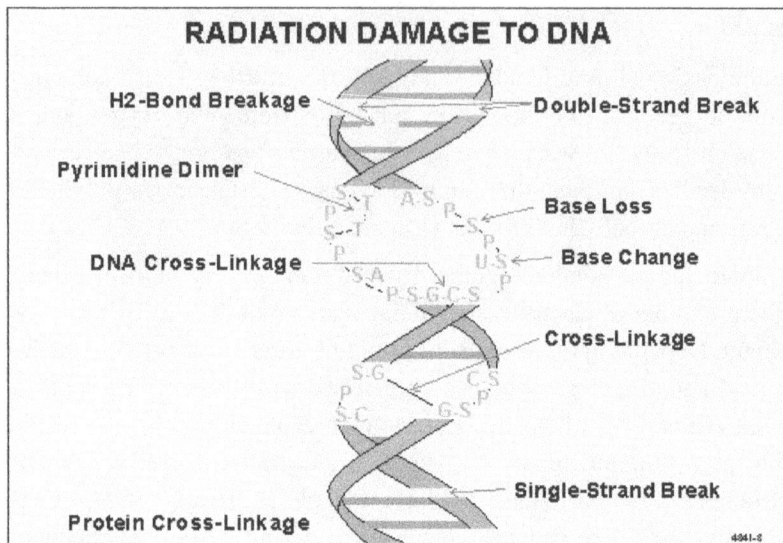

RADIATION DAMAGE TO DNA

H2-Bond Breakage

Double-Strand Break

Pyrimidine Dimer

Base Loss

DNA Cross-Linkage

Base Change

Cross-Linkage

Single-Strand Break

Protein Cross-Linkage

Figure A.2 A Free Radical Damaged DNA. Like moths that shred your wool clothes to pieces or termites that gnaw away the inner workings of your house, uncontrolled free radicals can do the same to your genes and delicate tissues of your body.

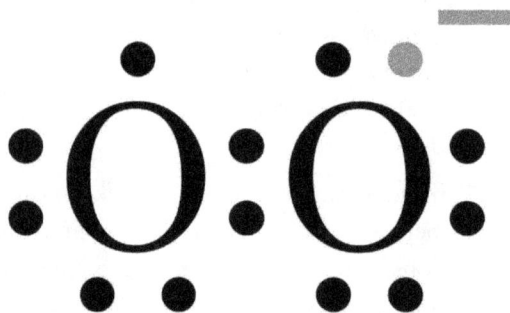

Superoxide (02, ● —)

This oxygen molecule known as superoxide radical is missing one electron. One of the byproducts of metabolic processes, superoxide free radical is very unstable and dangerous to the body tissues.

Figure A.3 An Illustration of a Free Radical

Missing electron (free radical) attacks any double bond such as in the fatty acids of intracellular membranes, DNA and other molecules.

Sources of Free Radicals

Inside the body, free radicals can be generated from normal metabolic processes and by white blood cells, which use them as a weapon to kill disease-causing foreign elements in the body. They can also be generated by oxidation of unsaturated fats, such as those found in the brain and other parts of the body.

Some of the environmental sources of free radicals are x-rays, ultraviolet light, chemical toxins in the air and water (such as lead, cadmium, mercury, copper and even iron) and nuclear radiation.

Cigarette smoking and dietary fats and oils—particularly those oils processed by the heat extraction method—are other common sources of free radicals. Barbecued and fried foods, such as those you buy at fast-food outlets, are also a great source of free radicals. The combination of high-temperature heated oils (used to prepare these foods) and oxygen is the ideal condition for the generation of enormous numbers of free radicals. The high temperature at the burning tips of cigarettes and the tar that results are also major sources of free radicals.

A single puff of cigarette smoke, for example, can contain up to 100 trillion free radicals, never mind the 3000 plus different aromatic compounds some of which are known carcinogens, it contains.

Perhaps the greatest source of free radicals is the oxygen we consume every day. It's reported that for every 25 molecules of oxygen we inhale, 1 free radical is produced. Considering that we consume trillions of oxygen molecules, with a single gulp of air, you can imagine how many free radicals can be generated every time you breathe in air.

In the mitochondria, during food metabolism, oxygen is reduced to water and carbon dioxide through an addition of electrons one at a time. Hence addition of one electron to a food-derived molecule generates the superoxide free radical (shown in Figure A.3) two electrons, the hydrogen peroxide free radical, and four electrons, water molecules. In the presence of energy such as UV light, x-ray, iron and copper the hydrogen peroxide converts to the hydroxyl free radical which is the most noxious of the radicals formed in the body. Hydrogen peroxide and hydroxyl free radicals are shown in Figure A.1).

It is important to note that free radical generation takes place throughout a person's lifetime but increases with age. Particularly vulnerable are brain cells and white blood cells because they are rich in unsaturated fats. A destruction of large numbers of white blood cells can lead to the weakening of your immune system. This is one of the reasons why you become more susceptible to diseases and infections as you get older.

Antioxidants

Luckily, we are not entirely without defense against these freaks of nature, free radicals. Through our bodies' manufacture of its own antioxidant enzymes and by the food we eat, we can help shield our tissues and organs from free radical damage. The three most powerful antioxidant enzymes are superoxide dismutase (SOD), glutathione peroxidase and catalase. These enzymes are manufactured by the body to promote good health.

Superoxide dismutase specifically works to help fight oxygen free radicals. Our body burns the food we eat by using oxygen through a process called metabolism. During this process, many oxygen free radicals are produced, the most common one being the superoxide free radical (see Figure A.3). The SOD helps neutralize this free radical before it attacks tissues and begins a chain reaction.

What is interesting is that there are two types of SOD—one that exists inside the mitochondria of the cell, the other outside but within the cell. The one inside the mitochondria has manganese as its component, and the one outside has zinc and copper in its structure. It has been shown that a small deficiency in any of these elements greatly affects the SOD activity in our body, thus speeding up our cellular attack by free radicals and our biological aging.

The minerals zinc, copper and manganese aid the body to manufacture its own SOD. Similarly, catalase is an antioxidant enzyme that is formed with and activated by iron. In collaboration with the other enzymes, it helps neutralize free radicals generated in the cell. Its function is primarily to neutralize the hydrogen peroxides.

The other antioxidant enzyme, glutathione peroxidase, is a very versatile molecule involved in a variety of activities in the body. This enzyme promotes the effectiveness of Vitamin C and Vitamin E and enhances the immune system. Glutathione peroxidase can also help neutralize the unhealthy effects of heavy metals such as cadmium, mercury, lead and aluminum. It saves cells from oxidation. Both white and red blood cells depend on this enzyme for their proper functioning. The power behind glutathione peroxidase comes from the mineral selenium, which is one of the major components of the enzyme. The importance of selenium in human health is discussed in Chapter 6.

Food-Derived Antioxidants

There are many well-documented antioxidants obtained from the food you eat. Some of the prominent ones are Vitamins A, C and E, beta carotene, minerals such as selenium, copper, zinc, manganese and iron, glutathione and the amino acids cysteine, methionine and lysine. And then you have the phytochemicals, as discussed on Page 105, found in many types of vegetables and fruits and the herbs and spices. As mentioned there, each one of these nutrients has many benefits to our health besides its role as an antioxidant. Let's look at each one separately.

Beta Carotene—Precursor of Vitamin A

"Eat your carrots. They can help you see better at night." Perhaps you heard your mother chirp this when you were little. And from that time on you have associated the absence of carrots in your diet with night blindness. You try to include a few sticks of these tuberous vegetables whenever you get a chance.

Perhaps you now know that carrots are good for you because they contain a substance known as beta carotene. It is beta carotene that converts to Vitamin A in the body and helps the *visual purple*—the pigment in the retina that enables your eyes to quickly adapt when you go from light to darkness.

For a long time, scientists had associated Vitamin A with night vision. Vitamin A is now known, however, to have many different functions and benefits for the human body. One of these functions is fighting free radicals. In the body the two most common free radicals are those that form from oxygen molecules and polyunsaturated fatty acids (PUFAs). PUFAs are an integral part of the cell membrane, body fat and some of the food you eat. Beta carotene is known to be an excellent scavenger of the PUFA-generated and singlet oxygen free radicals. Singlet oxygen free radical is one of the most damaging of the oxygen radicals in the body.

In test experiments, Vitamin A was also found to inhibit chemically induced cells from becoming cancerous. This, in itself, is very important because our body is constantly exposed to all kinds of chemical carcinogens found in foods as additives, e.g., preservatives, coloring and flavoring agents and texturizers. Vitamin A can also help fight the cancerous effect of drugs, cigarettes, radiation, water and air pollutants.

Vitamin C

Unlike vitamins A and E (the fat-soluble antioxidants), Vitamin C has the distinct advantage of being water soluble. Since nearly two-thirds of our body is water, it means this vitamin can go just about anywhere in the body. As an antioxidant, Vitamin C can travel freely in the bloodstream and aid the cells and tissues from the effects of free radicals.

Vitamin C, in effect, acts as your body's sacrificial lamb. A Vitamin C molecule gives up one of its electrons to a free radical substance, and in so doing, self-destructs. This battle between Vitamin C and free radicals takes place thousands, if not millions, of times a second (depending on the number of free radicals present in your body and the Vitamin C level in your bloodstream).

Free radicals, besides contributing to your aging process, are responsible for a variety of cancers. Vitamin C, by neutralizing these marauding chemical species and by boosting your immune forces (antibodies, white blood cells, lymphocytes), protects your body from bacterial and viral infections as well as from cancerous growth. In addition, Vitamin C is known to block the formation of nitrosamines—cancer-initiating compounds formed from proteins and nitrites (such as sodium nitrite), which are used as food preservatives.

Vitamin E

Vitamin E is the other food-based antioxidant that has important functions in the body. As one of the few fat-soluble vitamins, vitamin E's primary function is to protect fat molecules from free radical attack. These include the triglycerides and cholesterol in the circulatory blood and the polyunsaturated fats (PUFs) found in the cell membranes and the brain cells.

As said earlier, free radicals are generated during a normal metabolic process or are imported from outside via the water and foods we consume. These ravaging chemical species attack everything they encounter, but they have an affinity for the fundamental building units of your tissues and organs: the cells. A significant portion of the membrane that covers the cells and the sheath that coats nerve axons is made from proteins and substances known as polyunsaturated fatty acids (PUFAs).

As mentioned above, PUFAs are highly vulnerable to a free radical attack. Vitamin E is one of the few fat-soluble vitamins and lodges itself in the membranes of the cells and neutralizes the free radicals before they harm the membrane substances. In doing so, this vitamin averts the onset of many diseases and premature aging.

This effect of Vitamin E has been shown in several experiments. Researchers in one study showed the protective level of Vitamin E by giving a group of people 600 I.U. of the vitamin for ten days and then subjecting their red blood cells to oxygen and light. When they compared these results with that of the control group (those who had not received vitamin E), the red blood cells from the group who were supplemented with Vitamin E oxidized by only 8% while those of the control group were completely destroyed.

In another experiment, rats supplemented with Vitamin E had a greater resistance to the damaging effects of lead poison than those that weren't given the vitamin. Vitamin E in collaboration with Vitamin C has also been shown to counter the cancerous effects of several food additives (such as sodium nitrite) that lead to the formation of nitrosamines-well-known carcinogens. Nitrogen dioxide, a common pollutant and byproduct of automobile exhaust, is also known to be damaging to the lungs. There is evidence to show that vitamins C and E help prevent this problem, too.

The Mineral Antioxidants

The antioxidant property of the minerals copper, zinc, manganese, iron and selenium has largely to do to their function as part of the enzymes systems discussed earlier. Copper, zinc and manganese are part of the two superoxide dismutases that neutralize the superoxide free radical produced from the consumption of oxygen. Iron and selenium, as partners of catalase and glutathione peroxidase, respectively, help in destroying the hydrogen peroxide free radicals as well as free radicals generated from the breakdown of fats. Of course, as discussed in their respective sections, these minerals have many other functions and benefits to the body besides their antioxidant properties.

Selenium

Selenium has many great benefits to your health. As an antioxidant, selenium can function by itself or in conjunction with the enzyme glutathione peroxidase, a powerful enzyme that plays many important functions in the body, including fighting free radicals, boosting the immune system, cancer prevention and detoxification of heavy metals (such as cadmium, mercury, lead, arsenic) from the body. The mineral selenium is an integral part of this enzyme. Each molecule of the enzyme cradles four atoms of selenium. Many of the metabolic free radical fragments, such as hydrogen peroxides, and those generated from the breakdown of fats are neutralized with the help of this enzyme.

Selenium, together with vitamin E, has also been shown to fight the onset of two major killers: heart disease and cancer, so much so that the incidence of these diseases and the level of selenium in the soil have been correlated. In the areas of the country where there is a low level of selenium in the soil, there are more deaths from cancer and heart disease. (See Chapter 6 for the geographical distribution of selenium in the U.S. soil.)

This amazing mineral has many other benefits. The prevalence of cancer, for example, is equally consistent with the level and geographical distribution of selenium around the world. According to studies from many different countries, the use of selenium in the diet helps minimize the incidence of several types of cancer, including breast, uterine, lung, pancreatic, rectal, mouth, prostate, lymph gland, liver, thyroid, colonic and ovarian cancer. Selenium was found to be equally effective against cancer of the bladder, skin, cervix, esophagus, intestine, pharynx and kidneys.

Interestingly, even those who have already succumbed to cancer seem to realize improved survival time, fewer malignancies or metastases and less recurrence of lesions when they received sufficient selenium.

A study in which mice were infected with a virus that induces mammary cancer showed a reduction by eightfold in the occurrence of the tumor with a selenium-containing diet. This is a dramatic improvement considering that these mice ordinarily develop tumors in a purported 95% to 100% of the time when infected with the same virus.

Because of the close similarity to the way breast cancer develops in humans, the scientist who did the above study feels that the incidence of breast cancer in this country would be reduced significantly if women took 250 to 350 micrograms of selenium supplements daily.

Selenium is also very important for the proper functioning of the sex organs. The production of sperm cells, as well as their strength and motility, is aided by the level of selenium in these organs. More than half of the body's selenium is found in the testicles and seminal ducts. This means that every time men have sex, they lose a fair amount of it. To maintain an adequate body level of this mineral, they have to keep replenishing it.

In other areas, selenium has been found to be beneficial in the efficient production of energy, in relieving arthritis and in reducing the incidence of cataracts. All these, incidentally, have something to do with selenium's ability to fight free radicals.

Selenium is, indeed, a remarkable mineral.

Cysteine, Glutathione, Methionine and Lysine

In addition to vitamins and the mineral selenium, there is a group of amino acids that are well-known antioxidants. Glutathione is a small peptide molecule consisting of glutamic acid, cysteine and glycine.

Glutathione helps in the synthesis of the enzyme glutathione peroxidase. This enzyme, as was discussed earlier, has many protective benefits in your body. Glutathione, in collaboration with selenium, helps fight free radicals, guards against cirrhosis of the liver, boosts the protective power of vitamins E and C, assists in removing toxic metals from the system and helps in the production and fortification of immune cells.

Cysteine and methionine are the two sulfur-containing amino acids that are known to be good antioxidants. These amino acids, besides functioning as building components for the regeneration of tissues, are great at mopping up accumulated toxins, such as metabolic by-products, tobacco and alcohol derivatives and heavy metals, such as mercury, lead and cadmium, from the body.

All these are deleterious to the body's organs and tissues. Lysine is known to help boost the immune system by encouraging the production of antibodies. In addition, a daily dose of 1,000 mgs of lysine was shown to reduce herpes breakout in those who carry the virus.

Herbal Antioxidants

Over many years now, the phytochemicals or phytonutrients have been toted, after vitamins, as the next group of substances that may have many beneficial properties in our health. These compounds, which are extracted from the green, red, blue, black and yellow of vegetables and fruits, are not exactly nutrients (at least so far as we know), in the sense that they don't get involved in energy production or in repairing and building of tissues, but they apparently have many influences in the health and wellness of our bodies. One of these influences is in serving as antioxidants. The other is by interacting or interfering with certain enzymes and substances in our tissues in ways that enhance and maintain the health and well-being of our bodies.

Some of these compounds are sulforaphane (from broccoli), lycopene (from tomatoes), lutein (from alfalfa), allylic sulfides (from garlic), genistein (from soybeans) and capsaicin (from red peppers). There are many other compounds found in different herbs and spices that have been shown to have beneficial properties in our bodies. (Read the information on phytochemicals and herbal antioxidants).

A Team of Antioxidants for Maximum Health

If you notice, in a well-formulated supplement, all antioxidant vitamins, minerals and phytonutrients appear together. There are reasons for this:

1. All the antioxidants do not necessarily have the same function; that is to say, certain antioxidants are more effective than others in neutralizing certain types of free radicals. For example, beta carotene and selenium (as part of the enzyme glutathione peroxidase) are more powerful neutralizers of the singlet oxygen free radicals. This means, for instance, that during a strenuous physical exertion, like exercise or physical labor, you tend to use up a higher volume of oxygen, which consequently increases the metabolic activities of your cells and the production of the singlet oxygen free radicals. Taking the recommended amounts of these nutrients prior to your physical activity can thus minimize the damage these radicals can cause.

Vitamin E and selenium, on the other hand, are great suppressors of fat peroxidation. Fat peroxidation (the rupturing of fat molecules leading to the formation of free radicals) can be initiated by a number of agents, including radiation, toxic metals and chemicals, singlet oxygen free radicals and a number of other substances. Tissues that are highly vulnerable to some of these agents are the lungs, the digestive tract and the liver.

As you must know, the lungs and the digestive tract are the primary contacts of everything that enters the body, including the various chemicals and pollutants that come along with food, water and air. The liver, besides serving as main distribution center, is the place where many of the body's toxins accumulate. Consequently, these three organs take the brunt of many of the effects posed by substances that come in from outside as well as by those generated from within the body. The vitamins E and C and the mineral selenium are known to be excellent protectors of these tissues.

The phytoantioxidants also have their own special functions in the body. Some of them activate enzymes that are intimately involved in the health and proper function of the cell. Hence, for instance, while sulforaphane induces the synthesis of enzymes that are closely involved with the proper function of the cells, others like coumaric acid and cholorogenic acid help remove unfriendly substances from them. There are also phytoantioxidants involved in the health of certain tissues of the body. For example, the anthocyanosides (in bilberry) help with the health of the retina, and leucoanthocyanin (in grape seed extract) is important for the well-being of the blood capillaries. Likewise, the flavonoid molecules found in ginkgo biloba are important for the health and proper function of the brain and circulatory system.

2. When antioxidants are present together, besides enhancing your issues, they protect one another and other nutrients from the effects of the free radicals. For instance, Vitamin A protects vitamin C, which, in turn, protects vitamins A and E and some of the B complex vitamins from free radicals or other oxidative process. Vitamin E, similarly, can serve as a "bodyguard" for vitamins C, D and F[15] and the B complex vitamins.

As you can see, you should have not only high concentrations of the antioxidants in your tissues but also all of them together so that each one will adequately complete its specific job without getting destroyed before it reaches its destination—usually the cells. As an illustration, think of military airplanes that are on a bombing mission. Unless these planes are adequately shielded from enemy air fire by an escorting aircraft, they may never reach their target.

Inside your body, at a microcosmic level, a raging battle goes on between the free radicals and antioxidants. As in the real world, who wins this battle depends on the number and strength of the forces involved.

---

15   Essential fatty acids like omega-3 and omega-6 fatty acids.

APPENDIX B

The Importance of Good, Clean Water to Your Health and Longevity

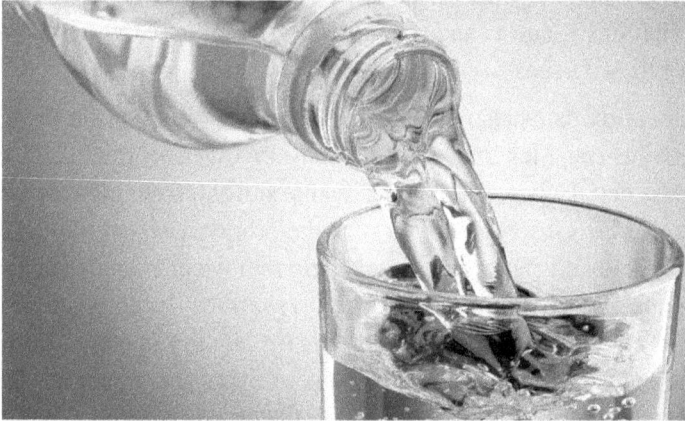

Throughout this book, we have talked about how good nutrition is the basis of good health, well-being and longevity. Good, clean water is an integral part of good health and nutrition. In fact, considering that about two-thirds of your body consists of water and that water is the medium in which nearly all the metabolic processes take place, the quality or integrity of this medium is very important indeed.

Some of the degenerative diseases such as cancer, arthritis, atherosclerosis (hardening of the arteries), kidney stones, cataracts, hearing loss, diabetes and a number of others that come with age could be caused by a lifelong consumption of bad water, as much as by bad nutrition. Unfortunately, as long as the water we use or drink every day satisfies our thirst, tastes reasonably OK and is readily available, many of us don't think twice about it.

In reality, as you can see below, the water you use from your tap, well or river can be the harbinger of many health hazards. These health problems are not cholera, typhoid, dysentery or any number of other water-borne diseases that have caused devastations in various parts of the world throughout history. The modern versions of these once fatal diseases are subtle, and in most cases, causes and symptoms may not be directly correlated. This is because many of the maladies that can be attributed to pollutants in water can also come from other sources.

From a number of disease-causing chemicals that are often found in our drinking waters and from the continuous rise in many degenerative diseases, as well as from specific correlational findings[16], our drinking water has indeed come to be a growing threat to our health. For example, radioactive minerals such as strontium 90, radium 226 and 228 and common chemicals such as chlorides and nitrates are known to be carcinogens. Yet all these and many other substances can commonly be found in our drinking water, albeit some in tolerable amounts.

The Environmental Protection Agency (EPA) has called the water pollution problem "the most grievous error in judgment we as a nation have ever made." Dr. Patrick Quillin, in his book *Healing Nutrients*, writes that those who still drink normal tap water are either "uniquely blessed with an isolated pocket of clean water" or "very cavalier about (their) health."

What Could Be Wrong With Your Drinking Water

Besides the inorganic minerals that naturally abound in most ground and river waters, there can be countless chemicals, bacteria, viruses and even radioactive stances contained in the water you use every day. Some of these pollutants come from agricultural runoffs. These can be pesticides, herbicides and fungicides, and fertilizers such as nitrates, sulfates and chlorides. Industrial and power plants emit a lot of waste (which includes radioactive substances) into the atmosphere and the water supply above or under the ground. Similarly, hydrocarbons and pollutants from auto exhaust fumes can find their way into the lakes, rivers and reservoirs from which your city draws your drinking water.

Moreover, because water is highly mobile and interactive (many organic and inorganic chemicals can dissolve in it), the pollutants that may exist in your drinking water may have come from far away. Because of this and the above reasons, the quality of the water you use for consumption should be of paramount importance[17]. Unfortunately, most of us are indeed cavalier about our drinking water. The sad thing about it is that our water pollution problem is not getting better. One writer refers to this worsening situation as a "scourge of major proportion (that could become) our legacy."

---

16   For example, people who live in New Orleans, near the delta of the Mississippi River are found to have a higher incidence of kidney and bladder cancers, as well as other urinary tract disorder. Nitrates from farmland runoffs that often contaminate the water supply in the Midwest, are probable culprits, and are known to be a major health hazard to babies and adults alike."

17   Even in a situation in which the quality of the water is closely monitored, the allowable level for each contaminant has been determined without the availability of studies of their long-term, chronic ingestion even at these "low" levels.

Here is a list of some of the substances that can be found in your drinking water:

- EDBs
- Strontium 90
- Algae
- Thorium
- Tannins
- Magnesium
- Petroleum solvents
- Copper
- Benzene
- Cadmium
- Nitrates
- Rust particles
- Chlorides
- Nickel
- Zinc
- Bacteria
- Silver
- Aluminum
- Mercury
- Pesticide
- Iron
- THMs
- Calcium
- Sulfates
- Arsenic
- Chlorine
- Sand
- Carbon 14
- Viruses
- Sodium
- Lithium
- Radium 226 & 228
- Herbicides
- Lead
- PCBs
- Chromium
- Sulfides
- Barium
- Fluorides
- Silt
- Cesium 137
- Radon

Because of these and many other inorganic and organic substances, your water can sometimes look unappetizingly murky, taste heavy and muddy and smell stale and swampy.

The heavy metals—cadmium, lead, mercury and others from the list above also known to generate free radicals, those chemical renegades that create havoc in chlorinated chemicals can generate free radicals on their upon by the enzymes in your body or can combine with water, hydrogen peroxide and hypochlorite (a compound found in most make the dangerous singlet oxygen free radicals. These chemical species, as mentioned, earlier, are believed to be one of the causes cancer.

Similarly, nitrates are a problem because when they combine with the amino acids in your diet, they create nitrosamines—also well-known carcinogens. Then have you have the radioactive elements such as carbon 14, strontium 90, radon and thorium that can collect in the bones to become a health threat. As you probably know, radioactive materials are carcinogenic as well.

Contrary to popular belief, the inorganic minerals such as calcium and magnesium that you find in most drinking waters may actually have a negative impact on your health. Some of these minerals, for example calcium, can settle out in the arterial walls, causing them to harden, collect cholesterol and impede the normal blood flow. The technical term for this is atherosclerosis, which is one of the causes of heart attacks and stroke. The reason why they can be bad when found in water but good when found in food or nutritional supplements is discussed further on in this section.

Minerals can also collect in the joints, kidneys, pancreas and inner ears, as well as eyes and tissues, leading to arthritis, kidney failure, diabetes, hearing loss and cataracts. According to Dr. Allen Banik, because of the impact they have on many vital functions of the body, too many minerals in your drinking water can "destroy every fond hope you have by striking you down . . . and will draw your activities from the great out-of-doors, into creaking rocking chairs and finally into bedridden old people's homes."

Considering how important minerals are to our health, the above statements may come as a total surprise to you. As discussed in Chapter 5 and 6, minerals are very, be very important indeed! Among other things, your muscles, heart, brain and many other body processes depend on minerals for their proper functioning. You need, however, only the minerals you get from organic sources, from the food you eat or from supplements.

Studies have shown that the amount of minerals the body metabolizes from drinking water (whether it be mineral, tap or well water) is less than 5%. And according to the American Medical Journal, "the body's need for minerals is largely met through foods, not drinking water." Similarly the National Water Quality Association has remarked: "The amounts of minerals found in water are insignificant when compared to those found in the food we eat."

To understand how waterborne minerals behave in your body, you can think of a river that carries sand, silt and many other organic and inorganic matters in it. This river, as it flows from higher grounds to the lower, flat lands, leaves behind much of what it carries along its course, banks and delta. Over a period of time, a lot of the material could collect so high and wide that it could cause the river to divert its course.

The blood in your arteries is similar to such a river in that it, too, tends to deposit any excess material along its path until, after some point, the sludge of minerals and fat harden and begin to interfere with the normal flow of blood. In your body, excess cholesterol, fat and mineral sedimentation are some of the major causes of circulatory disorders.

Amazingly, the average person could consume roughly 450 pounds of inorganic minerals from tap and well water in his/her lifetime. Where do you think some of this gunk ends up? Your kidneys try to get rid of as much as they can. What's left may slowly accumulate in the blood vessels, joints, lungs and other tissues in your body, leading to some of the diseases that come with age.

The Solution

Your best solution is to drink pure water, free of any of these substances. This means distilled water. Distillation, in combination with pre-carbon filtration, give you water that is 99.9% pure. Despite popular belief, this is the kind of water that is ideal for drinking. Your food and supplements, not your drinking water that can provide you with the minerals your body needs.

Reverse osmosis (RO) is perhaps the next best method of water purification. Manufacturers of RO systems claim that their devices can remove anywhere from 85% to 95% of substances found in water, but these percentages go down over time. Some critics have put the figures as low as 50% to 70% after a few operations. In either case, RO filters seem to have more problems than the manufacturer or door-to-door RO water filter salesperson would be willing to admit to.

Such problems include quality, variability in the filtered water, short service of the membrane, carbon and sediment filters (lasting only 1 to 2 years) water wasting. With steam distillers, you have none of these problems.

Let's now see how the city purifies the water you drink daily. The most common methods of water purification (carbon filtration and sediment filtration) remove only 20% and 5%, respectively, of matter contained in water. These two methods are used by most cities and towns to bring you filtered drinking water.

Depending on where you live and the type of water (soft or hard, lake or river or ground water) that exists there, your city may use different treatments and filtration process. Most of these treatments are designed to make the water safe (free of disease-causing bacteria and viruses) and to reduce unwanted smell, taste and appearance.

In typical filtration, a combination of several processes may be used. For starters, long-term storage is used to settle much of the suspended matter and bacteria.

This may be followed by aeration to reduce taste and odor and by coagulation and sedimentation to enhance the color and lower the material content. Because coagulation often entails the addition of several chemicals, such as ferrous sulfate, lime, sodium aluminate and ferric chloride, the resulting water can become hard and corrosive.

The last three steps of purification involve softening, filtration and disinfection. The softening process uses ion-exchange resins to remove most of the calcium and magnesium. The filtration process can be accomplished using either fine sand, underlaid with gravel or just large grains of sand. Both of these processes are used to improve the appearance as well as to reduce the mineral and bacterial content of the water. The final stage of the purification involves disinfection. This step most commonly uses chlorine, but ozone and ultraviolet radiation are also used to kill bacteria and to disable viruses. In addition, copper sulfate, to control algae growth, and activated charcoal, to trap odor and organic chemicals, may be used.

After all these steps, the maximum your town's filtration systems can do is to remove only up to 25% of the substances contained in your drinking water. This means that from the list of substances you saw earlier, the sediment filtration stage removes mainly sand, silt and rust particles, while the others and the activated carbon filter help remove bacteria and organic substances such as benzene, THMs, PCBs, petroleum solvents and some of the pesticides and herbicides. The activated carbon filtration can also remove bad taste, odors and chlorine. Otherwise, nearly 75% of what you see on the list, if they already exist in the water being processed, can end up in your tap water.

The other problem, often not apparent to the average consumer, is old, corroding water pipes. In fact, your city's water purification centers may have done the best they could in filtering your water supply. What they often don't have control over are the leaching metals such as copper, lead, nickel, cadmium and others that may be found in the network of underground water pipes.

Depending on the condition of the water itself (acidic or basic), the duration of contact it has had with the pipes since it left its source and the age of the pipes, you could have various levels of leaching and contaminations as a result of the above metals. For instance, a significant level of leached copper can change the appearance of your water to blue. A high level of lead in drinking water can cause a number of physical and neurological disorders, particularly in children. It can affect a child's mental development and learning abilities. The heavy metals listed also are known to be free radical generators, as we said in earlier chapters, and can initiate a number of diseases and speed up aging. To deal with these problems, you have a few choices.

The first option is to purchase distilled water for drinking and cooking. It may cost you considerably less than what you ordinarily pay for bottled water.

The second option is to buy and install your own steam distillation or reverse osmosis system. A distillation system, as we said earlier, is the best. You consistently get top quality water, and the system can last you a long time compared to an RO system. If this is too expensive, find a water company that at least uses reverse osmosis and purchase your water from it. In the long run, though, you might be better off owning a purification system.

The third option is to use tap water cautiously. If your piped water has not been in use for some time, such as overnight or when you've been on vacation, turn the faucet on and let the water run for at least 3 to 5 minutes. This will help flush any accumulated leached-out minerals in the water.

If you depend exclusively on your tap or even bottled and spring water for your drinking and cooking, eat foods that are a good source of antioxidants. Vitamin A, for instance, as retinol or beta carotene, is a great neutralizer of singlet oxygen free radicals. So are selenium and vitamin E. As mentioned earlier, singlet oxygen free radicals are some of the commonly produced chemical species in the presence of salt, sodium, chlorine and water.

Vitamin C and the amino acids cysteine and methionine are good in removing many of the toxic metals that may exist in your drinking water." Best of all, make your Four Pillars drink and consume it with all your meals. For the times you have not made the drink and as an added protection , find a good multi-vitamin supplement and take it regularly.

In summary, your overall health will greatly depend on both good nutrition and the quality of the water you drink. Since water occupies the largest volume in your body and since the multitude of biochemical processes that takes place in it happen in a water medium, the purity or integrity of this medium is very important for the efficiency and consistency of these processes.

Because polluted drinking water tends to depress your immune system, replacing your water supply with pure water will help you feel healthier and stronger.

When your body fluids are "uncluttered (as they are when you drink pure water), hormones can zip around the body quicker, oxygen and nutrients are transported faster and the enzymes and other chemicals work with higher efficiency. All these, in turn, can make you feel healthier and stronger. Pure water is truly a gift of nature. And you should give it to your body every day.

APPENDIX C
The Importance of Physical Exercise

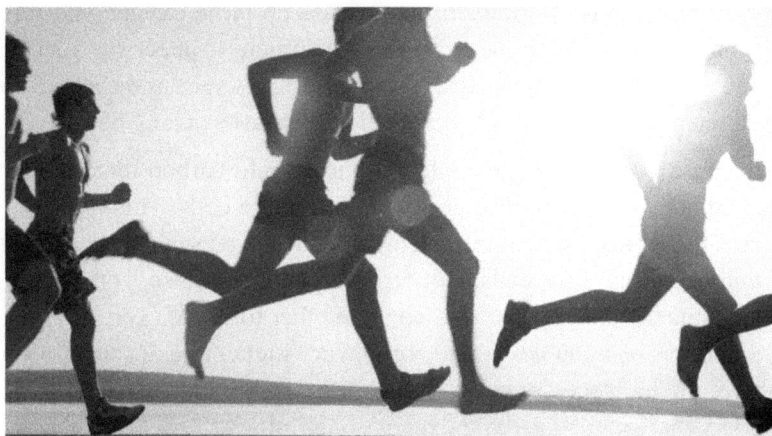

Understanding Exercise

This book cannot be complete without including a section on exercise. Physical exercise is a spice of life. Just as food can be pretty bland, dull and boring, life without regular exercise can be equally dull and boring. It's not food, it's not water, and your body doesn't depend on it for its survival. Yet, for those who want to live longer and look and feel better and younger, exercise can make a world of difference in their health. It's the last piece in the puzzle that completes and optimizes one's picture of health.

Perhaps the first and immediate benefit of exercise is that it can help you release stress, depression and any other matters that may be clouding your mind at the time. Exercise heightens your awareness of your environment, how you think and feel about it and how you appreciate it. With exercise, you can also think more clearly, react more quickly and accomplish tasks more efficiently. Finally, exercise enables you to manifest fully the power of good nutrition in your health.

How it Works

There are a few different kinds of exercises, and each one affects your body and mind differently. The aerobic ones—like long-distance running, swimming, cycling, cross-country skiing, climbing stairs and rowing—help you by maximizing your cardiac output. With exercise, you use up more oxygen and force your heart to pump a higher volume of blood per minute to meet the fuel demands placed upon it by the various tissues. Aerobic activities such as the above therefore help strengthen your heart muscles. Aerobic exercise has many benefits:

1. Because the food gets completely burned into carbon dioxide and water, there is less buildup of toxic substances in the cells. This type of exercise uses the Krebs cycle almost exclusively. The Krebs cycle takes place in the mitochondria of the cells. During this type of exercise, you use up greater amounts of calories than you would in other forms of exercise (see below). Since aerobics enables you to burn fat at a higher rate, it can help you minimize the incidence of heart-related diseases. By increasing your HDL (the good cholesterol), aerobic exercises can protect you against heart attack and atherosclerosis (fat deposits in the arterial walls). For those who want to lose weight, aerobic exercise is indeed very effective. The key is doing it regularly and in conjunction with other weight-reduction methods.

2. Aerobic exercise is perhaps the best for making you feel good and especially euphoric afterwards. During exercise a variety of brain chemicals called endorphins and norepinephrine are produced. It is these chemicals that give you the heightened sense of wellbeing, keenness of mind and euphoria. As a neurotransmitter, epinephrine also enhances your memory and learning ability. When you are mentally sharp, you can accomplish a lot more in life[18]. That is what good, vigorous, regular exercise will do for you.

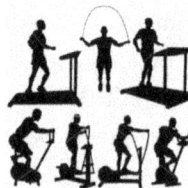

---

18 In an experiment to show the benefit of exercise to human health, three groups of people were studied. Over a four-month period, one group did aerobics, another did strength exercises like weight lifting and the third (the control group) did nothing. It was found that all those who exercised had an improved reaction time, higher recall rate and improved analytical and reasoning abilities than those who did not exercise. Furthermore, the aerobics group performed even better than those who did strength exercises.' Incidentally, in a similar experiment, children who exercised performed better academically and in other tests that measured their mental and physical abilities.

3. Because exercise in general, and aerobics in particular, pumps more blood through your circulatory system, more oxygen and nutrients are being delivered to the various tissues of your body. It's these nutrients and oxygen that enhance your looks and mental acuity. Notice how those who exercise regularly have something special about the way they look and relate to the world around them. Their skin may be clearer, smoother and more attractive than that of those who don't exercise regularly. These people also seem to be happier and have a higher energy level than their counterparts. As you can deduce from the above information, exercise indeed revitalizes and enhance the quality of your life. Since aerobic fitness enables you to burn more fat, it can also minimize the chance from death related to fat.

4. In another way, exercise rejuvenates your body by neutralizing free radicals—those molecular sharks that annihilate your body tissues at a cellular level. It's thought that since oxygen is used up in greater quantities when you exercise, it must also help neutralize the radicals that form during metabolism. This seems contradictory since we discussed in Appendix A that the most deadly of the radicals (singlet oxygen and peroxides) are formed from oxygen.

When the body is at rest, more of such radicals are formed than neutralized. With exercise, the numbers that are formed are equal to those that are neutralized. Since the oxygen molecule is a rich electron source, those generated from other sources get squelched by the oxygen molecules that bathe the tissue cells.

5. Finally, exercise can induce the release of an important substance known as growth hormone (GH). GH is your body's natural anabolic steroid that helps build muscle mass and strength. Unfortunately, like many other important substances that stop or slow down with age, the production of GH (by the pituitary gland in the brain) wanes after age 30. In those over 30, however, the amino acids arginine and ornithine with vitamin B5 and choline cofactors were shown to increase the production and release of GH.

Strength exercise like weight lifting, sprinting, short putting and discuss throwing, on the other hand, work by helping you build strengthen and tone certain muscles. Although not as vigorously, the heart and lungs also work hard at this type of exercise to bring food and oxygen to meet the energy demands of those specific muscles.

This type of exercise tends to depend less on the Krebs cycle for extraction of energy from foods. Thus such exercises are called anaerobic (without oxygen) exercise. The problem with this form of energy utilization is that food products are not completely burned, and as a result, lactic acid and other chemicals often collect in the muscle tissues. That is why weight lifters and sprinters commonly experience fatigue and cramps in their muscles when they engage in fast and highly intense exercise. . If you want to lose weight or be in good shape, aerobic exercise is your best choice. Anaerobics are good for building strength and for increasing bone and muscle mass.

Another form of exercise that does not affect muscle endurance or the cardio-vascular system is isometric. This type of exercise strives to strengthen or firm muscles by pushing or pulling on a fixed object like a doorframe or parallel bars.

Isotonic is a similar form of exercise in which the body works against gravity (i.e., push-ups or free weights). Calisthenics and weight training are examples of isotonic exercise, and they can help you build endurance, muscle strength and muscle mass.

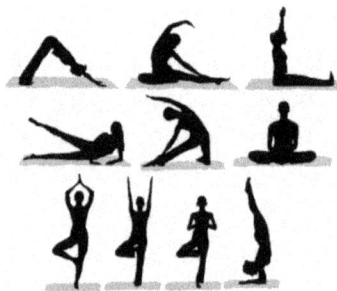

Although they began in Far Eastern countries, where the people practiced them as a way of purifying their minds and bodies through a series of mental and physical exercises, yoga and tai chi have found popularity in the West in the recent past. In these exercises, individuals attempt to attain maximum flexibility and coordination by stretching and breathing properly while simultaneously inducing the mind to free itself from unhealthy thoughts and desires. These exercises are unique in that they deal with the spiritual component of the body. To have a whole and totally integrated body and mind, it's important we work on our spiritual or subconscious mind. In most cases, our subconscious is more powerful in controlling our lives and destiny than any amount of muscles we are able to amass.

To build stamina and endurance and improve your cardiovascular efficiency, you need to do aerobics at least three times a week. Because this type of exercise strengthens the capillaries and encourages the formation of new ones, many of the remote tissues (like skin and scalp) will have more nutrients and oxygen delivered to them. As you must know, this is very important for the appearance of your skin and hair. This type of exercise can also increase the number and size of the mitochondria, the cells energy factories, which enables you to use more oxygen and burn more fuel.

When your heart is fit and strong and it pumps more blood (reportedly 25% and 50% per minute more blood while at rest and during exercise, respectively) and beats less frequently—60 to 70 times per minute as opposed to 80 to a 100 times per minute when you're unfit. Besides making you feel good afterwards by relieving stress and depression, aerobics also minimizes the incidence of cardiovascular diseases such as stroke and heart attack.

To build strength and increase muscle mass, do weight lifting, sprinting and a number of other similar exercises that develop and tone the specific muscle tissues. These exercises will enable you to lift, carry a load and push or pull on an object with power and strength. Simply speaking, these are your power exercises.

On the other hand, to improve flexibility and coordination, do isometric exercise, like gymnastics and calisthenics. These improve your joints' and body's ability to do a whole range of motions—bending, stretching, rotating, etc. These exercises enhance the mechanical efficiency of the body. Unexercised muscles and joints become cranky and stiff—particularly as you get older. Thus, to maintain your youthful attributes and delay the process of aging, do these exercises regularly.

Finally, to achieve a fully integrated mind and body, include yoga, tai chi, meditation, visualization in your daily routine. These exercises will enable you to reach deep within yourself and release mental and spiritual toxins. No matter what you are able to do for your physical self (through various exercises discussed above), you're not completely fit unless you also do the same thing for your mental/spiritual self.

Visualization is perhaps one of the most powerful techniques in achieving almost anything you want, including good health, power and strength, as well as in maintaining your youthful attributes.

In fact, true freedom (whatever that means to you) comes through the spiritual/ mental components of your "self". The relief or freedom you experience after intense workout lasts only through the duration of endorphins and epinephrine that your body produces during these physical exertions—and that is not very long. When you combine the mechanical/physical aspects of body fitness with your spiritual self, you en joy and appreciate life, and you will look and feel your best.

Nutrition and Exercise

Exercise without a good nutrition program is like driving your car with very of little oil and fuel in it. You may be able to drive it for a little while, but you're not going to get very far. Once all the oil or fuel is used up, the car will come to a grinding halt. This analogy is a good departure point for discussing your nutrition requirements while you pursue your exercise and fitness regimen. Let's follow the analogy a little further.

For your car to run properly, it needs fuel, oil and water. For fuel, you have regular, unleaded and supreme (a high-octane fuel). For oil you can get differ- ent grades: 40, 30, 10-40. Similarly, you can also use different water: tap, water (which is bad because the minerals in the water can corrode the water tank and engine overtime) or demineralized or distilled water (which is the best because it has no contamination and does little damage to your car.)

Your body has identical requirements. It needs fuel (food), oil (vitamins and minerals) and water. Like your car, although it can run on regular (proteins) unleaded (fats), its fuel of choice is supreme (carbohydrates—your body's high octane fuel). Strictly as an energy source, proteins are not a good option. Just as regular gas releases lead and other pollutants into the atmosphere, protein burning can release ammonia[19] and other toxins. Ammonia can be very deadly if allowed to build up to a significant level. Fortunately, your body has a built-in safer mecha- nism by which it can quickly convert this dangerous substance into harmless urea and uric acid. These and other by-products are just as quickly filtered through your kidneys.

The other problem with excessive protein intake is the associated excessive loss of much water. This happens as the body naturally tries to purge itself of the protein-induced pollutants. Incidentally, this problem also burdens your kidneys with extra work—often a prelude to kidney-related diseases that may come later in life. So, when you plan to exercise, avoid eating protein-rich foods beforehand.

---

19   The form that could temporarily build up is really not ammonia the gas but rather the water-soluble version (ammonium). It is this that the body quickly converts into uric acid. Bear in mind also not all the amino acids from protein can be used as an energy source.

Fats would seem an ideal fuel source for individuals who exercise and do body training—because each molecule of fat has more than twice as much energy stored in it as a similar protein or carbohydrate molecule. (Each gram of fat contains 9 calories, while each gram of protein or carbohydrate contains only 4 calories.) Unfortunately, not only are fats metabolized differently in the body, but also they are very cumbersome substances that have many bad health consequences[20].

Your best fuel supply is carbohydrates. These food groups are the cleanest (highest octane) and most readily available fuel. When athletes like sprinters, gymnasts or weight lifters or when you (in a fight-or-flight situation) need a burst of energy, you depend entirely on glucose—the smallest carbohydrate molecule, derived from foods like rice, pasta and potatoes and other food sources during digestion. This conversion is almost exclusively anaerobic (requiring no oxygen), and it happens in a flash.

The problem with the anaerobic process is that glucose is not completely oxidized, which leads to potential buildup of lactic acid. These acids cause muscle cramps and fatigue when you engage in long and arduous weight lifting or repetitive sprints. They also waste energy because only 5% of the potential energy is extracted from food in this process.

This energy is transferred to ATP (adenosine triphosphate), which serves as a temporary storage medium. Remember, though, that this is very temporary indeed. A sprinter's body, for instance, extracts energy from glucose, transfers it into ATP and uses this same ATP as his source of energy—all of which is done while he is still in motion.

The aerobic (oxygen-dependent) process, on the other hand, involves several steps and takes a little longer, comparatively speaking. This process uses the Krebs cycle solely and is the one in which 95% of the energy is extracted from each glucose molecule. In this reaction, all food molecules are completely oxidized into carbon dioxide and water. Long-distance runners, swimmers and cyclists who need a steady source of energy use the aerobic process almost exclusively.

The other benefit of the aerobic process is that your cells can burn other foods besides carbohydrates. Fats and proteins are equally "combustible" fuels that can be added to the furnace of the Krebs cycle. In endurance exercises like long-distance running, swimming and cycling, however, what becomes a limiting factor is the availability of enough oxygen.

---

20 Since it's not water soluble, it does not get around the body very easily. It needs carrier mediums like HDLs (high density lipoproteins). So, eating large quantities of fat to get your concentrated energy can be a dangerous affair. Some of the fats are free radical generators, others clog the blood vessels leading to cardiovascular diseases.

Just as it takes a strong hand to fan and make a big fire for cooking or heating, it takes a strong heart that can beat steadily and pump large quantities of oxygen-carrying blood per stroke to the furnaces of the mitochondria. Your cardiovascular system has to be free of artery-clogging fats, not only to carry oxygen and nutrients but also to remove the "soot" (carbon dioxide and other waste matter) from the cells.

As you can see from the foregoing discussion, you need aerobic exercises not only to build stamina and endurance but also to lose weight and feel emotionally and physically good. As to shedding extra pounds, the problem most people have is how not to regain it once they lose it.

Traditionally, many weight-loss programs used the Krebs cycle theory to help people lose weight. Since carbohydrates are one of the three competing fuels in the aerobic reactions, it was believed that if you restricted your intake of pasta, rice and other starchy foods, your body would rely on its own fat for energy. By this method, it was thought that over a period of time you could literally melt your fat away.

Although those who endured the agony of this approach may have eventually dropped their extra baggage, they also found it difficult to maintain their new weight. The brain, in normal circumstances, is entirely dependent on glucose for its fuel supply. When you restrict your carbohydrates, you put the brain under a terrible stress. That is why most dieters have a tremendous craving for sweets and feel fatigued and exhausted when they are on a calorie-restrictive program.

Unfortunately, what happens 98% of the time is that these people either end up abandoning the program when they can no longer stand the ordeal or, once they have lost all they want and start eating normally once more, regain all their dearly paid for poundage. Often, they may even add more, because their body wants to store as many calories as possible in the event they starve it again. It might also possibly be interpreted as the body's punishment to them for putting it through this ordeal.

The best solution is to combine aerobic exercise with a high-carbohydrate diet. Carbohydrate-rich diets not only keep your mind sharp and full of energy but also will enable you to undertake your exercise regimen without feeling exhausted. Carbohydrate-based diets also encourage the burning of your body fat, as opposed to contributing to storing it. The key is, once you lose all the pounds you want to lose, keep exercising regularly. This will enable you to maintain your new weight and have overall good health.

APPENDIX D
Losing and Managing Your Weight

Causes of Obesity

Nearly 68% of the American population is either obese or overweight. People have taken many different measures to lose or manage their weight, most without much success. One of the common methods is dieting.

Crash or fad diets deprive the body of key nutrients, reduce lean muscle mass and put the body and mind under enormous stress. This type of dieting, ironically, is also the worst way to try to lose or manage your weight. This is because when important vitamins and minerals are scarce (as they are when you reduce your caloric intake), the body's metabolic processes will be depressed. As a result, not only will your body struggle to mobilize body fat to the mitochondrial furnace of the cell, but it will also have difficulty in efficiently processing the food you consume.

This type of weight loss can be psychologically and emotionally devastating to the individual. When the ordeal becomes unbearable, the person often abandons the program and goes on with life as usual. What do you think is the cause of the weight problem in this country?

Think about it. Save for a few exceptions, people don't just become too fat.

Most often they bring it upon themselves. Here are some of the common reasons why people become overweight.

1. Consuming Too Much Fat

If you are a typical American, chances are you obtain over 40% of your calories from fat and fat-based foods. As much as this food substance is your body's secondary source of energy and offers more calories than similar amounts of carbohydrates and proteins combined, it is also one of the most easily stored substances in the body.

While nearly 25% of the calories from carbohydrates or proteins can be used to convert them into body fat, hardly any calories are expended to convert food fats into body fat. In other words, your body has an "open-door" policy with regard to fats. Hence, as long as you consume too many grams of fat and you have a sedentary lifestyle, these fats simply roll in and get stored in your body tissues.

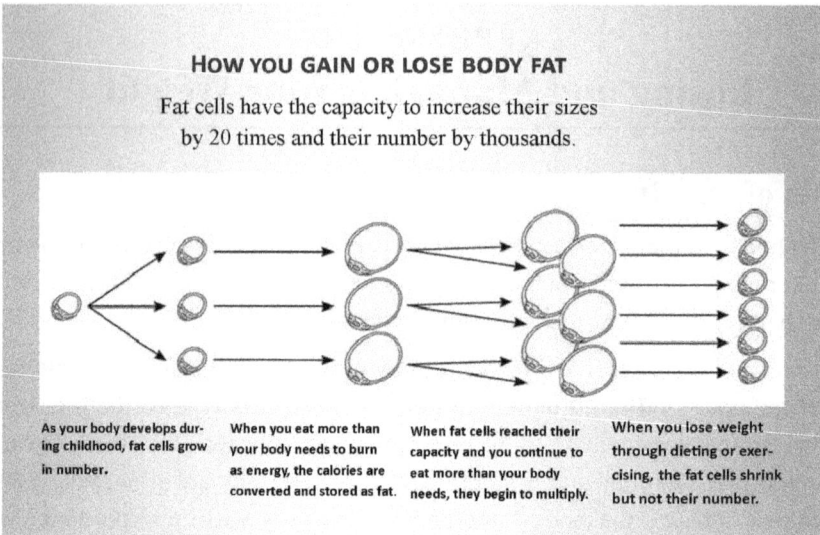

HOW YOU GAIN OR LOSE BODY FAT

Fat cells have the capacity to increase their sizes
by 20 times and their number by thousands.

| As your body develops during childhood, fat cells grow in number. | When you eat more than your body needs to burn as energy, the calories are converted and stored as fat. | When fat cells reached their capacity and you continue to eat more than your body needs, they begin to multiply. | When you lose weight through dieting or exercising, the fat cells shrink but not their number. |

This is the reason why parents should never let their children to gain weight...Eating junk foods and consuming high-calories soft drinks are the main causes of cardiovascular diseases, cancer, diabetes and a number of other degenerative diseases that afflict us as we get older. Managing our caloric intake and keeping our weight to normal level is very important.

To minimize this problem, experts recommend that you keep your fat calories to below 20% of your total calories.[21]

2.   Consuming Too Many Refined Foods

Processed and refined foods such as sugar and white bread are some of the major culprits regarding the accumulation of excess body fat. Since these foods contain hardly any fiber, they get processed and enter the bloodstream quickly. Because the body's tolerance level for large quantities of sugar is low, this sugar is quickly brought to your body's cells. There, if not used for energy production, it will be converted into and stored as fat.

The consumption of sugar in this country is bad business. Just to show you how bad it has gotten, the per capita consumption of sugar has gone up from 19 pounds per year in 1970 to nearly 70 pounds in 1989.5 This is an amazing 370% increase.

---

21   The American Heart Association and the National Cancer Institute have recommended that we keep our fat calories to below 30% of our total calorie. But for those who have weight problems, experts recommend that fat calories be below 20%.

Where do you think all that sugar ends up? Of course, most of it ends up in your fat cells. As you may know, there are many hidden and visible sugar- based foods. And the problem with an excessive intake of sugar is not limited just to the problem of obesity. You may also have to be concerned about dental cavities, hypertension, hypoglycemia and even adult-onset diabetes.

3.   Sedentary Lifestyle

The average American not only consumes high-calorie foods but also exercises very little. The automobile is omnipresent, and walking even a few hundred yards to a neighborhood store may be viewed as walking a long way. A combination of high calories and no exercise means a higher conversion of those calories into body fat.

As you must know, exercise is one of the great mobilizers of body fat. When your body is at rest, it uses up minimal calories to run the basic bodily functions, such as respiration, digestion and circulation. This so-called basal metabolic rate has been shown to increase with exercise. This means that those who exercise not only burn high calories during the activity but also increase their body's ability to burn fat when at rest.

4.   As You Age Your Metabolism Slows Down

One of the great mysteries of nature is the process of aging. As our bodies age, not only do our skins wrinkle and lose their moisture and our hair thins out, but also the absorption of nutrients from the digestive tract and their metabolism in the cells are compromised. During this time, fat and other calories tend to collect in the tissues at a greater rate than when we were younger. This problem, of course, will cause us to be too fat along with becoming predisposed to degenerative diseases, such as heart diseases, cancer and diabetes.

Things You Can Do About Obesity

From the above discussion, you can see that obesity is largely associated with our consumption of high-calorie foods (fats and too many sweets) as well as from our body's improper utilization of the food we eat (because of a lack of exercise or slowed metabolism). You can also see that the long-term solution to this problem does not come from a crash or fad diet program. It is something we can accomplish by combining well-established weight management techniques with state-of-the-art nutritional ingredients and technology.

1.   Reducing Your Caloric Intake

For a sedentary person, all calories (whether from carbohydrates, fats or proteins) can be fattening when consumed in high amounts. Particularly crucial, however, are those you get from fats. Fat calories, as mentioned above, are treated differently by the body than are other calories. Unlike the calories you get from carbohydrates and proteins, a quarter of which are used up before they turn into body fat, nearly all the fat calories that enter the body go directly into storage. In a country in which over 40% of our calories come from fat, the problem we have with obesity becomes readily apparent.

The best solution to this problem is, obviously, to reduce your daily fat calories to at most 20%, to eliminate or keep to an absolute minimum your daily consumption of sweets and to include regular exercise as part of your weight reduction effort. (You can be generous with your consumption of complex carbohydrates that come from whole foods (teff, brown rice, whole wheat flour and others). These foods can give your body a steady supply of energy.) If you are familiar with the traditional method of weight loss, you can see that the approach described above is revolutionary.

2.   Managing Your Caloric Intake

Along with reducing your consumption of fats and sweets, you may also want to learn how to manage your daily calories. This is to say that although you now have lowered your caloric intake, unless you know how to properly distribute those calories through the day, you may have difficulty in achieving your new weight.

Let's see what this means.

First, remember that any calories that are not used to run your basic bodily functions or your other energy needs are converted into and stored as fat. For example, let's say you have reduced your daily calories from 2,000 to 1,500. Unless you use these new calories wisely, you may not notice a great difference in your weight. How does this happen? Very simply.

Suppose you obtain a significant portion of the 1,500 calories from your evening meal. Since you are less likely to engage in physical activity at night, those calories not utilized by the basal metabolic process will end up in the fatty tissues. Once stored, fat calories are not readily available. (That is why, as discussed below, it takes at least four hours of walking at the rate of 3 miles an hour to lose a pound of body weight.)

Second, when you consume a large portion of your daily calories at night, you will have difficulty containing your hunger during the day and consequently maintaining or reducing your weight. How so? Once calories are stored, the body prefers to keep them for a "rainy day," so to speak. Thus, when the calories from the circulating fluids are depleted as a result of usage or storage, your brain sends hunger signals to the stomach, which you notice when you wake up in the morning or at other times during the day. Often what happens at such times is that you end up eating more at a meal or snacking more frequently on the wrong foods to satisfy the hunger. Neither of these options is going to help you in your weight reduction or maintenance efforts.

To circumvent this problem, you may want to consume a large portion of your 1,500 calories during the day. Since most of us are physically active during the day, we tend to expend a significant proportion of our caloric intake during this time. Thus, at dinner, you may want to have fewer calories but highly nutritious foods. Meals that are rich in protein, vitamins and minerals are preferable.

3.   Using the Four Pillars Drinks and State-of-the-Art Nutritional Ingredients and Supplements

The high mineral and vitamin content in The Four Pillars drinks as well as the fiber and phytonutrient in it should help metabolize fat in your tissues and purge the excesses in foods from the GI tract. Additionally, you may also include nutritional supplements.

In recent past, advances in nutritional science and technology have opened the door to unique and exciting nutritional ingredients and technologies which, if properly used, may enable us to have greater control of our health and well-being. For instance, substances like chromium picolinate and L-carnitine which find in some supplements, are excellent mobilizers of your body's two major fuels: carbohydrates and fats. While chromium picolinate enhances your body's ability to efficiently process and burn sugar and fats, 8 L-carnitine specializes in rounding up fat molecules and dumping them into the mitochondrial furnace. With the availability of these nutrients in your food, less of the sugar and food fat will be converted and stored as body fat. Reportedly, these two substances not only aid you in burning fat but also may help to maintain lean muscle mass.

Equally important in the metabolism of fats and sugars, as mentioned above, is the availability of key vitamins and minerals. In the previous paragraphs, very simplistic terms and analogies were used to describe the mobilization and burning of fats and sugar molecules. What actually goes on in your billions of cells to accomplish the conversion or mobilization of these substances is a very complex process involving millions of chemicals and chemical reactions. For these reactions to come to completion smoothly and efficiently, the availability of sufficient enzymes, minerals and vitamins is crucial.

4.   Exercising Regularly

For losing or controlling weight, as well as for overall good health and a good mental outlook, exercise can make a world of difference in your life. As was briefly mentioned above and is thoroughly discussed in Appendix C, exercise helps the body burn fat during the activity as well as afterwards.

Through a process called lipolysis, exercise encourages the release of fat molecules from their storage sites. This, according to experts, could go on for as long as 24 hours after exercise. Covert Bailey, author of Fit or *Fat,* says that exercise does this by inducing your cells to step up their production of the fat-burning enzymes.

Thus, when you exercise regularly, you will increase the synthesis of these enzymes, which in turn will increase the burning of fat from your body. Aerobic exercises such as running, cross-country skiing, swimming, cycling and climbing stairs are excellent mobilizers of fat deposits. Furthermore, with exercise, you not only build strength and stamina but also increase your lean body mass.

Bear in mind, however, that unless you also include other weight reduction methods, such as taking the fat-mobilizing nutrients discussed above, the amount of poundage you shed through exercise alone over a short period of time can be frustratingly small. For example, to lose just one pound you may need to expend roughly 3,500 calories. This translates into five hours of walking at the rate of 3 miles per hour or four and a half hours of running at 9 miles per hour. Nonetheless, the best way to lose weight is to do it gradually. When you do it slowly, your body is unstressed and the loss can be permanent, as long as you don't overindulge in fattening foods and keep exercising.

What is the best exercise?

For minimizing bodily injuries and for sustaining long-term weight loss, the low-impact types are often considered the best. These are swimming, cycling, walking, climbing stairs, low-impact aerobics, cross country skiing and weight lifting. High-impact exercises—such as downhill skiing, running or jogging, racquetball or basketball—can be stressful to an unconditioned body.

Regardless of the type of low-impact exercise you choose to pursue, bear this in mind: the frequency of the activity is more important than the length of the activity. This, in turn, is more important than the intensity of the activity.

Let me explain this further. Although almost all cells manufacture and store triglycerides (or fat), the ones that synthesize and store them the most are the adipocytes or fat cells (illustrated in Figure D.1). When one is obese, as much as 95% of an adipocyte's volume can be occupied by fat. Hence, when you exercise, the triglycerides are broken down by the lipase enzyme and the free fatty acids diffuse out of the cells and enter the bloodstream which brings them to the working muscles where they are burned as fuel.

As you increase your exercise, more and more blood will flow into the adipose or fat tissues, removing even greater fatty acids. The lipase enzyme is activated by a molecule called cyclic AMP (adenosine monophosphate) which in turn is regulated by the hormones, epinephrine, norepinephrine, glucagon and growth hormones. These hormones are secreted in greater amounts during exercise.

The Importance of Good Digestion

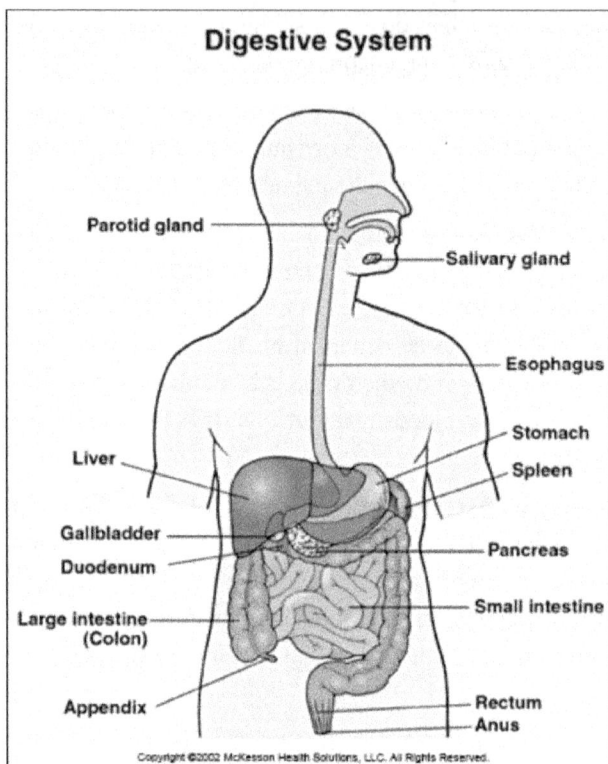

Digestive System

Parotid gland
Salivary gland
Esophagus
Stomach
Liver
Spleen
Gallbladder
Pancreas
Duodenum
Large intestine (Colon)
Small intestine
Appendix
Rectum
Anus

Copyright ©2002 McKesson Health Solutions, LLC. All Rights Reserved.

Proper Digestion: The First Step to Good Health

Someone once said that one of the greatest pleasures in life comes from filling and emptying an organ. Regarding this notion, eating is perhaps one of the most pleasurable activities we all engage in every day. It is also a crucial activity because our health and well-being are dependent on the food we eat. Yet most of us have little clue as to what happens to the food we eat once it gets past our lips and into our digestive tract. Like a sunrise or the change of seasons, we take this important, life-giving daily activity of ours for granted. This lack of interest or understanding is perhaps one of the reasons why we have such an unprecedented proportion of food-related degenerative diseases in this country.

In order for us to be intimately involved in our health and well-being, we should have a good understanding of the food we eat and how it is processed by the digestive system and the rest of the body. It is amazing how easy it is for us to spend time and money on things that may have no inherent value to our health or long-term survival and do so little for the physical and biochemical self.

Every aspect of our physical, emotional and intellectual well-being is as much a reflection of a properly working digestive system as the variety and diversity of nutrients that enter our bodies. It is with the digestive system that our health's glory or breakdown begins.

The complex and differentiated machinery we call the digestive system functions by reducing long chain and branched food molecules (also known as polymers) into their individual components, so that they are small enough to be absorbed by cells that line the gastrointestinal wall. Let's see how the digestive system breaks down long chain and branched food molecules and readies them for absorption.

The Digestion and Absorption of Nutrients

The first stage of digestion begins in the mouth. Here, the tongue whips the food into a moist mass while the teeth pummel, knead and masticate it. Certain enzymes in the saliva (lipase, amylase and others) begin the initial chemical breakdown of starch and some fat molecules. After the chewing or mastication is complete, the food is turned into a spherical mass known as the bolus, which, with a squeeze and wavelike motion of the throat, is pushed down the esophagus.

The bolus arrives in the stomach. Here a strong acid (called hydrochloric acid) and a medley of enzymes that specialize in snipping and splitting protein, fat and carbohydrate molecules takes action. The stomach, a J-shaped, pot-like organ, is also good at agitating and churning the food as the acid and enzymes untangle and rupture every morsel of food they come in contact with. From here, the food passes down to the small intestine, where, upon its entrance into the upper portion (the duodenum), it is drenched by another medley of digestive juices that come from the gallbladder and the pancreas.

The enzymes trypsin and chymotrypsin function as splitters or reducers of intact or partially digested protein chains. Their job is to reduce them to a size (as amino acids or short peptic chains—as two or three amino acid fragments) that will make it possible for the individual molecules to easily slip across the intestinal wall.

As you will see below, much of our day-to-day mental well-being, as well as our long-term health or demise, is dependent not only on the type of foods we put in our bodies but also on how well these foods are digested or processed once they enter our digestive tract.

First, as was mentioned elsewhere in the book, for food to be of any benefit to us, it has to be reduced or broken down to its basic components—proteins to amino acids, fats into glycol and fatty acids and carbohydrates into glucose and other simple sugars. At a microscopic or molecular level, it is these simple molecules that are capable of being transported across the gastrointestinal wall and into the bloodstream. The nutrients are then carried by the blood to the cells where they can be used to fuel, repair and build tissues.

Second, in order for the above nutrients as well as vitamins and minerals to be picked up and transported across the digestive tract, there have to be as few interfering factors as possible. These factors could be substances that trap nutrients and make them unavailable for absorption or those that suppress their transportation across the intestinal wall. Some of these suppressors could be alcohol, cigarettes, coffee and certain medications. Refer to the chapters on vitamins and minerals for specific absorption facilitators and suppressors.

Third, the nutrients that enter the circulatory system should be of the kind that won't upset or disturb the homeostasis ("steady state" conditions) of the body. This means that the foods we ingest should not only have the right balance of nutrients but also be of the kind that won't upset the body's rigidly controlled conditions. It also means that we should eat little or no sugar, sugar-based foods or saturated fats and that we should limit our intake of various foods to the level at which our bodies can process them without too much effort or encumbrance. In this regard, eating small but frequent meals is often considered the best approach.

Here are some of the specific problems that could arise from eating the wrong kind of food. Too much sugar may upset the body's glucose level, which also creates wild mood swings. Saturated fats are bad for the circulatory system. Too much food can strain gastrointestinal walls as well as the various glands that produce the digestive enzymes and juices. In the tissues, excess amounts of these substances must either be converted into fat and stored or be burned or eliminated from the body. If some of these substances are allowed to build up in the circulatory system, they can lead to many unwanted complications.

The pancreatic amylase goes about finishing up all the partially digested carbohydrate molecules and maybe even chopping up those that managed to come down untouched by the previous enzymes. Another enzyme, called lipase, goes after fat molecules. The bile from the gallbladder is a handy fluid that helps emulsify or reduce fats to small droplets so that the lipase gets to the individual molecules.

As the food goes down the small intestine, more enzymes are added from the glands that line the wall. These enzymes tend to be those that cleave the last food fragments into individual units: amino acids, glucose and other small sugar molecules. It is these that finally get picked up by a layer of fingerlike projections of the small intestine called villi and microvilli. Because of these tiny microscopic outgrowths, the surface area of the small intestine is increased by over 600 times, which is actually equivalent to the size of a real tennis court. Its length may be only 12 to 15 feet.

It is on the intestinal surface that most of the food gets absorbed. The absorption process can be either by simple diffusion, by active transport (also called facilitated diffusion) or by engulfing. As you will see below, there can be many factors that interfere with this process. It depends largely on the kind of food you eat, the health of the digestive tract and the existence of interfering factors.

The large intestine serves as the place where large quantities of water get removed from waste matter. It also serves as a temporary repository of waste matter.

That, in a nutshell, is how the digestive system works as one whole and integrated unit and serves as a watershed to the cascade of metabolic events that take place later within the trillion of cells in your body. When you think that very little solid food gets past our digestive tract without being broken down by the digestive processes and that life cannot exist without food, you can appreciate the tremendous importance of this living food processor, which we undignified call our "gut." It is the digestive system that gives food meaning and purpose in our lives.

There can also be many disruptive factors that interfere with this process, so let's look at them closely.

Digestion Disrupters

The process of digestion we described above may not be smooth or consistent from day to day or person to person. There are many factors that can disrupt the physiological and chemical processes involved in the digestion of food. Let's start with you. Without being aware of them, there are many things you do just before ingesting food that inhibit the production and secretion of digestive juices as well as interfere with the absorption of nutrients.

One of these could simply be not having sufficient time to sit, relax and enjoy your meal. The process of digestion requires the engaging of all those organs involved in the mobilization and breakdown of food that is placed in the digestive tract. This often entails the activation of key organs along the digestive tract through hormonal stimuli. Sight, smell, taste or even the thought of food can start a whole series of events, which are all concerned in the reception and proper digestion of food that arrives in the digestive system.

Unfortunately, when you eat in a hurry, your focus and energy are not concentrated on your food. This means that not only are all those key digestive organs not activated properly but also the food you consume will be underutilized by your body. The food consumed under such circumstances often stays longer than usual in the digestive tract and causes cramps, distention, constipation or diarrhea.

Similarly, depression, anxiety, overexcitement or stress can cause you to temporarily lose interest in food. Even if you have no physical or emotional disturbances, such simple practices as eating sweets, drinking too many caffeine-based beverages or alcohol or smoking cigarettes and other stimulants can have an equally disruptive effect on your digestive system. They could lead to a whole range of temporary or permanent problems involving the health of the digestive tract, including infections, ulcers, food poisoning and chronic diseases.

Another important concern you may have is what happens to the digestive organs and processes as you age. Unfortunately, like everything else in your body that atrophies with age, the digestive tract and all the organs that contribute to its function reduce their output of digestive juices. This in itself can be a limiting factor in the absorption and utilization of nutrients by the body. Add to this the fact that because most of the food in this country is processed, canned and prematurely harvested, there is a low nutrient content in foods.

Thus, not only do you have many of the disruptive factors mentioned above, but also you are dealing with a situation in which you might not be getting enough nutrients even if you have a healthy lifestyle. Although the health-eroding aspects of all the above factors are not apparent to you now, as the years pass, you may start to feel their impact.

Your Solution

The best thing that you can do to deal with some of the problems is to treat the whole activity of eating like an event, a celebration of something important in your life. Treat it with respect. Enjoy the anticipation as well as the act of consuming your meals. Take your time or slow down when you sit down to eat your meals.

Nothing in life should be more important than your health and well-being. After a meal, relax for 15 to 30 minutes before you engage in any activity. By doing so, you can help your body concentrate its energy in processing the meal. This may enhance the digestion as well as the absorption of nutrients. If you are hungry but don't have time to sit down and have a relaxed meal, have something simple instead, like an apple or water. This option can help kill your hunger and sustain your body until you have time to sit down and enjoy your meal.

You may want to avoid or minimize your intake of the absorption-disruptive foods and drinks mentioned elsewhere in the book before your meals. Although you may have no control over certain infections or chronic digestive disorders, you should have control over such everyday problems as stress, depression, anxiety or overexcitement. Even a chronic condition and infection can be dealt with effectively if you have the right kinds and sufficient amounts of nutrients in your body.

Digestion Disturbances

One of the by-products of digestion is what we often euphemistically refer to as gas. It's largely produced when bacteria in the stomach work on an improperly digested food. This happens, for example, if you eat your food too fast—without thoroughly chewing it and allowing the hydrochloric acid (HCI) and enzymes to break it down in the stomach. This means that before you're ready to eat, think about food. Think of some of the succulent foods you have eaten in the past. These thought processes stimulate the secretions of all the digestive enzymes in the saliva, the stomach lining and the pancreas gland. HCI, the strongest chemical in your stomach, kills bacteria and viruses and helps break down many of the foods. It is also produced in greater quantities when you mentally stimulate the secreting glands along the stomach wall.

A food that is not properly digested can become food for the bacteria in your intestines instead of for your body. The bacteria can start to break down this food and use it, creating gas as a waste product. Often, you may have noticed that when you eat your food in hurry, you end up with cramps and discomfort in your stomach.

This food tends to stay longer in your system, causing pain and constipation. It's believed that one of the causes of colon cancer is when such food putrefies and the bacteria convert it into carcinogenic chemicals. High-protein and lower-fiber foods tend to linger longer and, as a result, putrefy and produce carcinogenic chemicals.

Some foods are more gas generating than others. Most protein foods, especially those rich in sulfur like eggs, cauliflower, beans and broccoli, can be converted into hydrogen-sulfide gas (the most offensive kind) by the intestinal bacteria. Most of the legume family (beans, peas, soybeans, etc.) have two soluble sugars called raffinose and stachyose that are equally gas forming and distending. Most grains, fibers and other plant foods convert into methane gas, which is not as penetrating and jarring to the nostrils.

Fibers can sometimes be a double-edged sword. They have many healthful properties in the digestive tract, but to some people, they can also be a nuisance because the bacteria in their intestines digest them and produce gas. There are some remedies to this problem, however. When you eat fiber-rich foods or supplements for the first time, try to take them in small quantities. The key is not to overwhelm your intestinal bacteria with too much fiber for the first time, in which case they begin to proliferate and start a feeding frenzy and produce large quantities of gas. Just start slowly and build up to the normal serving level.

There are also drugs you can take. The easiest and the safest remedy is activated charcoal, which you can buy from your local drug store or health-food outlet. It comes as a tablet or powder, and it's a powerful absorbent of stomach gases. Just take two to three tablets of this harmless substance with your meal and you should see an improvement.

You may also be one of those people who cannot properly metabolize milk, or rather, the milk sugar (lactose). The milk-processing enzyme, lactase, may be lacking in your digestive system, leaving the milk to be processed by the bacteria into gas. In this case, the easiest remedy is, of course, to avoid milk and milk products.

In summary, just remember that your overall health and well-being and even longevity are dependent on the nutrients that are processed and provided by your gastrointestinal tract. Without the proper functioning of this system, there is no there is no beautiful hair, skin or healthy and properly working body and mind.

APPENDIX F
Enzymes: The Keys of Life

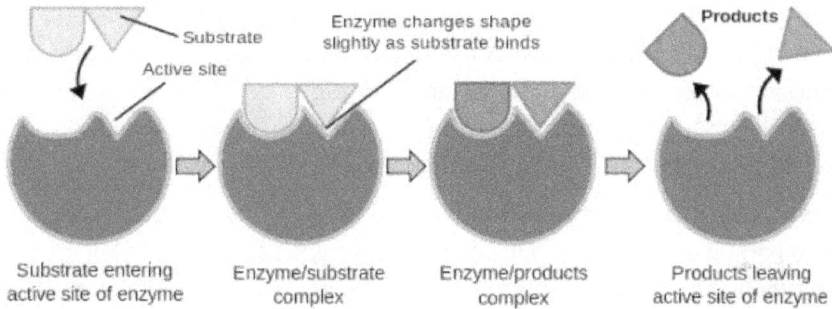

Substrate

Active site

Enzyme changes shape
slightly as substrate binds

Products

| Substrate entering active site of enzyme | Enzyme/substrate complex | Enzyme/products complex | Products leaving active site of enzyme |

Enzymes

We have now come to what is perhaps the most important and fundamental component of good health, wellness and longevity: enzymes. We have referred to Enzymes quite often in this book. Let's now take a close look at these wonders of nature a little closely.

Unlike vitamins, minerals and herbs, which directly or indirectly affect the function of the body, enzymes (as discussed in Appendix E), control the very fundamental processes or operations of the body. These range from the breakdown of foods in the digestive tract to their assembly or synthesis in the tissues and organs to their conversion into energy. In short, enzymes are the key that unlocks the essence of food in the body to give it strength, wellness, and vitality. This means that without enzymes, life would not exist and food would have no meaning or purpose.

What exactly are enzymes, and where are they made, you may ask. Enzymes are a special group of protein molecules that somehow behave as if they had a soul and a life of their own. They do what they do (break down food, synthesize or assemble food molecules, etc.) without instruction (at least as far as we know) from anywhere.

They are the architects and the laborers as well as the housekeepers of our body. Everything that we are and do is controlled or facilitated by enzymes. This can range from thinking to blinking our eyes to engaging in physical tasks as well as to building and repairing tissues.

The body contains two major classes of enzymes: digestive enzymes and metabolic enzymes. The digestive enzymes are synthesized in the pancreas and in the cell along the gastrointestinal tract as well as in other cells in the body. These enzymes are responsible for the breakdown or digestion of food. The metabolic enzymes are produced by every cell in the body and are involved in the conversion of food into energy or in using food to build and repair tissues.

Enzymes also can get involved in processing or converting toxins and pollutants into harmless substances. This is their scavenging function. Considering that many of us live in a polluted environment and consume food and water that may have been exposed to dubious chemicals, this housekeeping function of enzymes can be very important indeed.

Outside the body is a third class of enzymes, called food enzymes. As their name implies, these enzymes are responsible for all the activities that take place in plants, from germinating a seed to its growing and maturing into a plant to its blossoming and bearing fruit. Just as an organism decomposes after death with the help of its own enzymes, the enzymes in plants are responsible for making plants biodegradable. Most of the food enzymes are similar to the enzymes found in our bodies.

The Importance of Enzyme Supplements for Our Health

Before we discuss the significance of enzyme supplements to our health and well-being, let's talk about the specific functions of the different digestive enzymes found in our bodies. As you can see in the discussion on digestion in previous section, there are specific enzymes for the different classes of foods we consume every day. Hence, protease specializes in processing proteins; lipase, in breaking down fats; and amylase, lactase, cellulase in snipping and splitting starch, lactose and cellulose molecules, respectively. (Starch, lactose and cellulose are all carbohydrates.)

It can be said that nearly every single food molecule (or, for that matter, every chemical reaction) has its own specific enzyme that helps catalyze the conversion or breakdown of that food (or chemical substance).

It may be self-evident that without sufficient quantities of all the above enzymes, foods cannot be properly processed, and consequently our health and wellness could suffer. Does this mean that we need to be concerned about our supply of enzymes? Can there be a shortage or depletion of our enzyme supply? If so, could we benefit from an enzyme supplement? Let's answer each of these questions separately.

Our body's production of enzymes will depend on our age, the type of food we have been consuming throughout life and the stress and pollution levels we have subjected our bodies to.

Like everything else that happens to tissues and organs as we get older, our bodies' ability to secrete sufficient quantities of enzymes declines. For instance, in one study, the concentration of the enzyme amylase in the saliva of young adults was found to be 30 times stronger than in individuals over 69 years old. In another experiment, the concentration and strength of the same enzyme taken from the pancreas of a group of older men were found to be many times weaker than that taken from the pancreas of younger men.

Besides the normal aging process, extended consumption of processed, cooked and irradiated foods can deplete the body's reserve of both metabolic and digestive enzymes. As mentioned above, when consuming foods that have been processed and altered, (i.e., foods whose enzymes have been destroyed), the body has to produce a large quantity of its own to digest and utilize such food. Interestingly, like muscles that increase in mass from the challenge of physical exertion, glands and organs responsible for the secretion of digestive juices and enzymes enlarge when repeatedly burdened with a large quantity of processed and cooked foods. This fact has been demonstrated by comparing the pancreas of wild mice (mice that feed on raw food) with the pancreas of laboratory mice that were fed processed and cooked food.

Likewise, when our body is exposed to pollution or extraneous chemicals such as pesticides and food additives (preservatives, coloring and flavoring agents), it will use (and therefore waste) a large quantity of its own enzymes. This happens because, our liver, kidneys and other organs and tissues use enzymes to process or turn some of these chemicals (as well as viruses) into harmless substances. As these organs and tissues are stressed or burdened with the production of a large quantity of enzymes, they naturally enlarge to increase production and meet the demand placed upon them.

When we eat whole, uncooked foods, the enzymes that are naturally found in them can help break down those foods in the digestive tract. Cooking or microwaving foods destroys enzymes. This habitual practice will lead to our being dependent on our own enzymes to process the food and consequently may lead to the depletion of our bodies' reserve of enzymes. The long-term consequence of this reckless usage of our bodies' labor force can be a decline in the bodies' function, a greater susceptibility to degenerative diseases and in general a higher compromise of our health and wellness.

The above piece of information is one reason why the Four Pillars drinks—all prepared from raw fruits, vegetables and herbs—become healthy alternatives to similar processed and cooked foods people consume often.

What is the solution to the above problem? The first solution to this challenge is to consume whole and uncooked foods as much as possible (like the Four Pillars drinks). Because the enzymes that are naturally found in uncooked foods can help digest such foods, the body will produce fewer of its own enzymes in the presence of these foods. In other words, to quote Dr. Edward Howell, author of Enzyme Nutrition, "If we depend solely upon the enzymes we inherit, they will be used just like inherited money that is not supplemented with a steady income." The uncooked, whole food may serve as a good source of that supplemental, steady supply of enzyme income.

The second solution, if for some reason you're not making your Four Pillars drink as often or don't bother making it, is to use prepackaged enzyme supplements. Because processed, cooked and chemically adulterated foods are omnipresent, augmenting your diet with quality enzyme supplement may be a good alternative. That way you may conserve your body's reserve of enzymes as well as help you process your food efficiently.

Use a supplement that has multiple enzymes, or enzymes that can help you process protein, carbohydrates and fat. Hence, for example, while protease, peptidase, help you to digest proteins, amylase, invertase, glucoamylase and lactase can help your body break down carbohydrates. Similarly, a lipase enzyme can help you process fat. As we said above, enzymes can very specific in their function. Thus, the above different protein and carbohydrate enzymes can help you digest some of the most common carbohydrates and proteins found in ordinary foods, when taken as part of a supplement.

Acknowledgement

My wife, Rosario, has been my ardent fan and supporter of my work. She has allowed me the quiet and secluded space I needed to write this book, for which I'm appreciative and thankful.

I extend my many thanks to Philip Howe for his artistic wizardry with this and my other books and for his patience and understanding of my need to make the illustrations as vivid and authentic as possible. I thank Greg Brown for his professional work in the formatting and designing of the book's interior. Finally, I would like to extend my thanks to Gordy Grundy and Anita Philips for proofing and editing parts of the manuscript.

Glossary

A

acid A substance that produces hydrogen ions (H+'s) when in solution.

adrenaline A hormone secreted by the adrenal gland. Also called epinephrine, adrenaline hormone is responsible for the arousal of the "fight or flight" response in the body.

aerobic metabolism The oxygen-dependent, final breakdown of food molecules occurring in the mitochondria to release energy, carbon dioxide, water and heat.

alkaloids A group of nitrogen-containing compounds that are of plant or animal origin and that have medicinal or pharmacological activity. Examples of alkaloids are morphine, nicotine and quinine.

alpha-tocopherol The most biologically active and widely distributed natural form of vitamin E.

alterarive A substance that has a restorative or balancing effect on the body.

amino acid A group of nitrogen containing compounds that serve as building block for protein molecules.

anabolism The building or synthesis of bigger molecules, such as proteins, fats and carbohydrates, from their respective simple precursor molecules by living tissues. Anabolism is an energy-requiring process, and it is provided by the adenosine triphosphate (ATP).

anaerobic metabolism The breakdown of glucose molecules without oxygen which occurs in the cytoplasm (of the cell). Through this process, only 5% of the energy is extracted from glucose; the other 95% is extracted when the partially processed glucose molecules enter the Krebs cycle in the mitochondria. Anaerobic metabolism takes place usually during intense short-duration physical exertion such as sprinting, weight lifting and downhill skiing.

antibiotic A substance that inhibits the production or growth of bacteria. Most medicinal antibiotics are undiscriminating in their destruction of bacteria. Herbal antibiotics such as garlic, on the other hand, do not harm helpful bacteria such as those found in the GI tract.

antibody A specialized group of protein molecules produced by the body to deactivate destroy or neutralize foreign or invading substances (antigens).

antioxidants Electron-rich chemicals or nutrients used to minimize or eliminate oxidation. A number of nonfood-and food-based chemicals are used for this purpose. For example, vitamins A, C and E and the amino acids cysteine, methionine and taurine are well-documented antioxidants used to neutralize the damaging effect of free radicals. Nonfood chemicals, such as butylated hydroxytoluene (BHT) and butylated hydroxyanisole (BHA), ate common anti-oxidants added to food to slow down the aging or spoiling of foods.

ascorbic acid An alternate name for vitamin C. Vitamin C helps the absorption of iron and is an excellent antioxidant. It is also important for the health, growth and normal functioning of teeth, bones, gums and muscles.

ascorbyl palmitate The fat-soluble form of vitamin C. This form of the vitamin stays longer in the body. ATP (adenosine triphosphate) Serves as temporary storage of food energy extracted during aerobic and anaerobic metabolism.

astringent An agent or substance that causes contraction of tissue.

B

basal metabolic rate The metabolic rate of the body at rest.

basal metabolism The minimum amount of energy needed by the body to maintain vital processes, i.e., circulation, respiration and digestion.

base A molecule that produces hydroxyl ions (-OH) when dissolved in solution.

beriberi A disease arising from vitamin B 1 deficiency.

beta-carotene Precursor of vitamin A found mostly in yellow and orange vegetables. Beta carotene is an excellent antioxidant, particularly against the singlet oxygen free radicals. This water-soluble vitamin also has many other healthful properties.

beta cells The cells in the pancreas that manufacture insulin.

bile A pigmented fluid secreted by the liver and stored in the gallbladder that helps with the digestion of fats upon entry into the duodenum (upper portion of the small intestine). Bile can be yellow, green or brown, depending on the relative concentration of salts, acids, cholesterol, lecithin (a fat-emulsifying agent) and a number of other colored compounds. When these pigmented chemicals mix with digestion by-products in the intestine, they give feces its brown color.

bilirubin A bile component that is a breakdown of hemoglobin of the red blood cells. Bilirubin is responsible for the brown appearance of stool.

bioavailability The amount of nutrient (or chemical) that is available to the body in relation to the total ingested amount.

biochemistry The study of the chemical processes that takes place in living things.

bioflavonoids A group of related compounds that act as special helpers of Vitamin C. These pigmented substances team up with Vitamin C to help us maintain a healthy immune system as well as properly working muscular and other tissues.

biological aging The physical condition of a person compared to his/her chronological age.

biotin One of the B-complex vitamins that is involved in the metabolism of fat. Biotin is also vital for the health and growth of tissues.

blood-brain barrier A membranous tissue that prevents the passage of material from the blood into the brain.

Bromelain A protein-digesting enzyme obtained from pineapple.

C

caffeine A chemical substance obtained from coffee, tea and chocolate that serves as a stimulant to the nervous system.

calcium A major component of bones and teeth is also involved in muscle contraction, nerve impulse transmission and blood clotting.

calcium ascorbate A less acidic form of vitamin C that is also a highly absorbable form of calcium.

calmative A substance that has calming or sedative action.

calorie A measurement of energy that is equivalent to the amount of heat required to raise the temperature of one gram of water by one degree Celsius. In nutrition, "calorie" is used to indicate the energy value of foods. One calorie (also referred to as a kilocalorie) is equal to 1,000 calories.

capillary The smallest blood vessels that bring nutrients to the cells. In the capillaries, each blood cell passes through one at a time.

carbohydrates One of the three classes of food substances that provide the body with energy. There are !generally three classes of carbohydrates: monosaccharides (i. e., glucose, galactose and fructose), disaccharides (i. e., table sugar, lactose and honey) and 'polysaccharide (heat, corn, potatoes, etc.). Chemically, carbohydrates are made up of carbon, hydrogen and oxygen atoms.

carcinogen A substance that causes cancer in living tissues.

carminative An agent used to expels gas from the intestine.

carotene A fat-soluble plant pigment some of which can be converted into vitamin A in the body.

catabolism The breakdown of nutrients (carbohydrates, proteins and fats) or body tissues to provide energy and other necessary metabolic functions. (See also anabolism and metabolism) catalyst A substance that speeds up the rate of chemical reaction without being consumed itself.

catecholamines A group of substances generated by the brain and the adrenal glands that have important physiological functions. They include epinephrine, norepinephrine and dopamine, each of which has different functions, but mainly work as neurotransmitters and stimulators of the sympathetic and central nervous systems.

cell The basic building block of body tissues.

cell membrane The outer covering of a cell.

cellulose fiber A form of carbohydrate made up of thousands glucose molecules and is a major constituent of plants. Cellulose fiber is important for the healthy functioning of the digestive tract.

ceruloplasmins The combination of copper with plasma protein believed to protect the red blood cells from free radicals.

chelated minerals Amino acid (or other organic molecule) complexed (or bound) minerals to enhance their absorption across the digestive tract.

cholecalciferol A form of vitamin D-3 important for calcium absorption and in the calcification of bones.

cholesterol A fatlike substance found in the blood and in most animal tissues. Cholesterol is one of the important constituents of cell membranes and it serves as precursor to many hormones and bile salts. Cholesterol is not found in plants.

chronological age The age of an individual as measured by the passage of time.

coenzyme A nonprotein organic substance that assists enzymes in doing their job well. Coenzymes often contain B vitamins in their molecular structures.

cofactor Another nonprotein substance that is involved during an enzyme-catalyzed reaction. Certain minerals often function as cofactors.

cold pressed A process of extracting oils, without heat or chemicals, to preserve all the nutrients found naturally in vegetable oils. This process is also used to minimize damage to the nutrients found in vegetable oils. The chemicals are later removed.

colic Severe, spasmodic pain in the abdomen that comes in waves.

colitis Inflammation of the colon.

collagen A form of protein found throughout the body but which is highly concentrated in the skin, bone and cartilage tissues.

colostrum The first batch of a mother's breast milk, which is secreted shortly after, or sometimes before, birth. Colostrum is rich in antibodies and white blood cells, which serve as protection to the brand-new digestive tract of the baby.

compress Also known as fomentation, a compress is the application of herbal containing linen or gauze pad to increase circulation and relieve pain or swelling. The pad or gauze is usually socked in the tea of the herb and applied on the affected surface.

constipation An abnormally difficult or infrequent passage of stool. An increased consumption of dietary fiber, the use of laxatives or an enema can often be an effective solution to constipation.

cyanocobalamin A form of vitamin B12 that is important for the development of red blood cells, as well as for the proper function of the nervous system.

D

decoction A liquid extraction of a root, bark or leaves of a plant obtained by simmering either one of these plant materials in a closed container for 15-30 minutes

degenerative disease The gradual atrophying of organs or tissues in a biological system, which arises from the dysfunction or damage done to those organs or tissues.

demulcent A substance that soothes and softens inflamed tissues such as those found in the digestive tract.

diabetes A degenerative disease characterized by abnormally high blood sugar as a result of a malfunctioning pancreas and thus an insufficient production of insulin.

diarrhea A frequent and rapid passage of abnormally soft or watery feces. Diarrhea may be caused by a number of things, including intestinal inflammation, anxiety, malabsorption or infection.

diet The variety of foods that a person consumes habitually.

Dietary fiber The indigestible part of food (i.e., of fruits, vegetables and carbohydrates) that is not processed and absorbed for energy or other bodily purposes. Dietary fiber is divided into four groups: cellulose, hemicellulose, legnins and pectins. Dietary fiber is believed to be important in minimizing the incidence of colon cancer, diverticulosis, diabetes, obesity, constipation and a number of intestinal disorders.

digestion The breakdown of foods in the digestive tract into their simpler components for absorption and processing by the body.

digestive tract All the organs (mouth, esophagus, stomach, small intestine and colon) involved in the digestion and absorption of food.

disaccharide A form of carbohydrate consisting of only two sugar molecules.

diverticulosis An often painful ballooning or out pouching of the intestine or colon wall. It is believed to arise from eating foods low in fiber.

DL-alpha tocopherol Synthetic vitamin E. This forms of vitamin is less biologically active than d-alpha tocopherol.

DNA The genetic material found in the cells of nearly all living things, which controls the transmission of heredity or hereditary traits. DNA stands for deoxyribonucleic acid.

duodenum The first 12-inch portion of the small intestine that receives bile and pancreatic juice from the gallbladder and pancreas, respectively.

edema The accumulation of excess water in body tissues. This problem is often observed in protein deficiency conditions.

E

Eicosapentaenoic acid (EPA) A fatty acid found primarily in cold-water fish, flax seeds and primrose oil.

elastin The yellowish, elastic protein fiber found in the connective tissues.

electrolyte A substance that has dissociated into positively and negatively charged ions, which are capable of conducting electricity. For example, when table salt dissolves or melts, it gives rise to sodium (positively) and chloride (negatively) charged ions. These are capable of conducting electricity.

electron A negatively charged particle that revolves around the nucleus of an atom.

emetic A substance that causes vomiting.

emulsifier A fat- or oil-dispersing agent when added to water.

emulsify The breakdown of large fat globules into smaller uniform droplets enrichment.

enzyme A biological substance (usually a protein) that initiates and speeds up a biochemical reaction.

essential amino acids A group of (8 to 9) amino acids that are not synthesized by the body and that must be obtained from dietary sources.

essential fatty acids One group of unsaturated fatty acids that are not synthesized in the body and that are involved in many bodily functions and processes. essential oils Also called volatile oils or essences, essential oils are a complex mixture of organic compounds containing phenols, alcohols, ketones, acids, ethers, esters, oxides and aldehydes that evaporate when exposed to air.

Ester-C@ A highly bioavailable form of vitamin C.

estrogen A female hormone that is responsible for the sexual development, growth and function of the female sexual organs and secondary sexual characteristics.

extract A concentrated form of a natural product obtained by treating an herbal with a solvent and then completely or partially removing the solvent. In this manner a variety of extracts called liquid extracts, solid extracts, powder extracts, tinctures and native extracts can be obtained.

F

fats One of the three classes of nutrients that provide your body with energy. Fats can supply 9 calories per gram. There are three different types of fats: saturated (found mostly in animal products), monounsaturated and polyunsaturated(obtained from plants).

fat-soluble vitamin A vitamin molecule that is transported by fats in the body. Vitamins A, E, D and K are the only known fat-soluble vitamins.

fatty acid An organic molecule consisting of a chain of hydrogen-containing carbon atoms with a few oxygen atoms.

fiber See dietary fiber

flavonoid A term used to refer to a group of flavon-containing compounds or plant pigments such as anthocyanins, anthoxanthins, bigflavonols, flavonols, flavons and apeginens. It is now know that the flavonoids have a tremendous effect on the human body.

fortification The addition of one or more nutrients to foods to improve their nutritional quality. The nutrient added may already exist in the food to which it is added. Fortification is intended to increase the food's quality. (For example, vitamin D is added to milk and vitamin E is added to margarine.)

free radical A very unstable and highly reactive molecular fragment, which is known to cause a number of problems in the body, including aging.

frigidity Typically applied to a woman who lacks interest in sexual intercourse or has an inability to reach orgasm.

fructose One of the simple sugars found mostly in fruits and as part of honey and table sugar (sucrose).

G

galactose A monosaccharide that results from the breakdown of lactose (milk sugar).

gastric juice The colorless secretions of the gastric glands of the stomach. The major constituents of gastric juices are hydrochloric acid (which makes it very acidic, pH 2), pepsin, mucin and renin (in infants). The gastric juice is a very powerful neutralizer and deactivator of bacteria, viruses and a number of unwanted substances. It also is important for the absorption of minerals and vitamin B12.

glucose The most common monosaccharide found in fruits, sugars and starch. Glucose (sometimes called dextrose) is an important source of energy for the body and a primary source of fuel for the brain. In the blood, the optimal level of glucose is 5 milli-mole/liter. In a healthy person, the constancy of glucose is monitored by two hormones: insulin and glucagon. When there is an abnormally high level of glucose, insulin helps bring it down to normal by facilitating the cells' uptake of the sugar. Glucagon does the opposite: it helps break down glycogen (the body's stored sugar) when there is an abnormally low level of glucose in the blood.

glucose tolerance test (GTT) A test administered to determine how well a person's body utilizes sugar. GTT is usually given to someone who is suspected of having diabetes or hypoglycemia.

glutathione peroxidase A powerful free-radical quenching enzyme produced in the body from the sulfur-containing amino acid glutamine and the mineral selenium.

glycogen Often referred to as animal starch, glycogen is a polysaccharide made by the body from excess glucose. The conversion of glucose into glycogen and the storing of this energy source are nature's ways of dealing with excesses or shortages.

goiter An appendage or enlargement around the neck arising from an abnormal functioning of the thyroid gland due to a deficiency of iodine.

goitrogens Substances or agents that cause the onset of goiter when ingested. These substances or agents often interfere with the normal production or function of the hormone thyroxine (produced by the thyroid gland), thus creating goiters.

H

HDL (high-density lipoprotein) cholesterol A tightly "packaged" cholesterol that can easily and efficiently move through the blood vessels.

helper T cell A type of white blood cells that fight in the army of the immune forces.

hemoglobin The iron-containing protein made by the bone marrow that helps transport oxygen to the various tissues throughout the body.

homeostasis The process by which the body maintains many of its physiological components (body temperature, electrolytes, acid-base balance and blood pressure) within constant or near constant states.

hormone A chemical that is produced in one part of the body and transported by the bloodstream to another part of the body, where it can influence the function of a specific organ or tissue. Examples of such hormones are the epinephrine or glucagon secreted by the adrenal and pancreas glands, respectively, which influence the liver to convert glycogen into glucose whenever there is a low level of this sugar in the blood. Similarly, the pituitary gland at the base of the brain secretes (among many others) growth hormones, which help with development of muscle tissues and in the healing of wounds.

hydrogenation The addition of hydrogen to vegetable oils (i.e., unsaturated fats) to make them solid at room temperature. Examples are margarine and vegetable shortening hypoglycemia An abnormally low level of blood sugar resulting from the excessive production of insulin.

I

immunity The body's ability to fend off infections due to the production of specialized cells such as the white blood cells and antibodies.

immunoglobulin (Ig) A group of related proteins (so-called gamma globulins) that serve as antibodies in the body.

immunology The study of the immune system.

impulse In neurology, it refers to the transmission of electrical signals (i.e., information) from the cell body down the axon and on to the next neuron.

infertility In a woman, infertility means the inability to conceive a child; in a man, infertility means the inability to induce conception.

inflammation A localized defensive reaction by the body due to an infection, chemicals or abrasion. Inflammation is characterized by swelling, heat, redness, pain and a temporary loss of function by the affected tissue.

infusion The removal or extraction of the active ingredients of a plant material by steeping or immersing it in a liquid such as water.

inositol A quasi B vitamin and a six carbon alcohol found mostly in grain, brans and certain vegetables. When an inositol molecule combines with a phosphate molecule, it forms phytic acid, a substance believed to have anticolorectal-cancer properties. Some intestinal, carcinogenic bacteria thrive in the presence of high amounts of iron. Phytic acid, by combining with iron suppresses the proliferation of the offending microorganisms in the digestive tract.

insulin A sugar-metabolizing hormone that is secreted by the pancreas gland.

intercellular Something, such as fluid, that exists between cells.

interferon A group of proteins produced by the cells infected by a virus to coat and protect the neighboring, healthy cells. Interferons work only within the species that produces them.

intestinal flora Microorganisms found in the intestinal tract that are believed to have many useful functions, including the production of vitamin K, the blood-clotting nutrient.

intracellular Situated, or existing, inside a cell.

intrinsic factor A protein-based substance produced in the stomach that helps with the absorption of vitamin B12. Failure of its secretion by the gastric cells leads to pernicious anemia, a usually fatal disease.

in vitro Something that occurs outside a living organism and in an artificial environment.

in vivo Something that occurs in the living body of an animal or a plant.

K

keratin A fibrous protein found in hair, nails and the topmost layer of the skin.

ketone Any organic compound containing a ketone group (CO).

ketosis An abnormally high formation of "ketone bodies" in the body tissues. Ketones are produced from an incomplete burning (oxidation) of fats. During starvation or in diabetic conditions, however, ketone bodies can be the last energy source.

Krebs cycle An energy-producing process that occurs in the mitochondria of the cell. It's in the Krebs cycle that the maximum amount of energy is extracted from the food you eat. The other by-products of this process are carbon dioxide, water and heat.

L

lactic acid A by-product of glucose metabolism formed due to inadequate levels of oxygen in the cell. Lactic acid is generally formed during strenuous physical activities such as weightlifting, sprinting and other continuous, repetitive physical exertions.

lactose A sugar found in milk. Lactose consists of two disaccharide molecules, glucose and galactose. lactose intolerance An inability to metabolize lactose because of the absence of the enzyme lactase, which is responsible for the breakdown of lactose. The expressed symptoms are diarrhea and gas.

L-carnitine-L-tartrate The salt form of L-carnitine which helps transport long chain fatty acids across the mitochondrial membrane to be used for energy production.

LDL (low-density lipoprotein) cholesterol One of the forms in which cholesterol is transported in the blood vessels. LDLs are often regarded as "bad guys" because they are sluggish and tend to increase the risk of heart diseases.

lecithin A type of fat (containing phosphates) found in the cell membranes that serves as a fat-metabolizing agent in the liver. In commercial food products, lecithin is used as an emulsifying agent.

leukocytosis An abnormally high production of white blood cells, which often happens in the presence of antigens (foreign elements) in the blood.

liniment A thin medicinal liquid rubbed on the affected area of the body to relieve pain or a bruise.

lipid A group of organic substances consisting of fats, cholesterol, phospholipids, steroids and prostaglandins.

lipoprotein A complex of fats (lipids) and protein molecules found in the blood serum. Lipoprotein serves to transport cholesterol and fats to the cells for metabolism or to the liver for excretion. liver spots See age spots macronutrient Refers to foods that the body utilizes in large quantities.

M

malipant A condition in the body (such as cancer) that gets worse in time and eventually cause death.

malnutrition A nutritional condition in which the body is under- or over-nourished. Malnutrition can be subclinical, which means it cannot be detected through normal medical examination. It can be marginal, in which case there may be overt symptoms, such as unexplainable irritability depression or fatigue. Obesity is often the result of excessive intake of the wrong foods and is a form of malnutrition as well.

MAO see monoamine oxidase

MAO inhibitor A drug that interferes with the activity of the enzyme monoamine oxidase in the brain and that as a result affects a person's mood.

mast cells A group of cells found throughout the body that cause the allergic response of sneezing or inflammation by secreting histamine and other related substances.

medicinal A substance used to cure or treat a disease.

megaloblast An immature red blood cell with an enlarged nuclei. This occurs usually from a vitamin B 12 deficiency.

metabolism All the chemical and physical processes that take place within the body to ensure survival and proper development of the body.

minerals All the inorganic nutrients that are used during metabolism, as well as those that serve as structural components.

mitochondria A cellular power plant. In a process called the Krebs cycle, all oxygen-dependent reactions take place in the mitochondria.

monoamine oxidase (MAO) An enzyme that catalyzes the breakdown of mono-amines such as epinephrine, serotonin and norepinephrine. MAO is found in all tissues, but in particularly rich quantities in the liver and the nervous system. Drugs that inhibit the activity of this enzyme are effective in the treatment of depression.

monosaccharide A simple one molecule sugar such as fructose or glucose.

monounsaturated fatty acid A fatty acid that contains one double bond in its carbon chain. Because of its heat stability, monounsaturated fat is excellent for cooking: for example, olive oil, peanut oil and canola oil.

mucilage A substance that gels when placed in water to give rise to a soft and slimy product.

mucopolysaccharide One of a group of complex carbohydrates containing amino sugar. Mucopolysaccharid functions mainly as structural components in connective tissues such as tendons and cartilages. mucus The slimy fluid secreted by the **mucous** membrane to lubricate and protect it.

myelin A fatty tissue that covers the axon of a nerve fiber.

N

nerve impulse See impulse

neuron A single nerve cell containing a body, dendrites and an axon.

neurotransmitter A chemical messenger in the nervous system that transfers electrical activity (or information) from one neuron to the next.

niacinamide One of the B-complex vitamins that is essential for energy production. Also known as vitamin B3, this nutrient is important for healthy skin and proper functioning of the nervous and digestive systems.

nutrient A food substance that is essential for the growth, repair and maintenance of body tissues.

nutrient density The ratio of nutrients to calories obtained from a food source. If a food contains a small amount of calories in relation to its nutrient content, that food is thought to be nutrient dense.

O

obesity The accumulation of excess fat in a person's body. A person is said to be obese if he/she is 20% above the recommended weight for his/her height and build.

oil A fat that is liquid at room temperature.

organic foods Foods grown without the use of artificial fertilizers or pesticides.

osmosis The passage of particles or solvents through a semipermeable membrane from a high to low concentration. This will eventually bring the two solutions to an equilibrium.

osteomalacia The softening of the bones in adults arising from vitamin D deficiency or a loss of calcium from the body.

osteoporosis The depletion of calcium from the bones that causes them to become thin and porous. This leads to easy fracture or breakage of the bones. Osteoporosis is most frequency observed in postmenopausal women.

oxidation A chemical reaction in which oxygen is added to a substance or a hydrogen atom is removed from it.

P

papilla Any tiny nipple-like protrusion, or a clump of cells, that gives rise to hair.

pectin A dietary fiber that absorbs cholesterol and fats from the digestive tract. This helps lessen fat buildup in the blood vessels.

pepsin An enzyme in the stomach that breaks down protein into smaller chunks

peptide A molecule consisting of two or more amino acids linked by bonds between an amino group (-NH) and a carboxy group (-CO). This bond is referred to as a peptide bond.

peristalsis A wavelike muscular motion of the intestines which causes food to move through them.

pica A craving or desire for nonfood items such as clay, grass, chalk or clothes. This abnormal desire is normally experienced by pregnant women or by women who may have an iron deficiency.

platelets Tiny disc-shaped particles found in the blood. Their main fu placebo An inert substance used to test the efficacy of another substance. Its main function is to help stop bleeding when you have a cut.

polyunsaturated fatty acids Fatty acids containing two or more double bonds.

poultice A warm and soft herbal material spread over a thin clothe and applied on the skin to impart heat and relieve pain or serve as antiseptic.

powdered extract A solid extract that has been dried as powder.

polysaccharide A carbohydrate containing three or more glucose molecules.

protein One of the three classes of foods that are used for structural and functional purposes. Proteins are built from a chain of amino acids. Proteins differ from carbohydrates or fats by the nitrogen atom in their chain.

purgative A substance that causes vigorous bowl movement.

pyruvate A partially metabolized glucose molecule occurring during anaerobic metabolism.

prostaglandins Hormone-like substances synthesized in the body from omega-3 and omega-6 fatty acids. Prostaglandins have many healthful benefits, which include dilating blood vessels, lowering cholesterol and limiting the development of cancerous cells.

R
Recommended Dietary Allowance (RDA) Officially recommended amounts of various nutrients.

S
saccharide A sugar molecule.

salve A healing or relieving ointment.

saturated fat A fat molecule containing the maximum number of hydrogen atoms in its fatty acid portionssedative A substance the calms or tranquilizes the body.

serotonin A neurotransmitter made from the amino acid tryptophan, which induces sleep. Serotonin is also important for weight reduction

solid extract Extracts that have all their residual solvent removed.

stimulant An agent that temporarily hyperactivates a tissue or an organ.

subcutaneous Occurring or existing below the skin.

sucrose A sugar made of glucose and fructose, also known as table sugar.

suppressor T cells A group of white blood cell controlled by the thymus gland and that suppress the overproduction of other immune cells or antibodies.

synapse A contact point between two neurons where nerve impulses are transmitted.

T
tea An infusion made by adding hot water to an herb for use as medicine or as a beverage. Herbal tea is usually made by steeping one teaspoon of the herb in eight ounces of water.

T-cell A group of white blood cells that mature in and populate the thymus gland.

thiamine mononitrate A vitamin B complex (also known as vitamin B1) that is crucial for the extraction of energy from the food you eat. It acts like a spark plug that ignites carbohydrates and other foods in the body.

tincture An alcoholic solution of herbal active ingredients prepared by percolation or dilution of their corresponding fluid or native extracts. Although the alcohol amount may vary, the tincture strength is usually 1:10 or 1:5.

thyroxine A hormone produced by the thyroid gland, which is important for energy production.

tonic A substance that nourishes, restores and strengthens the entire body.

toxic A poisonous substance that can be of a plant or animal origin

Transfatty acid A type of fat such as margarine or shortening produced by applying hydrogen gas under a high pressure and temperature to vegetable oils.

triglyceride A fat molecule assembled from three fatty acids and an oily alcohol called glycerol. Nearly all the fats in foods and body tissues are made up of triglycerides.

U

unsaturated fatty acids A fatty acid containing at least one double bond.

urea A waste product of protein metabolism that is eliminated from the body through urine.

V

vegetarian A person who consumes vegetables and grains exclusively—anything but animal products

vein A blood vessel that brings blood to the heart (arteries take blood from the heart).

vitamin Essential nutrient that must be obtained from food sources for the proper growth and function of the body.

vitamin A palmitate One of the antioxidant vitamins that is also important for growth and the proper functioning of the eyes, healthy skin, hair and the lining of the digestive tract.

W

western diet A diet in Western societies that consists of high fat, low fiber and refined and processed foods.

water-soluble vitamin A vitamin that dissolves in water. All of the eight B vitamins and vitamin C are water soluble.

Ethiopian foods

berbere The base ingredient to many of the Ethiopian dishes made of toasted, dried red chili and a couple dozen spices.

alicha Spiced but mild stew usually made from vegetables or legumes but without berbere.

areqey Homemade whiskey.

awaze Red pepper paste made from several spices (ginger, nutmeg, cloves, onions, thyme, cinnamon, garlic, and red chili peppers which have been toasted and formed into a paste; adds heat to meat, seafood, and bread.

ayib Cheese harvested from heated butter milk, used as a side dish or added to other foods

Ferenge A white person.

injera Soft, stretchy, crepe-like flatbread, made of sourdough starter and teff and baked over clay griddle.

kitfo Finely chopped beef, seasoned with niter kibbeh (spiced clarified butter) and mitmita.

kurtet Cutting sensations in the stomach and intestines.

kurtmat Painful sensation in the joints and muscles, often experienced by people.

madd-bet Kitchen house (literally translated).

mitad Baking pan.

miser Lentils.

miser wot Lentils stew.

mitmita Very hot chili powder with spices, made from crushed bird's eye chili, cardamom, and salt.

netch White.

niter kibbeh Clarified butter made from fenugreek seeds, cumin, kewrerima, chopped onions, ginger, chopped garlic, ground turmeric, cardamom seeds and sacred basil.

siljo An aged dip made from either barely or fava beans flour and mixture of fenugreek, sunflower water, ginger, garlic , mustard powder, fresh rue leaves, salt and water.

sambusa Triangular, deep-fried pastry, stuffed with beef, chicken, or vegetables.

teff Tiny but hardy, gluten-free grain native to Ethiopia. It is the main flour used to make injera.

tej Ethiopian honey wine, brewed from raw honey and hops.

tella Homemade Ethiopian beer often brewed from barley and hops.

tibs Cubed beef, lamb or chicken sauteed with spices.

tikur or tikoor Black.

ye'abesha gomen Chopped collard greens cooked with minced onions, garlic, ground cardamom, fenugreek, and black cumin.

wot Ethiopia's spiced stew, made with vegetables, fish, chicken, lamb, or beef.

wugat Sharp pain in the chest or abdomen.

PART VIII
References

Chapter 2: Optimal Nutrition

- Schloss B: Possibilities for prologing life in the near future. Rejuvenation1981; 9 (20:30-32.

- Kinsella K: Changes in life expectancy 1900-1 990. Am J Clin N 1992;55: 1 196s-1202s.

- Lipschitz D, McClellan J: Impact of nutrition on the age-related decline in immune and hematologic function. Cont Nutr 1990; 15 (2): 1-2.

- Sacher, George A. " Life Table Modification and Life Prolongation." Handbook of Biology of Aging.

- Masoro E: Nutrition and aging: A current assessment. J Nutr 1985; 1 15 (7):842-848.

- Kushi, M., and Cottrell, M.C., M.D., AIDS, Macrobiotics and Natural Immunity. Tokyo, New York: Japan Publication, Inc., 1990.

- Schleettwein-Gsell D: Nutrition and the quality of life: A measure for the outcome of nutritional intervention? Amjclin N 1992;55:1263s-1266s.

- Quillin, Patrick. Healing Nutrients, Chicago, New York: Contemporary Books, Inc., 1987

- Block G, Dresser C. Hartman A, et al:Nutrient sources in American Diet:Quantitative Data from the NHANES I1 survey. 2. Macronutrients and fats. Am JEpidem 1985;122(1):27-40.

- Mendil, Earl. Earl Mindell Anti-Aging Bible, New York: Simon 81 Schuster, 1996 pp. 150-1 5 1.

- Cancer Research, 1994 April, 54(7 Suppl): 1976s-198 1s. R.W. and Castonguay. Antimutagenic effects of polyphenolic compounds, Cancer Letter 66, no.2 (Spetember 1992), 107- 1 13

- Proceedings of the National Academy of Sciences of the United States of America, 1994 April 12, 91 (8):3147-50.

- Hocaman, Gabriel. Prevention of cancer: vegetables and plants Comparative Biochemistry and Physiology 93B, no.2 (1989):210-212.

- Annals of the New York Academy ofsciences, 1992 Sept. 30, 669:7-20.

Chapter 3: Fat-soluble Vitamins

Vitamin D

- Garrison, R.H., and Somer, E., The Nutrition Desk Reference, New Canaan, Conn.: Keats Publishing, Inc., 1990, p. 215.

- Berger, Stuart M., How to Be Your Own Nutritionist, New York: Avon Books, 1987, p. 188.

Vitamin E

- Bosco, Dominick, The Peoplei Guide to Vitamins and Minerals, Chicago: Contemporary Books, 1980

- Lieberman, S., and Bruning, N. The Real Vitamin &Mineral Book, Publishers Group West, Garden City Park, N.Y.: 1990

- Bosco, Dominick, The People? Guide to Vitamins and Minerals, Chicago: Contemporary Books, 1980, p. 48. 1985,

- Jacobs. D.H., New EnglandJournalofMedicine, vol. 314, May 1986,

Niacin

- Lieberman, S., & Bruning, N., The Real Vitamin &Mineral Book, Bosco, Dominick, The People? Guide to Vitamins and Minerals, Chicago:

- Quillin, Patrick, Ph.D., Healing Nutrients, Chicago, New York: Contemporar Books Inc., 1987, p. 101.

- Anderson, R.A., et al., American Journalof Clinical Nutrition, vol. 36, Dec. Pantothenic Acid (Vitamin B5)

- Krombout. D., et al., American Journal of Clinical Nutrition, vol. 41, June

Chapter4: Bulk Minerals

Calcium

- Quillin, Patrick, Ph.D., Healing Nutrients, Chicago, New York: Contemporary Books Inc., 1987, pp. 307-3 14.

- Fisher, S., et al., American Journal of Clinical Nutrition, vol. 3 1, 1978, p 667.

Copper

- Quillin, Patrick, Ph.D., Healing Nutrients, Chicago, New York: Contemporary Books Inc., 1987, p. 318.

- Walker, B.C., et al., Agents and Actions, vol. 6, 1976, p. 454.

- Huber, W., et al., Clinics in Rheumatic Diseases, vol. 6, 1980, p. 465.

- American Journal of Medicine, vol. 74, 1983, p. 124.

- Frank, B ., Nucleic Acid and Antioxidant Therapy of Aging and Degeneration, New York: Rainstone Publishing, 1977.

The World of Herbs

- Lust, J.B. The Herb Book, New York, Toronto, London, Sydney, Aukland: Bantam Books, 1974, P.4
- Tierra, Michael. The way of Herbs, New York, London, Toronto, Sydney, Tokyo, Singapore: Pocket Books, 1990, xxiv – xxvii

Chapter 8 Herbal Samplers

- Hendler, S.S., The Doctors fitamin and Mineral Encyclopedia, New York: Simon and Schuster, 199 1, p.279.
- Murray, M.T., The Healing Power of Herbs, Roklin: Prima Publishing, 1992, p.121.
- Clostre, F., From the Body to Cellular Membranes: The different Level of Pharmacological Action of Ginkgo Biloba Extract. In Rokan (Ginkgo
- Biloba) - Recent Results in Pharmacology and Clinic. Funfgeld, E.W., ed., New York: Springer-Verlag, 1988, pp. 180-98.
- Schaffler, V.K., and Reeh, PW.: Double-blind Study of the Hypoxiaprotective Effect of Standarized Ginkgo Bilobae Preparation After Repeated Administration in Healthy Volunteers. Arzneim-Forsch 35:1283-6, 1985.
- Foster, S. Making wise choices in herbal energy boosters, in Better Nutrition for Better Living, Jan, 1995, 12 1.
- Shibata, S., Tanaka, O., Shoji, J., and Saito, H., Chemistry and Pharmacology of Panax, Economic and Medicinal Plant Research 1:217-84, 1985.
- Brekham I1 and Dardymov IV: New Substances of Plant Origin which Increase Non-specific Resistance. Ann. Rev. Pharmacol. 9:419-30, 1969.
- Brekham I1 and Dardymov IV: Pharmacological Investigation of glycosides from Ginseng and Eleutherococcus, Lloydia 32:46-5, 1969.
- Saito, H., Yoshida, Y. and Takagi, K: Effect of Panax Ginseng Root on Exhaustive Exercise in Mice. Jap. J. Pharmacol. 24: 1 19-27, 1974.
- Avakia E.V. and Evonuk, E., Effects of Panax Ginseng Extract on Tissue Glycogen and Adrenal Cholesterol Depletion During Prolonged Exercise. Planta Medica 36:43-8, 1979.
- Petkov, W. The Mechanism of Action of l? Ginseng. Arzniem-Forsch, 1:288-95, 418-22, 1961.
- 18. Foster, S.: Making Wise Choices in Herbal Energy Boosters, in Better Nutrition for Better Living, Jan. 1995, P.66.
- 19. Ritchason, Jack, The Little Herb Encyclopedia, Woodland Health books: Pleasant Grove, UT, 1994, p.214, 215.

Ethiopian spices

Chapter 13 Beso Bela (Sacred Basil)

- http://www.medicinehunter.com/holy-basil
- Singh N, Misra N, Srivastava AK, Dixit KS, Gupta GP. Effect of anti-stress plants on biochemical changes during stress reaction. *Indian Journal of Pharmacology.* 1991;23:137–142
- Evidence-Based Complementary and Alternative Medicine Volume 2012 (2012), Article ID 894509, 7 pages
- *Indian Journal of Experimental Biology,* Vol. 40, July 2002, pp. 765-773
- Sembulingam K, Sembulingam P, Namasivayam A. Effect of Ocimum sanctum Linn on the changes in central cholinergic system induced by acute noise stress.
- *J Ethnopharmacol.* 2005 Jan 15;96(3):477-82.
- Sembulingam K, Sembulingam P, Namasivayam A. Effect of Ocimum sanctum Linn on noise induced changes in plasma corticosterone level. *Indian J Physiol Pharmacol.* 1997 Oct;41(4):429-30.
- Archana R, Namasivayam A. Effect of Ocimum sanctum on noise induced changes in neutrophil functions. *J Ethnopharmacol.* 2000 Nov;73(1-2):81-5.
- Sen P, Maiti PC, Puri S, Ray A, Audulov NA, Valdman AV. Mechanism of antistress activity of Ocimum sanctum Linn, eugenol and Tinospora malabarica in
- experimental animals. Indian J Exp Biol. 1992 Jul;30(7):592-6.

Chapter 14

Dimbilal (Coriander)

- http://www.whfoods.com/genpage.php?tname=foodspice&dbid=70
- Ballal RS, Jacobsen DW, Robinson K. Homocysteine: update on a new risk factor. Cleve Clin J Med 1997 Nov-1997 Dec 31;64(10):543-9. 1997.
- Chithra V, Leelamma S. Hypolipidemic effect of coriander seeds (Coriandrum sativum): mechanism of action. Plant Foods Hum Nutr 1997;51(2):167-72. 1997. PMID:12610.
- Chithra V, Leelamma S. Coriandrum sativum changes the levels of lipid peroxides and activity of antioxidant enzymes in experimental animals. Indian J Biochem Biophys 1999 Feb;36(1):59-61. 1999. PMID:12590.

- Delaquis PJ, Stanich K, Girard B et al. Antimicrobial activity of individual and mixed fractions of dill, cilantro, coriander and eucalyptus essential oils. Int J Food Microbiol. 2002 Mar 25;74(1-2):101-9. 2002.

- Ensminger AH, Esminger M. K. J. e. al. Food for Health: A Nutrition Encyclopedia. Clovis, California: Pegus Press; 1986. 1986. PMID:15210.

- Fortin, Francois, Editorial Director. The Visual Foods Encyclopedia. Macmillan, New York. 1996.

- Gray AM, Flatt PR. Insulin-releasing and insulin-like activity of the traditional anti- diabetic plant Coriandrum sativum (coriander). Br J Nutr 1999 Mar;81(3):203-9. 1999. PMID:12600.

- Grieve M. A Modern Herbal. Dover Publications, New York. 1971.

- Kubo I, Fujita K, Kubo A, Nihei K, Ogura T. Antibacterial Activity of Coriander Volatile Compounds against Salmonella choleraesuis. *J Agric Food Chem.* 2004 Jun 2;52(11):3329-32. 2004. PMID:15161192.

- Wood, Rebecca. The Whole Foods Encyclopedia. New York, NY: Prentice-Hall Press; 1988. 1988. PMID:15220.

Chapter 15

Inslal (Anise)

- Anise. Review of Natural Products. factsandcomparisons4.0 [online]. 2005. Available from Wolters Kluwer Health, Inc. Accessed April 16, 2007.

- Anise (*Pimpinella anisum* L.) from Gernot Katzer's Spice Pages, How to Grow Anise from growingherbs.org.uk

- Philip R. Ashurst (1999). *Food Flavorings*. Springer. p. 33. ISBN 978-0-8342-1621-1.

- J.S. Pruthi: Spices and Condiments, New Delhi: National Book Trust (1976), p. 19.

- J "Anise History". *Our Herb Garden*. Retrieved 3 March 2013.

- Jack S. Blocker, Jr.; David M. Fahey; Ian R. Tyrrell (2003). *Alcohol and Temperance in Modern History: An Global Encyclopedia*. ABC-CLIO. pp. 478–.ISBN 978-1-57607-833-4. Retrieved 28 March 2013.

- John Gerard, *The Herball, or Generall Historie of Plantes*, 1597, p. 880, side 903

Chapter 16

IRD (Turmeric)

- http://www.whfoods.com/genpage.php?tname=foodspice&dbid=78
- Abbey M, Noakes M, Belling GB, Nestel PJ. Partial replacement of saturated fatty acids with almonds or walnuts lowers total plasma cholesterol and low-density-lipoprotein cholesterol. Am J Clin Nutr 1994 May;59(5):995-9. 1994. PMID:16240.
- Aggarwal B. Paper presented at the U.S. Defense Department's 'Era of Hope' Breast Cancer Research Program meeting in Philadelphia, PA, October 5, 2005,. reported in NUTRAingredients.com/Europe "Turmeric slows breast cancer spread in mice.".
- Ahsan H, Parveen N, Khan NU, Hadi SM. Pro-oxidant, anti-oxidant and cleavage activities on DNA of curcumin and its derivatives demethoxycurcumin and bisdemethoxycurcumin. Chem Biol Interact 1999 Jul 1;121(2):161-75. 1999. PMID:7690.
- Arbiser JL, Klauber N, Rohan R, et al. Curcumin is an in vivo inhibitor of angiogenesis. Mol Med 1998 Jun;4(6):376-83. 1998. PMID:7540.
- Asai A, Nakagawa K, Miyazawa T. Antioxidative effects of turmeric, rosemary and capsicum extracts on membrane phospholipid peroxidation and liver lipid metabolism in mice. Biosci Biotechnol Biochem 1999 Dec;63(12):2118-22. 1999. PMID:7550.
- Balasubramanian K. Molecular Orbital Basis for Yellow Curry Spice Curcumin's Prevention of Alzheimer's Disease.*J. Agric. Food Chem.*, 54 (10), 3512 -3520, 2006.
- Calabrese V, Butterfield DA, Stella AM. Nutritional antioxidants and the heme oxygenase pathway of stress tolerance: novel targets for neuroprotection in Alzheimer's disease. *Ital J Biochem.* 2003 Dec;52(4):177-81. 2003.
- Calabrese V, et. al. Paper on curcumin's induction of hemeoxygenase-1. Presented at the annual conference of the American Physiological Society, held April 17-21, 2004, Washington, D.C. 2004.
- Cruz-Correa M, Shoskes DA, Sanchez P, Zhao R, Hylind LM, Wexner SD, Giardiello FM. Combination treatment with curcumin and quercetin of adenomas in familial adenomatous polyposis. i>Clin Gastroenterol Hepatol. 2006 Aug;4(8):1035-8. Epub 2006 Jun 6. 2006. PMID:16757216.

- Deshpande UR, Gadre SG, Raste AS, et al. Protective effect of turmeric (Curcuma longa L.) extract on carbon tetrachloride-induced liver damage in rats. Indian J Exp Biol 1998 Jun;36(6):573-7. 1998. PMID:7740.
- Dorai T, Cao YC, Dorai B, et al. Therapeutic potential of curcumin in human prostate cancer. III. Curcumin inhibits proliferation, induces apoptosis, and inhibits angiogenesis of LNCaP prostate cancer cells in vivo. Prostate 2001 Jun 1;47(4):293-303. 2001. PMID:16280.
- Egan ME, Pearson M, Weiner SA, Rajendran V, Rubin D, Glockner-Pagel J, Canny S, Du K, Lukacs GL, Caplan MJ. Curcumin, a major constituent of turmeric, corrects cystic fibrosis defects. *Science*. 2004 Apr 23;304(5670):600-2. 2004. PMID:15105504.
- Ensminger AH, Esminger M. K. J. e. al. Food for Health: A Nutrition Encyclopedia. Clovis, California: Pegus Press; 1986. 1986. PMID:15210.

Chapter 17
Kewrerima (False Cardamom)

- *Aframomum corrorima* was published in *Spices, Condiments and Medicinal Plants in Ethiopia, Their Taxonomy and Agricultural Significance.* (Agric. Res. Rep. 906 & Belmontia New Series) 12:10. 1981. The specific epithet was taken from its basionym,*Amomum corrorima* A.Braun GRIN (April 9, 2011). "*Aframomum corrorima* information from NPGS/GRIN". *Taxonomy for Plants*. National Germplasm Resources Laboratory, Beltsville, Maryland: USDA, ARS, National Genetic Resources Program. RetrievedJune 19, 2011. Synonyms: (≡) *Amomum corrorima* A.Braun (basionym)

- *Amomum corrorima* A.Braun, the basionym of *Aframomum corrorima* (A.Braun) P.C.M.Jansen, was originally described and published in *Flora* 31:95. 1848 GRIN. "*Amomum corrorima* information from NPGS/ GRIN". *Taxonomy for Plants*. National Germplasm Resources Laboratory, Beltsville, Maryland: USDA, ARS, National Genetic Resources Program. Retrieved June 19, 2011.

- Bernard Roussel and François Verdeaux (April 6–10, 2003). "Natural patrimony and local communities in ethiopia: geographical advantages and limitations of a system of indications" (PDF). *29th Annual Spring Symposium of Centre for African Studies*. Archived from the original (PDF) on 2006-11-26. This Zingiberaceae, *Aframomum corrorima*(Braun) Jansen, is gathered in forests, and also grown in gardens. It is a basic spice in Ethiopia, used to flavor coffee and as an ingredient in various widely used condiments (berbere, mitmita, awaze, among others).

- J Jansen, P.C.M. (2002). "Aframomum corrorima (Braun)". Archived from the original on 2008-11-20. P.C.M. Jansen. Record from Protabase. Oyen, L.P.A. & Lemmens, R.H.M.J. (Editors). PROTA (Plant Resources of Tropical Africa / Ressources végétales de l'Afrique tropicale), Wageningen, the Netherlands.

Chapter 18
Koseret (Lippia Javania)

- Van Wyk, B., Van Oudtshoorn, B., Gericke, N. 1997. Medicinal Plants of Southern Africa. Briza, Pretoria.
- Van Wyk, B., Gericke, N. 2000. People's plants: A guide to useful plants of Southern Africa. Briza, Pretoria.
- Pooley, E. 1998. A filed guide to Wild Flowers. Kwazulu-Natal and Eastern Region. Natal Flora Publications Trust, Durban.
- Van Wyk, B., Malan, S. 1997. Field guide to the Wild Flowers of the Highveld. Struik, Cape Town.
- Fox, F.W., Norwood Young, M.E. 1983. Food from the Veld: Edible wild plants of Southern Africa. Delta Books, Cape Town.
- Mitchell Watt, J., Breyer-Brandwijk, M.G. 1962. The Medicinal and Poisonous Plants of Southern and Eastern Africa. E. & S. Livingstone Ltd., Edinburgh and London.
- Roberts, M. 1990. Indigenous Healing Plants. Southern Book Publishers.

Chapter 19

Kundo Berbere (Black Pepper

- http://www.whfoods.com/genpage.php?tname=foodspice&dbid=74
- Abila B, Richens A, Davies JA. Anticonvulsant effects of extracts of the west African black pepper, Piper guineense. J Ethnopharmacol 1993 Jun;39(2):113-7. 1993. PMID:16400.
- Ao P, Hu S, Zhao A. [Essential oil analysis and trace element study of the roots of Piper nigrum L.]. Zhongguo Zhong Yao Za Zhi 1998 Jan;23(1):42-3, 63. 1998. PMID:16370.
- Calucci L, Pinzino C, Zandomeneghi M et al. Effects of gamma-irradiation on the free radical and antioxidant contents in nine aromatic herbs and spices. J Agric Food Chem 2003 Feb 12; 51(4):927-34. 2003.

- Dorman HJ, Deans SG. Antimicrobial agents from plants: antibacterial activity of plant volatile oils. J Appl Microbiol 2000 Feb;88(2):308-16. 2000. PMID:16390.
- Ensminger AH, Ensminger, ME, Kondale JE, Robson JRK. Foods & Nutriton Encyclopedia. Pegus Press, Clovis, California. 1983.
- Ensminger AH, Esminger M. K. J. e. al. Food for Health: A Nutrition Encyclopedia. Clovis, California: Pegus Press; 1986. 1986. PMID:15210.

Chapter 20
Mitmita (Bird's Eye Chili)

- https://ethnomed.org/clinical/nutrition/the-traditional-foods-of-the-central-ethiopian
- Agren, G., A1mgard,G., Mellander, 0., Vahiquist, B., Bjornesjo, K.B., Hofvander, Y., Jacobsson, K., Knutsson, K.E., Mellbin, T., and Selinus, R.: Children's Nutrition Unit - an Ethio-Swedish project in the field of health. Ethiopian Medical Journal, 1966:5, 5-13.
- Agren, C., Gibson, R.: Food Composition Table for use in Ethiopia. SIDA, Stockholm 1968.
- 3.Hofvander, Y.: Haematological investigations in Ethiopia with special reference to a high iron intake. Acta Med. Scand. Suppl. 494, 1968
- Analysis carried out in the Jones and Amos Laboratory in London.
- Levine, D.: Wax and gold. London 1965
- Knutsson, K.E., Selinus, R.: Fasting in Ethiopia-an Anthropological and Nutritional Study. American J. Clin. Nutr. June 1970.

Chapter 21
Netch Azmud (Bishop's Weed)

- http://www.drugs.com/npp/bishop-s-weed.html
- Boskabady MH, Shaikhi J. Inhibitory effect of Carum copticum on histamine (H 1) receptors of isolated guinea-pig tracheal chains. J Ethnopharmacol . 2000;69:217-227
- Chopra RN. Chopra's Indigenous Drug of India . 2nd ed. Calcutta: Academic Publishers; 1982:93-94.
- Biswas NR, Gupta SK, Das GK, et al. Evaluation of Ophthacare eye drops—a herbal formulation in the management of various ophthalmic disorders. Phytother Res . 2001;15:618-620.
- Thangham C, Dhananjayan R. Antiinflammatory potential of the seeds of Carum copticum Linn. Indian J of Pharmacol . 2003;35:388-391.

- Khan MA. Protective effects of Arque-Ajeeb on acute experimental diarrhoea in rats. BMC Compl Altern Med . 2004;4:8.
- Ishikawah T, Sega Y, Kitajima J. Water-soluable constituents of ajowan. Chem Pharm Bull . 2001;49:840-844.
- Garg S, et al. A new glucoside from Trachyspermum ammi . Fitoterapia . 1998;6:511-512.
- Ethiopia and their indigenous uses. J Essent Oil Res . 1993:5:465-479.
- Nagalakshmi S, et al. Studies on chemical and technological aspects of ajowan (Trachyspermum ammi syn. Carum copticum). J Food Sci Technol . 2000;37:277-281.
- Choudhury S, et al. Composition of the seed oil of Trachyspermum ammi (L.) Sprague from northeast India. J Essent Oil Res . 1998;10:588-590.
- Chialva F, et al. Essential oil constituents of Trachyspermum copticum (L.) Link fruits. J Essent Oil Res . 1993;5:105-106.
- De M, Krishna De A, Banerjee AB. Antimicrobial screening of some Indian spices. Phytother Res . 1999;13:616-618.

Chapter 22
Netch Shinkoort (Garlic)

- http://lpi.oregonstate.edu/mic/food-beverages/garlic
- Lawson LD. Garlic: a review of its medicinal effects and indicated active compounds. In: Lawson LD, Bauer R, eds. Phytomedicines of Europe: Chemistry and Biological Activity. Washington, D. C.: American Chemical Society; 1998:177-209.
- Block E. The chemistry of garlic and onions. Sci Am. 1985;252(3):114-119. (PubMed)
- Blumenthal M. Herb Sales Down 7.4 Percent in Mainstream Market. HerbalGram: American Botanical Council; 2005:63.
- Tapiero H, Townsend DM, Tew KD. Organosulfur compounds from alliaceae in the prevention of human pathologies. Biomed Pharmacother. 2004;58(3):183-193. (PubMed)
- Lawson LD, Wang ZJ. Allicin and allicin-derived garlic compounds increase breath acetone through allyl methyl sulfide: use in measuring allicin bioavailability. J Agric Food Chem. 2005;53(6):1974-1983. (PubMed)
- Germain E, Auger J, Ginies C, Siess MH, Teyssier C. *In vivo* metabolism of diallyl disulphide in the rat: identification of two new metabolites. Xenobiotica. 2002;32(12):1127-1138. (PubMed)

- Lachmann G, Lorenz D, Radeck W, Steiper M. [The pharmacokinetics of the S35 labeled labeled garlic constituents alliin, allicin and vinyldithiine]. Arzneimittelforschung. 1994;44(6):734-743. (PubMed)

- de Rooij BM, Boogaard PJ, Rijksen DA, Commandeur JN, Vermeulen NP. Urinary excretion of N-acetyl-S-allyl-L-cysteine upon garlic consumption by human volunteers. Arch Toxicol. 1996;70(10):635-639. (PubMed)

- Jandke J, Spiteller G. Unusual conjugates in biological profiles originating from consumption of onions and garlic. J Chromatogr. 1987;421(1):1-8. (PubMed)

- Kodera Y, Suzuki A, Imada O, et al. Physical, chemical, and biological properties of s-allylcysteine, an amino acid derived from garlic. J Agric Food Chem. 2002;50(3):622-632. (PubMed)

- Steiner M, Li W. Aged garlic extract, a modulator of cardiovascular risk factors: a dose-finding study on the effects of AGE on platelet functions. J Nutr. 2001;131(3s):980S-984S. (PubMed)

- Gebhardt R, Beck H. Differential inhibitory effects of garlic-derived organosulfur compounds on cholesterol biosynthesis in primary rat hepatocyte cultures. Lipids. 1996;31(12):1269-1276. (PubMed)

Chapter 23
Senafich (Mustard Seed)

- http://www.whfoods.com/genpage.php?tname=foodspice&dbid=106

- Ensminger AH, Ensminger, ME, Kondale JE, Robson JRK. Foods & Nutriton Encyclopedia. Pegus Press, Clovis, California. 1983.

- Ensminger AH, Esminger M. K. J. e. al. Food for Health: A Nutrition Encyclopedia. Clovis, California: Pegus Press; 1986. 1986. PMID:15210.

- Fortin, Francois, Editorial Director. The Visual Foods Encyclopedia. Macmillan, New York. 1996.

- Grieve M. A Modern Herbal. Dover Publications, New York. 1971.

- Thimmulappa RK, Mai KH, Srisuma S et al. Identification of Nrf2-regulated genes induced by the chemopreventive agent sulforaphane by oligonucleotide microarray. Cancer Res 2002 Sep 15;62(18):5196-5203. 2002.

- Wood, Rebecca. The Whole Foods Encyclopedia. New York, NY: Prentice-Hall Press; 1988. 1988. PMID:15220.

Chapter 24
Shinkoort (red, yellow, and white)

- http://www.whfoods.com/references/index. php?tname=foodspice&dbid=45

- Ali M, Thomson M, Afzal M. Garlic and onions: their effect on eicosanoid metabolism and its clinical relevance. Prostaglandins Leukot Essent Fatty Acids. 2000 Feb;62(2):55-73. Review. 2000.

- Azuma K, Minami Y, Ippoushi K et al. Lowering effects of onion intake on oxidative stress biomarkers in streptozotocin-induced diabetic rats. J Clin Biochem Nutr. 2007 Mar;40(2):131-40. 2007.

- Borjihan B, Ogita A, Fujita KI et al. The Cyclic Organosulfur Compound Zwiebelane A from Onion (Allium cepa) Functions as an Enhancer of Polymyxin B in Fungal Vacuole Disruption. Planta Med. 2010 May 19. [Epub ahead of print]. 2010.

- Brat P, George S, Bellamy A, et al. Daily Polyphenol Intake in France from Fruit and Vegetables. J. Nutr. 136:2368-2373, September 2006. 2006.

- Chun OK, Chung SJ, and Song WO. Estimated dietary flavonoid intake and major food sources of U.S. adults. J Nutr. 2007 May;137(5):1244-52. 2007.

- Dorant E, van den Brandt PA, Goldbohm RA. A prospective cohort study on the relationship between onion and leek consumption, garlic supplement use and the risk of colorectal carcinoma in The Netherlands. Carcinogenesis 1996 Mar;17(3):477-84. 1996. PMID:13660.

- Eady CC, Kamoi T, Kato M et al. Silencing onion lachrymatory factor synthase causes a significant change in the sulfur secondary metabolite profile. Plant Physiol. 2008 Aug;147(4):2096-106. 2008.

- El-Aasr M, Fujiwara Y, Takeya M et al. Onionin A from Allium cepa inhibits macrophage activation. J Nat Prod. 2010 Jul 23;73(7):1306-8. 2010.

- Fukushima S, Takada N, Hori T, Wanibuchi H. Cancer prevention by organosulfur compounds from garlic and onion. J Cell Biochem Suppl 1997;27:100-5. 1997. PMID:13650.

- Galeone C, Pelucchi C, Levi F, Negri E, Franceschi S, Talamini R, Giacosa A, La Vecchia C. Onion and garlic use and human cancer. *Am J Clin Nutr*. 2006 Nov;84(5):1027-32. 2006. PMID:17093154.

- Galeone C, Pelucchi C, Talamini R et al. Onion and garlic intake and the odds of benign prostatic hyperplasia. Urology. 2007 Oct;70(4):672-6. 2007.

- Galeone C, Tavani A, Pelucchi C, et al. Allium vegetable intake and risk of acute myocardial infarction in Italy. Eur J Nutr. 2009 Mar;48(2):120-3. 2009.
- Gates MA, Tworoger SS, Hecht JL, De Vivo I, Rosner B, Hankinson SE. A prospective study of dietary flavonoid intake and incidence of epithelial ovarian cancer. Int J Cancer. 2007 Apr 30; [Epub ahead of print]. 2007. PMID:17471564.
- Gautam S, Platel K and Srinivasan K. Higher bioaccessibility of iron and zinc from food grains in the presence of garlic and onion. J Agric Food Chem. 2010 Jul 28;58(14):8426-9. 2010.
- Imai S, Tsuge N, Tomotake M et al. Plant biochemistry: an onion enzyme that makes the eyes water. Nature. London: Oct 17, 2002. Vol. 419, Iss. 6908; p. 685. 2002.
- Kim JH. Anti-bacterial action of onion (Allium cepa L.) extracts against oral pathogenic bacteria. J Nihon Univ Sch Dent. 1997 Sep;39(3):136-41. 1997.
- Kook S, Kim GH and Choi K. The antidiabetic effect of onion and garlic in experimental diabetic rats: meta-analysis. J Med Food. 2009 Jun;12(3):552-60. 2009.
- Matheson EM, Mainous AG 3rd and Carnemolla MA. The association between onion consumption and bone density in perimenopausal and post-menopausal non-Hispanic white women 50 years and older. Menopause. 2009 Jul-Aug;16(4):756-9. 2009.

Chapter 25
Tena Adam (Rue)

- http://www.drugs.com/npp/rue.html
- Furniss D, Adams T. Herb of grace: an unusual cause of phytophotodermatitis mimicking burn injury. J Burn Care Res . 2007;28(5):767-769.
- lChevallier A . The Encyclopedia of Medicinal Plants . New York, NY: DK Publishing; 1996:262-263.
- Conway GA , Slocumb JC . Plants used as abortifacients and emmenagogues by Spanish New Mexicans . J Ethnopharmacol . 1979;1(3):241-261.
- Pollio A, De Natale A, Appetiti E, Aliotta G, Touwaide A. Continuity and change in the Mediterranean medical tradition: Ruta spp. (rutacecae) in Hippocratic medicine and present practices. J Ethnopharmacol .
- Duke J . CRC Handbook of Medicinal Herbs . Boca Raton, FL: CRC Press; 1989:417-418.

- Minker E , Bartha C , Koltai M , Rózsa Z , Szendrei K , Reisch J . Effect of secondary substances isolated from the Ruta graveolens L. on the coronary smooth muscle . Acta Pharm Hung . 1980;50(1):7-11.
- Tyler VE . The New Honest Herbal: A Sensible Guide to the Use of Herbs and Related Remedies . Philadelphia, PA: GF Stickley Co; 1987.
- Wolters B , Eilert U . Antimicrobial substances in callus cultures of Ruta graveolens . Planta Med . 1981;43(2):166-174.
- Verzár-Petri G , Csedö K , Möllmann K , Szendrei K , Reisch J . Fluorescence microscopic investigations on the localisation of acridone alkaloids in the organs of Ruta graveolens [in German]. Planta Med . 1976;29(4):370-375.
- Spoerke DG . Herbal Medications . Santa Barbara, CA: Woodbridge Press; 1980.
- Haesen JP , Vörde Sive Vörding JG , Kho KF . Isolation and identification of xanthotoxin from the underground parts of Ruta graveolens . Planta Med . 1971;19(3):285-289.
- Zobel AM , Brown SA . Determination of furanocoumarins on the leaf surface of Ruta graveolens with an improved extraction technique. J Nat Prod . 1988;51(5):941-946.
- Paulini H , Popp R , Schimmer O , Ratka O , Röder E . Isogravacridonchlorine: a potent and direct acting frameshift mutagen from the roots of Ruta graveolens . Planta Med . 1991;57(1):59-61.
- Montagu M , Petit-Paly G , Levillain P , et al. Synchronous fluorescence spectrometry and identification of dihydrofuro[2,3-b]quinolinium alkaloids biosynthesized by Ruta graveolens cultures in vitro. Pharmazie . 1989;44:342-34

Chapter 26
Tikur Azmude (Black Cumin)

- http://healthimpactnews.com/2014/
  black-cumin-seeds-better-than-drugs-a-look-at-the-science/
- Ahmad A1, Husain A, Mujeeb M, Khan SA, Najmi AK, Siddique NA, Damanhouri ZA, Anwar F, Kishore K.; "A review on therapeutic potential of Nigella sativa: A miracle herb," Asian Pac J Trop Biomed., 2013 May, PMID: 23646296.
- Salem ML.; "Immunomodulatory and therapeutic properties of the Nigella sativa L. seed," Int Immunopharmacol. 2005 Dec, PMID: 16275613.

- Entok E1, Ustuner MC, Ozbayer C, Tekin N, Akyuz F, Yangi B, Kurt H, Degirmenci I, Gunes HV.; "Anti-inflammatuar and anti-oxidative effects of Nigella sativa L.: 18FDG-PET imaging of inflammation," Mol Biol Rep. 2014 May, PMID: 24474661.

- Vanamala J1, Kester AC, Heuberger AL, Reddivari L.; "Mitigation of obesity-promoted diseases by Nigella sativa and thymoquinone," Plant Foods Hum Nutr. 2012 Jun, PMID: 22477645.

- [Hasani-Ranjbar S1, Jouyandeh Z, Abdollahi M.; "A systematic review of anti-obesity medicinal plants – an update," J Diabetes Metab Disord., 2013 June 19, PMID: 23777875.

- Farzaneh E1, Nia FR2, Mehrtash M2, Mirmoeini FS3, Jalilvand M1.; "The Effects of 8-week Nigella sativa Supplementation and Aerobic Training on Lipid Profile and VO2 max in Sedentary Overweight Females," Int J Prev Med., 2014 February, PMID: 24627749.

- Oysu C1, Tosun A1, Yilmaz HB2, Sahin-Yilmaz A3, Korkmaz D1, Kara-aslan A1.; "Topical Nigella Sativa for nasal symptoms in elderly," Auris Nasus Larynx. 2014 Jun, PMID: 24398317

Chapter 27
Timiz (Long Pepper)

- http://en.wikipedia.org/wiki/Long_pepper
- Sesha Iyengar, T.R (1989). "Dravidian India". ISBN 9788120601352.
- Rawlinson, H. G (2001-05-01). "Intercourse Between India and the Western World: From the Earliest Times of the Fall of Rome".ISBN 9788120615496.
- J Barnett, Lionel D (1999-01-01). "Antiquities of India: An Account of the History and Culture of Ancient Hindustan".ISBN 9788171564422.
- Maguelonne Toussaint-Samat, Anthea Bell, tr. *The History of Food*, revised ed. 2009, p.
- Philippe and Mary Hyman, "Connaissez-vous le poivre long?" *L'Histoire* no. 24 (June 1980).
- "Novel compound selectively kills cancer cells by blocking their response to oxidative stress". Science Daily. July 15, 2011.

Appendix A
Free Radicals and Antioxidants

- Halliwell, B. and Gutteridge John M.C. Free Radicals in Biology and
- Medicine, Oxford: Clarendon Press, 1989, pp. 454-458.
- Quillin, Patrick, Ph.D., Healing Nutrients, Chicago, New York: Contemporary Books Inc., 1987, p. 335.
- Ershoff, B.H., American Journal of Clinical Nutrition, vol. 27,1974, p. 1395.
- Ershoff, B.H., American Journalof ClinicalNutrition, vol. 41, 1976, p. 949.

Selenium

- Bosco, Dominick, The People? Guide to fitamins and Minerals, Chicago:
- Contemporary Books, 1980, p. 249.

Ethiopian Traditional and Herbal Medications and their Interactions with Conventional Drugs[22]

Herb/Spice	Common Uses	Drugs Affected	Mechanism	Consequences
Basil *Ocimum basilicum* Besobila (A) Zahahene (O)	• Mostly culinary • Medicinal: headache, insect repellent, malaria	• Anticoagulants • Hypoglycemic agents	• Oil extract has been found to increase clotting time • Synergistic interaction with insulin and oral hypoglycemic agents	• Increased chance of bleeding • May further lower blood glucose
Black Mustard *Brassica nigra* Senafitch (A) (T) Senafitcha (O)	• Culinary use • Medicinal use: stomach ache, constipation, bloating, amoebic dysentery and abortifacient • Also used for wound dressing.		• Mustard seeds and oil- may increase production of stomach acid • Allyl thiocyanate is an irritant that can cause severe burns and tissue necrosis (Fullas 2003) • High concentration of Vitamin K	• Interferes with antacid treatment • Antagonizes effects of Warfarin
Black seed *Nigella sativa* Tiqur azmud (A) Awoseta (T) Gura (O)	• Culinary uses • Medicinal: headache, stomachache, abortifacient		• Platelet aggregation inhibition • Increases pancreatic insulin secretion • Evidence in animal studies of reduced arterial blood pressure by increasing vasodilation and inhibiting contraction. • Evidence of pregnancy inhibitor in rats (Fullas, 2003)	• Increased risk of bleeding • Synergistic action with medication that lowers blood pressure and blood glucose
Capsicum pepper **Cayenne pepper** *Capsicum annum* Berbere (A)	• Mostly culinary • Medicinal: stomach ache, antimicrobial		• Capsaicin may inhibit platelet aggregation • Increases production of catecholamines • Decreases blood glucose levels and stimulates insulin release	• Increased risk of bleeding • May counteract mechanism of anti-hypertensives • Recorded incidences of increased cough when combined with ACE inhibitors
Cinnamon *Cinnamomum zelanicum* Qarafa (A) Crefte (T) Carafu (O)	• Culinary • Medicinal: treatment for cold symptoms		• Claimed to increase stomach acid • Experimental evidence of tetracycline dissolution rate interference	• May counteract antacids • May inhibit tetracycline action

22   Author(s): Alevtina Gall, BS, BA; Zerihun Shenkute, RPh
Reviewer(s): David Kiefer, MD; J. Carey Jackson, MD, MPH, MA
Date Authored: November 03, 2009

Herb/Spice	Common Uses	Drugs Affected	Mechanism	Consequences
Coriander *Coriandrum sativum* Dimbelal (A) Zagada (T) Shucar (O)	• Mostly culinary • Medicinal: stomach ache and colic		• Unknown, but has been shown to be effective in treating stomach upset (Fullas 2003)	• *Lowers blood sugar levels;
Cumin *Cuminum cyminum* Ensilal (A) Kemano (T) Hawaja (O)	• Mostly culinary		• May have hypoglycemic properties • May have anticoagulating properties	• *Hypoglycemia • *Increased risk of bleeding
Dingetegna(A) *No common English name* Taverniera abyssinica	• Medicinal only for stomach upset • Fever reduction		• Antispasmodic properties may affect absorption of medication	• Decreased absorption of medication
Fenugreek *Trigonella foenum-graceum* Abish (A) Halbata (O)	• Mostly culinary • Medicinal: stomachache, antispasmodic, powder used for wound dressing		• Studies have shown that fenugreek acts synergistically with blood glucose lowering drugs • Decreases total cholesterol and LDLs • Alters T3 and T4 levels • Anticoagulating properties	• *Hypoglycemia • *Lower cholesterol • *Reduced intestinal absorbance of medication • *Increased risk of bleeding
Flaxseed and flaxseed oil *Linum usitatissimum* Telba (A) Lina (T) Konfur (O)	• Medicinal: purgative, diuretic, laxative		• Flaxseed and oil decrease platelet aggregation, increase effects of lipid lowering and hypoglycemic agents • Lignans (phyto-estrogens) from flaxseed (not oil) possess hormonal effects • As a bulk forming laxative, flaxseed may bind to cardiac glycosides and other orally administered medications and prevent absorption • Flaxseed enhances laxative effects of stool softeners	• *Increased risk of bleeding • Reduced intestinal absorbance of oral medication; as any fiber source • Increased risk of hypoglycemia • Possible dehydration from increased laxative effects of flaxseed (Due to absorption of liquid by fiber. It is important for patient to drink enough water.)

Herb/Spice	Common Uses	Drugs Affected	Mechanism	Consequences
Garlic *Allium sativum* Nech shinkrut (A) Tsada shgurti (T) Qullabbiiadii (O)	• Culinary • Medicinal: common cold, malaria, cough, pulmonary TB, hypertension, wounds, STDs, asthma, parasitic infections, toothache, diabetes, hemorrhoids		• May be additive with cholesterol-lowering drugs • Hypertensive activity but it is not known if this effect is antihypertensive drug additive • Decreases T3 and T4levels • May have blood thinning properties	• *Possible increased risk of bleeding; • *Reverses effects of orally administered thyroxine
Ginger *Zingiber officinale* Zingibil (A) (T)	• Culinary • Medicinal: stomachache, cough, fever, influenza		• Irritates gastric mucosa • Decreases platelet aggregation	• *Inhibits antacid therapy • *Increased risk of bleeding
Khat *Catha edulis* Chat (A) Ciut (T) (O)	• Mostly recreational • Medicinal: stimulant, mental illness, gonorrhea, common cold		• Cathinone (active ingredient) may act synergistically with amphetamines • Tannins (component of Khat) complexes with ß-lactam antibiotics	• Possible additive effect with amphetamines • Decreases absorbability of b-lactam antibiotics • Lowers seizure threshold, • Increases b.p and heart rate and induces cardiac arrythmias.
Peppermint *Mentha piperita* Nanna (A) (O) Semhal (T)	• Medicinal: common cold, headache		• Inhibits gut wall metabolism of felodipine and simvastatin • Decreases absorption of non-heme iron • Reduces Warfarin internal normalized ratio to sub-therapeutic levels	• Increased risk of clots if patient is in a hypercoagulable state • Non-absorption of felodipine, simvostatin and iron • Increases GERD symptoms unless taken as enteric-coated capsules
Rue *Ruta chalepensis* Tenadam (A) (T) Talatam (O)	• Medicinal: common cold, stomachache, diarrhea, influenza		• No major interactions reported • 5-methoxy psoralen content of rue may increase phototoxic response • May interact with Warfarin	• Anticoagulant effects maybe additive
Turmeric *Curcuma longa* Ird (A) (O)	• Mostly culinary • Medicinal: used topically for "crying eyes" in children		• Has been shown to inhibit platelet aggregation *in vitro* • Curcuminoids and sesquiterpene components of turmeric have hypoglycemic	• Increased risk of bleeding (theoretical risk; has not been demonstrated) • Reduces blood sugar levels

Language key: (A) – Amharic   (T) – Tigrinya   (O) – Oromo

Ethiopian Spice and Teff flour suppliers

Brundo Ethiopian Spices
6419 Telegraph Ave.
Oakland, CA 94609
(510) 298-7101
www.brundo.com
info@brundo.com

Selam Import
2294 S. Bascom Ave.
Campbell, CA 95008
Phone: 408.377.3090
Fax: 408.377.1099
selamimport@yahoo.com

Ethio Imports, LLC
EthiopianSpices.com
2804 Taylorsville Rd.
Louisville, KY 40205
502-459-6301
502-243-5472
Order@ethiopianspices.com

Workinesh Spice Blends
3451 W. Burnsville Parkway
Minneapolis, MN 55337

Abyssinian Market
500 Woodcroft Parkway
Durham, NC 27713
www.abyssiniamarket.com
CustomerService@AbyssiniaMarket.com

For a more extensive list, go to:
http://www.pitt.edu/~kloman/markets.html

Cook books:

Exotic Ethiopian Cooking
by Daniel Mesfin

Cooking with Imaye:
Ethiopian Cooking Straight from Mom's Kitchen
By Lena Deresse

Ethiopian Cooking in the American Kitchen
by Tizita Ayele

PART IX
Index

A

Abesh 184-187
    health benefits of 185-187
acetylcholine 52, 59
acid/alkaline foods 93-94
acrodermatitis enteropathica 90
alcohol 3, 7-8, 20, 300
allspice 188-189
Amharic 173
amino acids 9, 11, 43-44, 178
anise 141, *see* inslal (196-198)
anthocyanidins 155
antioxidants 268-275
    body-borne 268
    food derived 268-275
    herbal 274-275
    mineral 269, 271-273
    a team of 274-275
    vitamin 269-271, 19-53
appendices 261-308
astragulus 125-126

B

baptisia 126
base blend, The Four Pillars, 163
basil 142, *see* beso bela (190-192)
bay 142
beans, soy 112
berbere, blend 238-240
berries 109-110
beso bela 190-192
beta carotene 21
bilberry 126-127
    and its compounds 127
bioflavonoids 106, 109-110
    compounds of 110
biotin *see* vitamin H
bird's eye chili, *see* mitmita (213-215)
Bishop's weed aka ajwain, *see* netch
azmud (216-217)
black pepper 142, *see* kundo berbere
(208-212)
black cumin, *see* tikur azmud (229-232)
broccoli 110
burdock 127

C

cabbage 111
    Phytochemicals in, 111
CDC 153
caffeine 312
calcium 62-66
    absorption suppressors 66
    absorption facilitators 66
    and absorption rates 64
    and bones 62-64
    and osteoporosis 64
    and colon cancer 65
    food sources of 65-66
    toxicity range of 60
caraway 143
carbohydrates 312
cardamom 137, 202-205
carob 137-138
catnip 138
cayenne 113, 155, 209, 344
calcium rigor 59
catalase 222, 268, 271
celery 97, 11, 143-144, 158, 160
Center for Disease Control, *See* CDC
chamomile 137, 138, 235
cherries 109-110
chicory 127-128
cholesterol 270, 279, 313
choline 52-53
    absorption suppressors 53
    absorption facilitators 53
    function/benefit 52
    and the brain/memory 52
    food sources 53
chromium 74-75
    absorption suppressors 75
    absorption facilitators 75
    food sources of 75
    and food utilization 75
    and glucose tolerance 75
chromium picolinate 75, 295
    body function of 295
    and weight management 295

cigarettes 45, 99, 267, 302
    as source of free radicals 267
    and health risks xiii, 267
cinnamon 144, 188, 157, 204
citrus fruit 109-110
citrus peels 138
cloves 144
cobalamin *see* vitamin B12
cold drink, The Four Pillars, 157
comfrey 121, 128
copper 76-77
    absorption suppressor 77
    absorption facilitators 77
    and amino acid synthesis 76-77
    food sources of 77
    and the skin 76
    and SOD 76
    toxicity range of 77
coriander 144, *see* dimbilal (193-195)
cretinism 78
cuisine, Ethiopian 173-177
cumin 144
curves, survival 4

D

Daily Reference Value, *see* DRVs
decoction 122-123
deep earth blend, The Four Pillars 159
digestion 298-304
    and absorption 298-300
    disturbances 300-301
    problems with 299-300
    solution to problems with 301-302
dill 144-145
dimbilal 193-195
diseases
    cancer, heart, diabetes, etc 84, 93,
    107, 109
dong quai 128
DRVs = Dietary Reference Values
dunaliella salina 129

E

echinacea 129
enzymes 305-308

supplemental 306-307
essential fatty acids 11-12, 30-3,22, 315
    omega-3 fatty acids 30-31, 135
    omega-6 fatty acids 79
Ethiopian, map of 181
Ethiopians 173
exercise 283-290
    the meaning of 283-287
    and nutrition 287-290
extraction 123-124
    quantification and
    standardization of 124

F

false cardamom, *see* kewrerima (202-203)
fennel 129-130
fenugreek *see* abesh (184-187)
Fibers 97-101
    benefits of 98
    and environmental pollution 99
    and blood pressure 99-100
    and blood sugar 99
    and heart disease 98
    and weight loss 99-100
flax seeds 315
Folacin 46-47
    absorption suppressors 47
    absorption facilitators 47
    function/benefit 46
    DNA/NA/proteins synthesis 46
    food sources 43
    and megaloblastic anemia 46
    and the nervous system 46
    deficiency symptoms 47
    food sources 47
food, Ethiopian 175
    benefits of 175-176

G

garcinia cambogia 130
garlic 112, 124, 145, *see* also netch shinkoort (218-220)
Ge'ez 173

Gibbon, Edward 173
ginger 146, 155, 156, 191, 199
ginkgo biloba 130-131
   as antioxidant 130
   and the brain cells 131
ginseng 131-132
   as an adaptogen 132
   and energy production 132
   and physical performance 132
glossary 310-325
glucose tolerance test 316
glutathione peroxidase 85, 222, 268, 272, 273, 274
   function of 222
   and the immune system 268
   and other vitamins 268
goiter 78-79
goldenseal 132-133
gomen 259-260
green drink, The Four Pillars 158

H

hibiscus 139
hot drink, The Four Pillars 157

I

infusion 122
injera 247-251
Inositol 51
   absorption suppressors 51
   absorption facilitators 51
   function/benefit 51
   food sources 51
iodine 78-79
   absorption suppressors 79
   absorption facilitators 79
   and cretinism 78
   and goiter 78
   food sources 78
   ird 199-209
   the science behind ird 200
   health benefits of 201
iron 79-82
   absorption suppressors 82

   absorption facilitators 82
   and anemia 80
   and the elderly 81
   and low income people 81
   and pregnant women 81
   food sources 82-83
   and teenagers 81
   toxicity range of 83
inslal 196-198

K

Kewrerima 202-203
kita, The Four Pillars 167
kitfo 256
Keshan's disease 182
Koseret 206-207
kundo berbere 208-212

L

leucoanthocyanin 275
life expectancies 3, 5
   in United States 3
   in other countries 3
lippia Javanica, *see* koseret (206-207)
loaf, The Four Pillars 166
long pepper, *see* timiz (233-234)

M

magnesium 68-70
   absorption suppressors 70
   absorption facilitators 70
   and diabetes 69
   and mental disorders 69
   and muscles 68-69
   and the heart 70 -71
   food sources of 70
   toxicity range of 70
malnutrition xvi, 6-10
   causes of 9-10
   marginal 6, 7
   obesity 6, 7
   subclinical 6,7
manganese 87-88
   absorption suppressors 88

absorption facilitators 88
as an antioxidant 87
and the immune system 87
as cofactor of enzymes 87
food sources 88
marigold 133
marjoram 146-147
master dough 164
megaloblastic anemia 46
mekelesha blend 241
milk thistle 133
minerals 57-92
role in the body 57-61
as antioxidants 271
and biological processes 58-59
bulk 62-73
as cofactors 58
electrolyte 58-61
and muscles 59
and nerve transmission 59-60
trace 74-92
mitmita 213-215
blend 241-241
benefits of 214-215
molybdenum 83-84
absorption suppressors 84
absorption facilitators 84
and different cancers 83
and food preservatives 84
food sources 84
mustard seeds, *see* senafich 221-223

N

netch azmud 216-217
netch shinkoort 218-220
niacin *see* vitamin B3
Niter kibbeh 245
nutmeg 232-233
nutrition, xiii
continuum 10
current status of 7-10
density 10, 12, 177
level of 10-12
and diseases xiii, 19

optimal 10-12
and the public xiii
for those with special needs 12
for health & longevity 10-12, 13-15
nutritional deficiencies, 7-12

O

obesity 6-1, 291-297
causes of 291-293
solution to 293-297
onions 196-1 97
and bloating 225, 224-225
oregano 147, 148, 155
osteoporosis 23, 62, 64-69, 93, 321

P

PABA 53
absorption suppressors 53
absorption facilitators 53
function of 53
pantothenic acid *see* vitamin B5
para-aminobenzoic acid, *see* PABA
parsley 148,155
passion flower 134
pellagra 41
peppermint 137, 139
peppers 155, 213-215
phosphorus 67
absorption suppressors 67
absorption facilitators 67
food sources of 67
toxicity range of 67
phytochemicals 105-115, 218, 234, 269, 274
definition of 107
function of 106-108
sources of 108-115
various names of' 107
Pizza, The Four Pillars 168
pollution 99, 265, 277
potassium 70-72
absorption suppressors 72
absorption facilitators 72
food sources 72

and the heart 70-712
and muscles 70
prostaglandins 30-32, 322
pyridoxine *see* vitamin B6

R

RDA 322
Recommended Dietary Allowance, *see* RDA
red onions, *see* shinkoort (224-225)
riboflavin *see* vitamin B2
rose hips 110,140
rosemary 140-149
rue, *see* tena adam (226-228)

S

sage 149
St. John's Wart 134
salad, Ethiopian 261
savory, *see* tosign (235-236)
schisandra 134-135
selenium 84-87
    absorption suppressors 87
    absorption facilitators 87
    body stores of 85
    and cancer 84-87
    food source of 86-87
    geographical distribution of 86
    and heart disease 85
    and heavy metals 85
    and the immune system 86
    and sex organs 273
    and vitamin E 272
sem-ena worq 173
senafich 221-223
    benefits of 223
shinkoort (red, yellow or white) 224-225
shiro, mitten 243-245
    netch 244-245
sodium 72-73
    absorption facilitators 73
    absorption suppressors 73
    food sources 73

soil
    depletion in mineral content of 20
    variation in mineral content of xvi,
    84-87
soup, The Four Pillars 169
soybean 112
spearmint 140
spices 141-150, 184-236
spirulina 135
sulforaphane 110, 274, 275
Super blend, The Four Pillars, 163
Superoxide dismutase (SOD) 268
    function of 268
    and the immune system 272

T

tea 131, 136
    herbal 137-140
teff 178-180
tena adam 226-228
    medicinal properties of 237
thiamin, *see* vitamin B1
thyme 150
tikur azmud 229-232
    benefits 230
tincture 123
timiz 233-234
tobacco, *see* cigarettes
tomatoes 113-114
    pytochemicals in 114
tosign 235-236
turmeric, *see* ird (199-201)

V

valerian 135
vegetables 105-115
    mixed, Ethiopian 259
vitamin A 21-22
    absorption suppressors 22
    absorption facilitators 22
    deficiency symptoms 21
    forms of 21
    food source 22

vitamin D 23-24
  absorption suppressors 24
   absorption facilitators 24
  function/benefit of 23
  and the bone xv,23
  calcium absorption 23
  synthesis of 23
  food sources 24-25
  toxicity 24
vitamin E 25-28
  absorption suppressors 28
  absorption facilitators 28
  function/benefit 25-26
  and breast cancer 27-26
  and sex 25
  synthesis of 23
  food sources 27-28
vitamin K 126-127
  absorption suppressors 127
  absorption facilitators 127
  function/benefit 28-29
  forms of 28
  deficiency of 29
  food sources 127
  toxicity 29
vitamin F 30-32
  function/benefit 30-32
  forms of (omega-3 and omega-6
  fatty acids) 30
  and prostaglandins 32, 319
  and insulin 30
  and heart attack 31
  food sources 32
vitamin C 33-36
  absorption suppressors 36
  absorption facilitators 36
  adequacy of 35
  as an antioxidant 34
  food sources of 36
vitamin B complex 37-53
  function of 37
  and metabolism 37
  and the nervous system 37
vitamin B1, 38-39

absorption suppressors 39
absorption facilitators 39
function/benefit 38
deficiency of 38
food sources 38-39
vitamin B2, 39-40
  absorption suppressors 40
  absorption facilitators 40
  function/benefit 39-40
  food sources 40
vitamin B3, 40-42
  absorption suppressors 42
  absorption facilitators 42
  deficiency of 41
  function/benefit 40-41
  food sources 41-42
vitamin B5 42-43
  absorption suppressors 43
  absorption facilitators 43
  function/benefit 42-43
  and stress 42
  food sources 43
vitamin B6 43-45
  absorption suppressors 45
  absorption facilitators 45
  function/benefit 43-44
  and diabetes 44
  and the nervous system 44
  and PMS 43-44
  and toxins 45
vitamin B12 47-49
  absorption suppressors 49
  absorption facilitators 49
  function/benefit 48
  and old age 47
  food sources 48-49
vitamin H (biotin) 49-50
  absorption suppressors 50
  absorption facilitators 50
  function/benefit 49-50
  deficiency symptoms 50
  food sources 50

W

wax and gold 173
wot
    doro 252-253
    sega 254
    alicha, doro 255
    shiro, 256-257
    miser 257-258
    kik 258

Y

Yared, 173
yellow, The Four Pillars 162

Z

zinc 89-92
    absorption suppressors 92
    absorption facilitators 92
    function/benefit 89
    and health of skin, hair and nails 89
    and the immune system 89
    and the reproductive system 89
    food sources 91-92

Want to learn about the Ethiopian people and their culture? Read the *Desta* series!

www.amazon.com or www.gettyambau.com

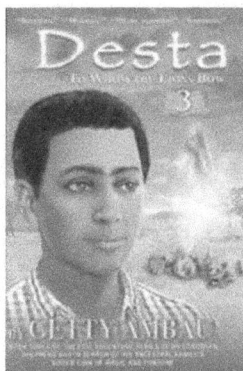

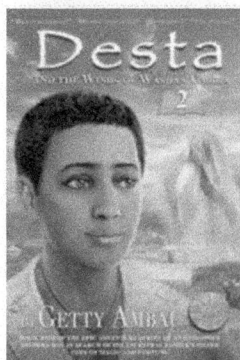

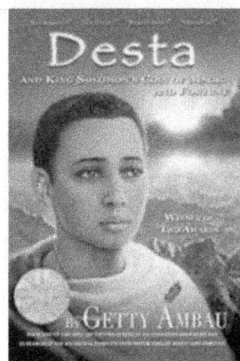

About the Author

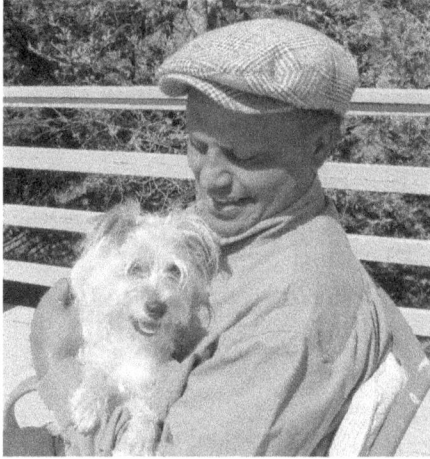

Author Getty Ambau was born in Ethiopia. He first came to the United States as a foreign exchange student, where he studied one year at a high school in Ohio. Later he entered Yale University, where he majored in molecular biophysics and biochemistry and Economics. After he graduated, he worked as a research chemist, earned a graduate degree in business and ran his own companies, but above all, writing has always been his inner calling. He is the author of two health and nutrition books, which became international bestsellers.

Getty is also the creator of the Desta series (novels), which have received recognition and won three awards. He lives in San Francisco Bay Area with his wife and an adorable terrier named, Scruffy.

www.ingramcontent.com/pod-product-compliance
Lightning Source LLC
Chambersburg PA
CBHW031144270326
41931CB00006B/138